AI in Mental Health:

Innovations, Challenges, and Collaborative Pathways

Maria Efstratopoulou
United Arab Emirates University, UAE

Agathi Argyriadi
Frederick University, Cyprus

Alexandros Argyriadis
Hellenic Mediterranean University, Greece

IGI Global
Scientific Publishing
Publishing Tomorrow's Research Today

Vice President of Editorial Melissa Wagner
Director of Acquisitions Mikaela Felty
Director of Book Development Jocelynn Hessler
Production Manager Mike Brehm
Cover Design Jose Rosado

Published in the United States of America by
IGI Global Scientific Publishing
701 East Chocolate Avenue
Hershey, PA, 17033, USA
Tel: 717-533-8845
Fax: 717-533-7115
Website: https://www.igi-global.com E-mail: cust@igi-global.com

Library of Congress Cataloging-in-Publication Data

Names: Efstratopoulou, Maria A. editor | Argyriadi, Agathi, 1987- editor | Argyriadis, Alexandros, 1982- editor
Title: AI in mental health : innovations, challenges, and collaborative pathways / edited by Maria Efstratopoulou, Agathi Argyriadi, Alexandros Argyriadis.
Description: Hershey, PA : IGI Global Scientific Publishing, [2025] | Includes bibliographical references and index. | Summary: "This book explores the transformative role of AI in reshaping educational practices and mental health support systems. It addresses the intersection of AI-driven innovations in learning environments, mental health interventions, and how these advancements present both opportunities and challenges for educators, health professionals, and policymakers"-- Provided by publisher.
Identifiers: LCCN 2025026197 (print) | LCCN 2025026198 (ebook) | ISBN 9798337350721 h/c | ISBN 9798337350738 s/c | ISBN 9798337350745 ebook
Subjects: LCSH: Mental health services--Technological innovations | Artificial intelligence--Medical applications | Artificial intelligence--Educational applications
Classification: LCC RA790.5 .A435 2025 (print) | LCC RA790.5 (ebook)
LC record available at https://lccn.loc.gov/2025026197
LC ebook record available at https://lccn.loc.gov/2025026198
British Cataloguing in Publication Data
A Cataloguing in Publication record for this book is available from the British Library.

Table of Contents

Detailed Table of Contents

Health education is important for all children as it helps them develop a balanced and safe relationship with their bodies and gender. Especially for children diagnosed with Autism Spectrum Disorder (ASD), health education is a matter of priority, because they may experience difficulties in their psychosocial functioning. The objectives of a health education program for children with ASD are to acquire better understanding of their body, learn basic hygiene skills, to be informed about personal safety/issues of abuse, to improve their gender awareness and behavior, which in the long term will benefit their full social inclusion. The aim of this research is the implementation of a health education program for school-aged children with ASD based on video modeling and focused on body awareness and privacy as dimensions of health education. The results showed that all the children were able to respond to the program and understood which body parts they are able to expose in public and which they are required to keep in private.

The integration of artificial intelligence (AI) into mental health intervention programs for children has emerged as a promising avenue for enhancing emotional well-being. AI technologies can facilitate early detection of mental health issues. AI-driven applications can analyze behavioral data from various sources, including social media and mobile devices, to identify patterns indicative of anxiety or depression. By utilizing machine learning algorithms, AI programs can adapt therapeutic approaches based on individual responses, preferences, and progress. This personalized approach increases engagement in children, empowering them to take an active role in their mental health management. AI-powered tools, such as chatbots and virtual therapists provide 24/7 support, enabling children to seek help without the barriers often associated with traditional therapy settings. Moreover, gamification elements in these programs can make mental health management more engaging for children. Incorporating AI into mental health programs also allows for enhanced parental involvement.

Autism Spectrum Disorder (ASD) is a neurodevelopmental condition with rising global prevalence, driven by improved awareness and diagnostic practices. Early diagnosis and intervention are crucial for better outcomes, yet delays persist due to systemic inefficiencies and sociocultural disparities. Artificial Intelligence (AI), including machine learning (ML) and deep learning (DL), offers promising tools for accurate and efficient ASD detection, reducing diagnostic delays and human error. AI-driven tools like Canvas Dx and EarliPoint System show high accuracy, while hybrid models and explainable AI (XAI) enhance precision and interpretability. However, ethical concerns and equitable access remain challenges. AI integration can improve early diagnosis, personalized care, and long-term outcomes for individuals with ASD.

The integration of artificial intelligence nto occupational therapy and speech therapy marks a significant advancement in making therapeutic interventions more accessible, effective, and tailored to individual needs. Particularly in the realms of education and mental health, AI has demonstrated its potential to transform the delivery of care for individuals with disabilities, speech and motor impairments, and mental health challenges. In educational settings, AI-based tools have revolutionized the approach to personalized learning. For students with special needs, including speech and motor impairments or developmental delays, Ethical concerns and the risk of dehumanizing care must be addressed. Importantly, AI serves as a complementary tool, enhancing human expertise rather than replacing the critical empathetic role of therapists. Looking forward, AI's potential in OT and speech therapy is vast. From early diagnosis and intervention to cognitive rehabilitation and social-emotional development, AI's evolving capabilities promise to further enhance therapy outcomes.

Mental health issues among Filipino students have escalated since the COVID-19 pandemic, with studies reporting a significant prevalence of anxiety and depression among youth. Filipino schoolchildren face persistent challenges due to poverty, academic pressures, and cultural stigmas surrounding mental health. School guidance counselors play a vital role as mental health therapists, providing emotional support, psychoeducation, and crisis intervention. This chapter explores the potential of generative artificial intelligence (AI) to support mental health services in Philippine schools, particularly for high school and college students. AI-powered tools, such as chatbots, can assist counselors by addressing less complex issues and providing coping strategies.

Artificial intelligence (AI) can significantly contribute to improving the mental health of children with neurodevelopmental disorders, such as autism and ADHD (Attention Deficit Hyperactivity Disorder), by offering tools to monitor, diagnose and support their emotional state. Through behavioral and voice analysis systems, AI can recognize signs of anxiety, depression or other psychological challenges at an early stage, allowing for early intervention by specialists and caregivers. In addition, personalization-based AI applications can offer interactive exercises and stress management strategies, contributing to children's overall well-being and enhancing their psychological well-being. For this purpose, a semi-structured interview survey was conducted with 30 mental health specialists. Their responses were coded and the following channels emerged from their decoding: AI helps mental health through

use. For successful integration, ongoing research, funding, professional training, and interdisciplinary collaboration are essential.

This research study examines how artificial intelligence is shaping ground-breaking impacts on the essence of human existence. An extensive examination reveals how artificial intelligence has transformed multiple aspects of life, ushering in a new age marked by remarkable productivity and ease of use. This study explores the complex interplay between artificial intelligence and mental well-being, analyzing its contradictory effects of positive and negative influence. Artificial intelligence (AI) technology possesses significant potential to revolutionize mental healthcare, but inherent risks. This study article provides a thorough analysis of the complexity of artificial intelligence in relation to mental well-being. This paper provides insights to use its advantages while minimizing risks, finally establishing a comprehensive plan for mental health treatment in contemporary society.

The aim of this investigation is to review the integration of Artificial Intelligence (AI) into mental health therapy, specifically in Cognitive Behavioral Therapy (CBT). AI can provide support in CBT, aiming to improve therapy accessibility. The search included scientific studies and articles indexed in the electronic databases. The results were synthesized to highlight AI's potential in CBT, while providing a detailed understanding of its capabilities. Findings indicate that the integration of AI into CBT offers a new era of more efficient and personalized mental health interventions. Additionally, conversational agents and chatbots offer effective emotional support. Overall, the relationship between cognitive psychology and artificial intelligence is a fact. We may effectively take advantage of the potential of AI to enhance the efficacy and accessibility of mental healthcare. However, challenges and limitations in current AI applications persist because the excessive reliance on AI is dangerous.

The present chapter delves into the dual role of artificial intelligence (AI) in reflecting and modifying society institutions, with a special emphasis on its applications in mental health and education. This chapter will analyze how AI mimics ideals, power dynamics, and biases of society while actively altering these areas, using a historical and sociological lens. By examining important technological breakthroughs from the Industrial Revolution to the AI age, we will analyze the lessons learned from previous sociotechnical systems and their implications for modern AI tools. The chapter will also critically examine the ethical and sociological concerns offered by AI, such as bias, equity, and cultural competence, and provide recommendations for developing more inclusive and socially responsible AI technology.

The domain of mental healthcare has been transforming rapidly against the backdrop of a global pandemic. The scale of mental health crisis that exists in the world is very high with highly prevalent mental health conditions in all countries. In this scenario, incorporating AI systems into mental healthcare marks a significant milestone in addressing the global mental health crisis. This chapter discusses AI's potential in mental healthcare, the extent of AI's capability in supporting mental health, popular AI platforms and their applications, and the risks and regulations grounded in ethical principles. The chapter emphasizes the necessity of adhering to ethical standards in mental health practices while utilizing AI to elevate the mental health field to provide accessible, cost-effective, and readily expandable services. Establishing strong rules, ensuring transparency, validating AI models, and continuously investing in research and development are all necessary to fulfill this potential.

Preface

MENTAL HEALTH IN CHILDREN AND YOUNG ADULTS—THE CRISIS WE ARE IN

Mental health disorders are on the rise globally. At least 10% of the population is affected, with almost 15% of adolescents experiencing a mental health condition and suicide being the fourth leading cause of death among those aged between 15 and 29 in US today. No one seems to know exactly why depression and anxiety are so common nowadays. The rise is attributed to multiple contributing factors, from the demands of modern society to the impact of the COVID-19 pandemic that has aggravated existing mental health issues. Some experts even argue that what we see is just an increasing awareness of mental health disorders, resulting in a surge of people actively seeking treatment.

Indeed, the number of adults receiving inpatient or outpatient care or counseling has been steadily rising in the US in the last two decades. At the same time, access to care is still limited, says Mental Health America in its 2023 report. Almost 30 million US adults with a mental disorder do not receive any treatment. Today, AI is used to analyze electronic health records (along with blood tests and brain images), questionnaires, voice recordings, behavioral signs, and even information sourced from a patient's social media accounts. Data Scientists employ a variety of techniques, such as supervised machine learning, deep learning, and natural language processing, to parse patient data and flag mental and physical states—pain, boredom, mind-wandering, stress, or suicidal thoughts—associated with a particular mental health disorder

Chatbots operate using natural language, and they have gained a lot of traction recently because they have the potential to provide a multitude of services through one point of contact. Chatbots have been used in education, customer service innovations, and healthcare. Within the area of mental health, there has been a recent drive toward creating digital interventions that can either supplement or replace face-to-face mental health services. As access to mental health services remains an issue worldwide, with the mental health workforce insufficient to meet the growing demand for mental health services, automated procedures hold great promise for both mental healthcare providers and for those in need of mental health services.

Privacy is also a major concern for users of these applications, and developers need to ensure that data sharing will not expose users to privacy risks. Poor adherence seems to be another problem with digital mental health interventions, and for those people who do go on to maintain a relationship with these digital resources, the fear is that some vulnerable people may begin to rely on them too much, which may lead to anxiety when these applications are not available. Overall, there is a need for a wider discussion about how all mental health services can and should encourage the safe and ethical use of chatbots

Although, there is scepticism among mental health practitioners that artificial intelligence solutions for mental health will ever be able to provide emphatic care, which they believe is vital, people do like chatting with chatbots and can even develop an emotional connection with them. We are talking here about vulnerable people's willingness to pour their hearts out anonymously to an AI companion. People tend to believe that robots don't judge, are unbiased, and can provide instant answers to health-related questions.

Multiple meta-analyses have confirmed that computer-aided cognitive behavioral therapy (CBT) delivered via desktop or mobile apps is equivalent to or even more effective than standard CBT. Moreover, studies have shown that the AI chatbot experience of people struggling with mental health issues has been overwhelmingly satisfactory but more research is definitely required on the adoption of AI for mental health treatment.

ORGANIZATION OF THE BOOK

As underlined by the theme *AI in Mental Health: Innovations, Challenges, and Collaborative Pathways* the book is an opportunity to explore in depth the transformative power of AI and its great potential in Mental Health. The chapters in this book throw light on new developments that can inform prevention, therapies and innovating supporting strategies in the field of mental health as well as the challenges that exist in implementing AI ideas in real clinical settings. The authors in this Book draw from a range of experience, examples, case studies, research and clinical cases to present this engaging text on using AI in Mental Health.

Section I: AI in Children's Wellbeing & Health

The first section of this volume provides innovating ideas on using AI to support children's mental health and wellbeing. More specifically, Chapter 1 explores how the integration of artificial intelligence (AI) into mental health intervention programs for children with ASD using video has emerged as a promising avenue for enhancing body awareness and well-being. Chapter 2 explores how the integration of artificial intelligence (AI) into mental health intervention programs for children has emerged as a promising avenue for enhancing emotional well-being. Chapter 3 discusses about using Artificial Intelligence to support screening and accurate Diagnosis for children with ASD. Chapter 4 explores AI 's potential to transform the delivery of care for individuals with disabilities, speech and motor impairments, and mental health challenges. Chapter 5 explores the potential of generative artificial intelligence (AI) to support mental health services in Philippine schools, particularly for high school and college students. Finally, Chapter 6 focuses on how AI can recognize signs of anxiety, depression or other psychological challenges at an early stage, allowing for early intervention by specialists and caregivers.

Section II: AI in Therapeutic Interventions

The second Section of the volume shifts the focus towards the use of AI in Therapeutic Interventions discussing how AI can transform the process of prevention, assessment, diagnosis and therapy suggesting theoretical and practical ideas that will be of value to mental health professionals. More specifically, Chapter 7 discusses how AI can improve well-being by automating repetitive tasks, providing personalized healthcare solutions, and supporting employee engagement. In addition, the chapter highlights key challenges, including AI anxiety, job displacement, privacy concerns, and the ethical risks of bias in decision-making. Chapter 8 focuses on how Artificial Intelligence (AI) offers solutions such as early diagnosis, personalized therapies, through virtual platforms, and machine-learning database.

Chapter 9 explores the complex interplay between artificial intelligence and mental well-being, analyzing its contradictory effects of positive and negative influence. Chapter 10 discusses research findings indicate that the integration of AI into CBT offers a new era of more efficient and personalized mental health interventions. Chapter 11 explores the integration of artificial intelligence (AI) into education and healthcare through a multidisciplinary lens, emphasizing both the transformative potential and the complex ethical, infrastructural, and contextual challenges of implementation. Chapter 12 examines how Brain-Computer Interfaces (BCIs) are transforming communication and emotion recognition for individuals with conditions like Locked-In Syndrome (LIS), Autism Spectrum Disorder (ASD), and Amyotrophic Lateral Sclerosis (ALS). Chapter 13 delves into the dual role of artificial intelligence (AI) in reflecting and modifying society institutions, with a special emphasis on its applications in mental health and education.

Chapter 14 discusses AI's potential in mental healthcare, the extent of AI's capability in supporting mental health, popular AI platforms and their applications, and the risks and regulations grounded in ethical principles. Chapter 15 explores the risks from the constant use of AI platforms and applications which may reduce the need to engage deeply in intellectual tasks, shortens attention span, and discourages independent thinking. Chapter 16 examines the psychological and social effects of AI such as decreased motivation, resilience, and intellectual curiosity. Finally, Chapter 17 explores the multidisciplinary approaches to AI integration, focusing on how collaboration across fields such as data science, psychology, social sciences, and policy-making can ensure the successful deployment of AI technologies.

Maria Efstratopoulou
Agathi Argyriadi
Alexandros Argyriadis

REFERENCES

Tong, A. C. Y., Wong, K. T. Y., Chung, W. W. T., & Mak, W. W. S. (2025). Effectiveness of Topic-Based Chatbots on Mental Health Self-Care and Mental Well-Being: Randomized Controlled Trial. *Journal of Medical Internet Research*, *27*, e70436. DOI: 10.2196/70436 PMID: 40306635

Ware, S., Yue, C., Morillo, R., Lu, J., Shang, C., Bi, J., Kamath, J., Russell, A., Bamis, A., & Wang, B. (2020). Predicting depressive symptoms using smartphone data. *Smart Health (Amsterdam, Netherlands)*, *15*, 2020. DOI: 10.1016/j.smhl.2019.100093

Chapter 1
A Health Education Program for Children With Autism Spectrum Disorder Using Video-Modeling

Dimitra Maria Tomprou
https://orcid.org/0000-0002-0434-0999
Frederick University, Cyprus

Anna Christina Galani
Frederick University, Cyprus

Maria Georgiadi
University of Crete, Greece

Stefanos Plexousakis
Frederick University, Cyprus

Nataly Loizidou Ieridou
https://orcid.org/0000-0002-8988-4804
Frederick University, Cyprus

Olga Lyra
Frederick University, Cyprus

ABSTRACT

Health education is important for all children as it helps them develop a balanced and safe relationship with their bodies and gender. Especially for children diagnosed with Autism Spectrum Disorder (ASD), health education is a matter of priority, because they may experience difficulties in their psychosocial functioning. The objectives of a health education program for children with ASD are to acquire better understanding of their body, learn basic hygiene skills, to be informed about personal safety/issues of abuse, to improve their gender awareness and behavior, which in the long term will benefit their full social inclusion. The aim of this research is the implementation of a health education program for school-aged children with ASD based on video modeling and focused on body awareness and privacy as dimensions

DOI: 10.4018/979-8-3373-5072-1.ch001

of health education. The results showed that all the children were able to respond to the program and understood which body parts they are able to expose in public and which they are required to keep in private.

INTRODUCTION

Autism Spectrum Disorder (ASD) is a neurodevelopmental disorder with a complex etiological background, in which a combination of genes and environmental interactions seem to be involved (Kirk et al., 2021). The symptoms of ASD mainly include deficits in social communication and interaction, as well as restricted and repetitive patterns of behavior (APA, 2013; Holopainen et.al, 2019; Noel & Angelaki, 2023). In particular, the first main group related to social communication and interaction is associated with deficits in social-emotional reciprocity, extra-verbal communication behaviors, difficulties in the ability to develop, understand and maintain relationships, dysfunction in verbal and non-verbal communication, avoiding eye contact, not understanding gestures to a complete lack of expressions and communication methods (APA, 2022; Georgiadi, 2022; Xiong, et.al., 2019). The second group of deficits concerns certain and repetitive patterns of behavior, which may include stereotypes and repetitive movements, production of echolalia and other idiosyncratic expressions, insistence on similarity and strict commitment to regular routines, which affect the individual's adaptation to change (Kirk et al., 2021).

Autism has a prevalence of 1-1.5% with the onset of symptoms beginning in the early developmental period of the child's life (Pain et al., 2019; Rosenberg et.al. 2015). According to the Diagnostic and Statistical Manual of Mental Disorders (DSM-5) (APA, 2013), there are three levels of severity for ASD symptoms, and these deficiencies reflect major obstacles that a child has to overcome and that may affect critical facets of the child's life, including academic, social, and mental health (Tomprou et al., 2022). The etiological background of ASD seems to include hereditary factors and chromosomal abnormalities, neurology and brain development factors, infectious diseases, psychosocial factors and environmental influences (Tomprou, 2022; Xiong, et.al., 2019). This multitude of etiological factors potentially explains the different phenotypes and levels of severity of the disorder with current research data highlighting the interaction of genetic and environmental factors in the development of ASD (Shaw et al., 2014).

Each child with ASD manifests his or her intrinsic characteristics in a very different way and intensity and thus special education and individualized support that is carefully planned and subject to frequent assessment and reflection is essential (Tomprou et al., 2022). Intervention programs are therapeutic approaches that facilitate child's functioning. In many cases, a combination of interventions is applied that is perfectly in line with the child's needs. Intervention programs may be cognitive-behavioral, social, or may reinforce an alternative method of communication and they focus on enhancing social and functional skills, such as social adaptation, autonomy and quality of life, avoiding pervasive social deficits (Brignell et al., 2018).

The Importance of Health Education

Despite the growing research interest in the study of ASD, important aspects of these people's lives, such as health education and interpersonal relationships have been neglected. The inability to understand social situations, which can lead to social withdrawal, is the main cause of difficulty in developing skills (Zhao, et.al., 2021). It is not recognized that people with autism struggle to form and maintain close relationships and are often considered to have misbehavior. Many children and adolescents experience a loss of self-regulation due to nervous system overstimulation, which makes difficult for them to adjust to a social setting (Schilbach, 2022; Wood - Downie, et.al., 2021). For children diagnosed with a form of disability such as ASD, health education should be a priority because they are at serious risk of being sexually exploited, have difficulty understanding and verbally expressing an abusive behavior and may generally experience difficulties in psychosocial functioning (Ballan & Freyer, 2017; Dekker et. al., 2015).

It is worth noting that health education includes concepts such as body image, emotions, attitudes, behaviors, etc. (Plexousakis et al., 2011). The need for education in self-concept, understanding the words and intentions of others, and the demands related to relationships with others seem to play a crucial role in the health development of children with ASD (MacKenzie, 2018) from preschool onwards because evidence suggests that early intervention can lead to better self-protective behaviors such as understanding and management of personal boundaries, social interactions and appropriate behaviors (Walsh et al., 2015). In particular, the objectives of a health education program for children with ASD are to enable them to acquire a better knowledge tailored to their needs regarding the understanding of the anatomy and physiology of the human body, to know basic rules of personal hygiene, to be informed about issues related to personal safety/issues of abuse, boundary violation, to be informed about reproduction and pregnancy, to be informed about how to protect themselves from sexually transmitted diseases, to learn ways to establish healthy relationships, and improve body awareness and behavior, which in the long term will benefit the full social inclusion of people with ASD (Georgiadi et al., 2022; Davis et al., 2021. Littner et al., 2017). According to research, children with ASD frequently receive insufficient health education, which can lead to confusion about body autonomy, consent and personal safety (Holmes et al., 2016). The importance of health education is related to biological, emotional, moral and social aspects of human behavior (Kaestle & Halpern, 2005).

Health Education Through Video-Modeling

Health education for children with autism requires special methods that take into account the unique needs of people with ASD. Modeling is one strategy that can be used, in which one or more people demonstrate a behavior that a child is urged to imitate (American Psychological Association, n.d.). The behavioral model can be either live or videotaped, as in the case of video modeling, which is a method where children are shown how to perform a particular activity or how to react to a particular situation using video (Acar et al., 2016; Besler & Kurt, 2016). During video modeling interventions, a child watches videos of peers, adults, or themselves demonstrating a behavior that is being taught and research findings suggest that teaching children with autism a range of skills and behaviors through video modeling is effective (Delano, 2007; Halle et al., 2016; Qi et al., 2018).

During modeling process, the target behavior is modeled on screen by an adult, the instructor provides appropriate instructions and prompts to focus on the desired elements, and finally, the participant is reinforced to perform the target behavior through imitation of the model (Anderson et al, 2018). Videos are recommended to be short in duration (30 seconds to 4 minutes) and low in stimulation to allow children more easily perceive key cues (Chen et al., 2016). There are several types of video-modeling, such as video self-modeling (self-modeling using video), point of view video-modeling (video modeling from the person's point of view), and peer video-modeling (peer modeling) (McCoy & Hermansen, 2007).

For children with autism, who often respond positively to visual stimuli, videos can be an effective tool. Meta-analysis of Bellini & Akullian (2007) examined the effectiveness of video modeling interventions for children and adolescents with ASD and their findings imply that video modeling is an effective intervention strategy for teaching social communication and behavioral functioning skills are maintained over time. Similar findings highlighted Wang et al. (2011) in their meta-analysis about the effectiveness of peer-mediated and video-modeling approaches; both approaches used for social skills training of children with ASD were found to significantly improve the social performance of children with ASD.

Video-modeling is visually and audibly stimulating, which means that it is difficult to lose attention to the stimuli (Turner, 2017). Additionally, the presentation of concrete examples helps children to better understand the target behavior and generalize it, providing also the opportunity to replay the video until the child has acquired the target behavior (Mitsch et al., 2021). Furthermore, it seems to help children to engage with their peers and better cooperate with them (Alpaydın, 2020).

It is an approach that does not involve eye contact and is performed without the need for physical communication or interaction with another person, which reduces the chances of anxiety and fear (Alhuzimi, 2022; Besler & Kurt, 2016). Video-modeling is, moreover, very easy to implement and low in cost (Taheri-Torbati & Sotoodeh, 2019). Finally, watching videos on tablets and smartphones attracts children's attention (Mitsch et al., 2020) and simultaneously increases their motivation (Alhuzimi, 2022).

Several studies have demonstrated the significant contribution of video modeling to the acquisition of basic health education skills. Piccin et al. (2018) conducted a review of research that relied on video modeling to enable autistic children to help themselves regarding their hygiene skills such as learning to brush teeth correctly, hand washing and toileting and the findings demonstrated that video modeling is a useful tool in learning self-care skills. Godish et al. (2017) created a preventative intervention program for children with ASD that aimed to reinforce self-defense skills, such as saying no, walking away from a stranger and heading to a trusted person, and reporting to a trusted adult being lured or harassed. The intervention was deemed successful and it was felt that developing these skills could reduce exploitation and abduction rates (Godish et al., 2017). Meister & Salls (2015), finally, investigated the efficacy of point-of-view video modeling as an intervention strategy to improve self-help skills in children with ASD. Results suggested that video modeling was an effective technique for teaching students with ASD self-care and daily living skills with significant improvement in task performance during a six-week period (Meister & Salls, 2015).

Video-modeling, in addition to the above, has been shown to significantly improve visual attention skills and the children's ability to ask for something they want (Alpaydın, 2020; Rudy et al., 2014). Joint attention, in particular, is a key skill that is underdeveloped and needs to be cultivated in children with ASD, as it is a key skill that emerges from early infancy and appears to be a predictor of later language development (White et al., 2011). Joint attention refers to the child's ability to focus and share an interest (event or object) with another person (Lord et al., 2020). Several early intervention programs have been developed to enhance this skill; however, the importance of indirect teaching of joint attention skills during the therapeutic process is pointed out (White et al., 2011). The research by Ho et al. (2019) confirmed the contribution of video modeling to the rapid acquisition of joint attention and social engagement. Duenas et al. (2019) developed an intervention based on joint video-modeling to enhance spontaneous behaviors in joint play with peers. Results showed improvement in expressions during scripted games with typically developing peers (Duenas et al., 2019). Chen et al. (2016) created a video modeling-based intervention through a storybook, that aimed to improve perceptual and critical thinking skills from expressions and emotions to a broader social interaction. Results showed that children's attention was sustained and helped participants to understand facial expressions and emotions of storybook characters (Chen et al., 2016).

The purpose of the present study was to examine the effects of a video modeling health education program for school-aged children diagnosed with ASD. We aimed to extend current literature in this area by assessing the ability of school-aged children with ASD to acquire a better knowledge of the human body and to be informed about issues related to personal safety through video modeling. The main goal of this intervention program was to enhance health education focusing on body awareness and privacy as dimensions of health education, as well as on the permissible social involvement (communication and interaction) in these situations.

METHOD

Participants

Four children with ASD, three boys and one girl, between 7 to 10 years old, participated in this study. All children were diagnosed with ASD and mild to severe intellectual disability by doctors or public assessment services not associated with this study (see Table 1). Basic inclusion criterion was each child to demonstrate eye contact in response to having his name called or the instruction "Look". A questionnaire addressed to parents was also used in order to create a profile of the participants. It included information of personal history, developmental and medical history, school history and emotional and social development. The Basic Skills Checklist (Greek Ministry of Education-Pedagogical Institute, 2009), which focused on cognitive, psychomotor, emotional and oral language skills, were used as the basis for gathering data from teachers and observation of the children (see Table 2).

Table 1. Participants demographics

	Participant's gender	Age (in years)	Diagnosis
1	boy	9,1	ASD moderate intellectual disability
2	girl	10	ASD mild to moderate intellectual disability
3	boy	8,3	ASD mild to moderate intellectual disability
4	boy	7,6	ASD moderate to severe intellectual disability

Table 2. Participants characteristics according to basic skills checklist

Participant 1 Verbal skills: he uses single words and does not compose sentences. He gives single-word answers in simple questions and does not participate in discussions. He gets very anxious by loud noises. Psychomobility: he performs general mobility movements on his own. He takes care of his personal hygiene with the help of his mother. Fine motor skills are limited. He defines his position in space by sitting where he wants, but he does not have good balance. Cognitive skills: he learns by visualizing pictures. He does not identify similarities and differences and cannot connect temporal events. When is called, he responds and makes eye contact. He recognizes the names of some of his classmates. Emotional organization: he accepts familiar faces, but is distant with unknown faces; he does not have outbursts of anger.
Participant 2 *Verbal skills:* She answers in simple personal questions (e.g., where do you live, does you have siblings) and names familiar people but she does not promote dialogue. She communicates her simple needs. *Psychomobility:* She performs general mobility movements on her own. She takes care of her personal hygiene. Fine motor skills are good. She defines her position in space but does not orientate herself. *Cognitive skills:* She identifies simple similarities and differences and connects temporal events with guidance. When is called, she responds and makes eye contact. She has mastered basic academic skills *Emotional organization:* She seems to like friends, family and classmates, but does not respond positively to physical contact. She does not seem to be upset by loud sounds, only by loud rhythmically changing lights. She does not like changes.
Participant 3 *Verbal skills:* He answers in simple personal questions and names familiar people. He does not promote dialogue. He communicates his simple needs. *Psychomobility:* He performs general mobility movements on his own. He takes care of his personal hygiene but he needs supervision. Fine motor skills are good. He defines his position in space and he has good balance. *Cognitive skills:* He identifies simple similarities and differences and connects temporal events with guidance. When is called, he responds and makes eye contact. He has mastered basic academic skills. *Emotional organization:* He is usually alone and does not respond positively to physical contact. He seems to be upset by loud noises.
Participant 4 *Verbal skills:* he uses sometimes single words and does not compose sentences. He usually uses echolalia. He does not mention names and objects. Facial expressions are neutral. He gets very anxious by loud noises. *Psychomobility:* he performs general mobility movements on his own. He does not takes care of his personal hygiene without help. Fine motor skills are limited. *Cognitive skills:* he learns by visualizing pictures. He does not identify similarities and differences and cannot connect temporal events. When is called, he responds and makes eye contact, but he does not know the names of his classmates. *Emotional organization:* he accepts familiar faces, but is distant with unknown faces; he has outbursts of anger in loud noises and sudden changes.

(Greek Ministry of Education-Pedagogical Institute, 2009)

Intervention Design and Implementation

The video modeling intervention consists of four short videos (2 min to 2 min 30 sec), each focusing on specific health education topics, including body awareness and privacy/social involvement. Repetition to reinforce learning along with opportunities for practicing the skills demonstrated in the videos were essential and incorporated in this intervention program.

Specifically, the first group of two videos were related to body awareness, where the child watches each video with peers talking about the body parts that are male/female or common to both genders. Then, based on the video, the child proceeds to an assessment exercise, where he/she matches body parts according to gender. The second group of two videos focuses on privacy as a dimension of health education, but also on social involvement. The child watches relevant videos with peers showing a desired behavior according to situations in which one is allowed to expose private parts of his/her body. Videos shows people and private and public places where exposure of the private parts of the body is allowed and considered safe or not (e.g. being naked in places with privacy such as home bathroom or child's room/public places like school or playground where exposure of the private parts of the body is not safe). Then, based on video, the child proceeds to a related matching exercise on a computer-based environment. The duration of each individual session was 30 minutes (including videos an assessment exercises).

At Phase 1 of this research process, the researchers collected the data from the parents regarding child's history. All parents also were given a consent form for their child's participation in the intervention process. After obtaining informed consent to participate, all assessments, observations and interventions were completed for each child in Phase 2. Specifically, a non-participatory assessment of the participants was conducted within the school setting in order to create the profile of the participants (see above).

At phase 3, the main part of the intervention was initiated. A four-week and eight-session intervention program was implemented focusing on body awareness and privacy as dimensions of health education. The intervention took place in a structured setting, such as a school classroom for all of the participants. Each child entered the classroom accompanied by his/her teacher. During intervention sessions that involved video modeling, the participant was oriented toward the computer screen and the trainer said "*Watch this.*" When the video ended, the trainer facilitated the procedure with guided brief discussions following each video, reinforcing the concepts demonstrated and allowing children to express their understanding or ask questions. Then, the trainer said "*Now you do the exercise*" followed by brief and structured instructions. The duration of each individual session was 23-27 minutes (including videos an assessment exercises)

RESULTS

A four-week and eight-session health education intervention program was implemented in four children with ASD focusing on body awareness and privacy issues. Each session included four short videos; two videos focused on body parts that are male/female or common to both genders and two videos focused on privacy showing desired behaviors according to situations in which one might feel safe (being naked in places with privacy such as home bathroom or child's and not in public places like school or playground). Then, based on videos, all children proceeded to related assessment exercises.

Initially, all 4 participants responded positively during the observation phase, as they behaved typically and were not disturbed by the presence of the researcher in the classroom. Similarly, during the intervention phase they had a positive attitude towards the process and demonstrated good adaptation and engagement skills. All children required verbal guidance and appeared to respond positively to reinforcement and reward. However, the last participant, in almost all sessions, appeared to have difficulty in focusing his attention, as well as more time and continued redirection of attention was required.

Specifically, with regard to the first strand of the intervention concerning body awareness, all participants showed significant improvement and their performance in the assessment activities related to common body parts was very good in all sessions with an improvement trend. Specifically, the second child performed the best scores, while the first and third child scored 85%. The fourth participant although seemed to struggle in the initial sessions, scored 50%), was significant, reaching 80% by the end of the intervention (Figure 1).

Figure 1. Percentage of correct responding for all participants per session after the assessment exercise regarding common body parts in both boys and girls.

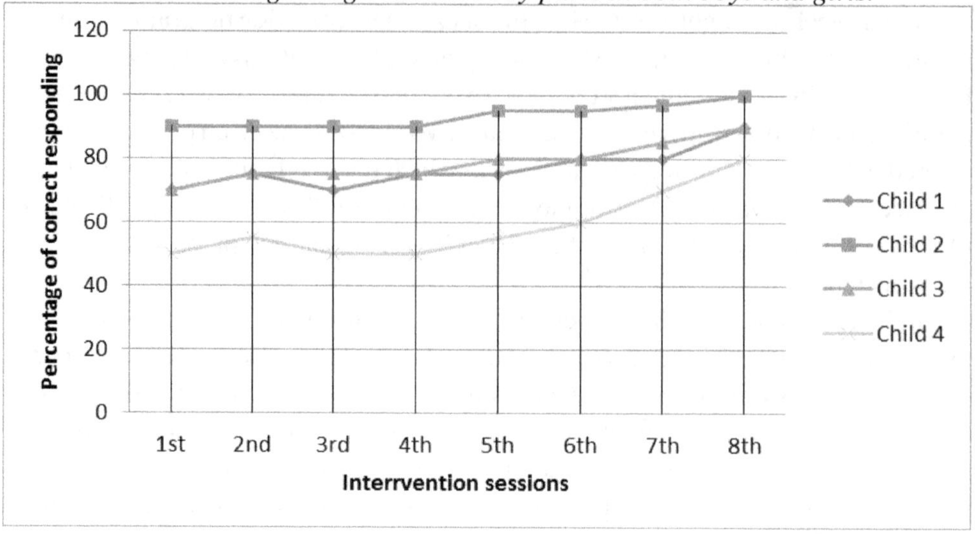

Similar results in children's performance were observed in terms of understanding the different body parts according to gender. As in the first evaluation exercise, the first participant had the higher scores (100%), while the fourth child appeared to have difficulty understanding this distinction during the initial sessions; however, he made significant progress as it began at 45% and improved to 75% by the final sessions. (Figure 2).

Figure 2. Percentage of correct responding for all participants per session after the assessment exercise about different body parts according to gender

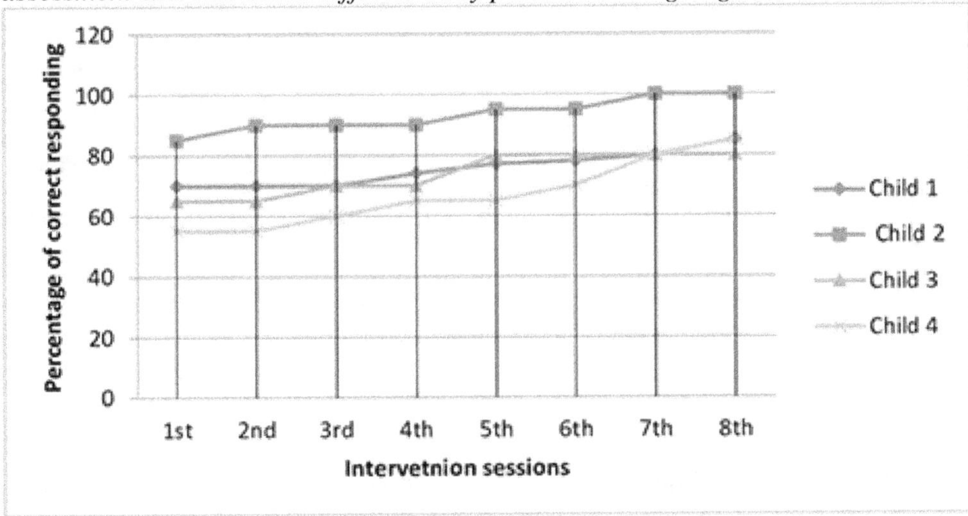

Regarding the second strand of the intervention concerning privacy and desired behaviors of exposing or not exposing body parts in order for a child to feel safe (being naked in places with privacy such as home bathroom or child's room and not in public places like school or playground), their performance in the initial sessions was obviously lower compared to the subsequent sessions of the intervention program. As shown in Figure 3, all four participants initially found it difficult to associate private or public places with permissible exposure of private body parts; yet, their performance improved significantly, with percentage increases from 30% to 80% across all participants.

Figure 3. Percentage of correct responding for all participants per session after the assessment exercise regarding the private and public places that the exposure of the private parts of the body is allowed and considered safe

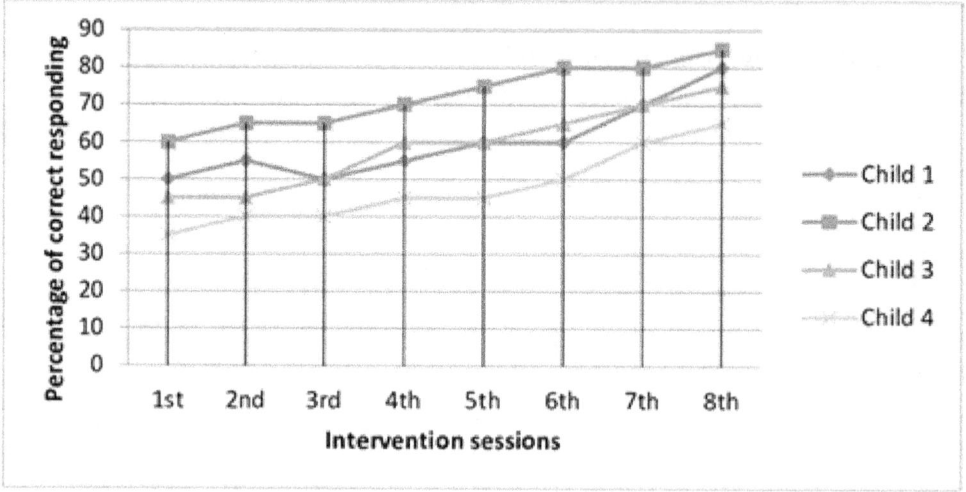

Correspondingly, in Figure 4 is shown children's progress in social understanding regarding the people to whom it is considered safe to expose private parts of their bodies. Again, this reflects the ascending trend in children's percentage of correct responding during the intervention program (from 30% to 90% across all participants).

Figure 4. Percentage of correct responding for all participants per session after the assessment exercise regarding who is considered reliable to expose private parts of the body

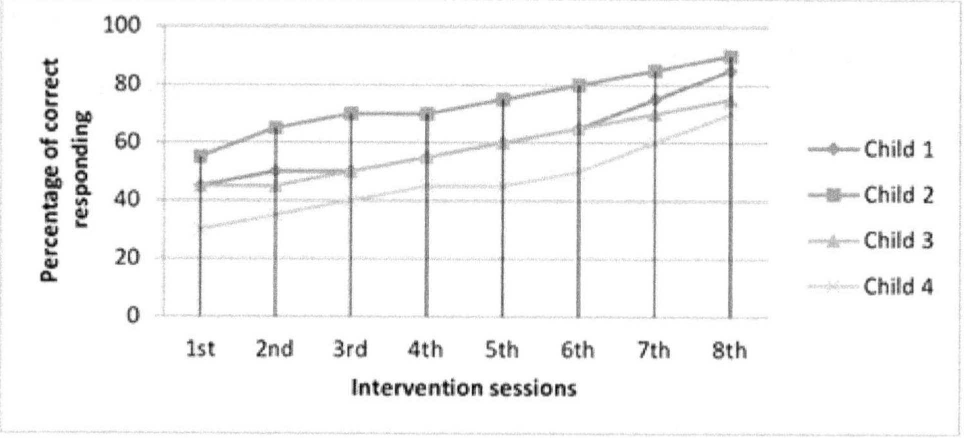

In conclusion, all participants responded positively to the process and appeared to improve the degree and quality of their engagement and joint attention skills through the video modeling intervention. The performance of the child with mild to moderate intellectual disability and less deficits in basic skill areas was higher in all phases of the program. In contrast, the student with the most severe degree of intellectual disability and the more deficits in functional skills recorded the lowest performance; yet it should me underlined that he performed significant intrapersonal improvement during the interventions. Respectively, the efficacy of video modeling interventions was further demonstrated by the four participants' notable intrapersonal improvement in the degree of achievement of program goals.

DISCUSSION

Health education skills are a complex set of skills associated with factors, such as biological, psychological and social. The primary means of expression include feelings, thoughts, and actions as well as the type of relationship that an individual develops with another (Chianese, et al., 2021). It is part of the personality and contributes to the maintenance of physical and mental health and balance (Schöttle et al., 2017). Primary goals of a health education program are to help a child understand his/her body an gender, to experience the choice of interpersonal relationships in a responsible and safe way and to be informed against possible violation of his/her rights (Pugliese, et.al., 2020).

Research suggests that children with ASD are more vulnerable because they often lack critical knowledge regarding personal safety and appropriate behaviors (Georgiadi et al., 2022). Age-appropriate health education is essential for promoting self-advocacy and positive interpersonal interactions. It has been demonstrated that video modeling is an effective educational technique for teaching children with ASD a variety of abilities, especially in social and behavioral contexts (Schreibman et al., 2015; Wilson, 2013). This approach utilizes children's with ASD's strength on visual learning and is considered a promising method for improving social awareness and imitation abilities in the context of health education.

The integration of video modeling in health education for children with ASD has several benefits (Solomon et al., 2019). Firstly, it supports different learning styles, especially visual learning which is known to be helpful for children with ASD (Tissot & Evans, 2003). Video modeling provides clear, concrete examples of social situations, behaviors, and concepts related to health education that may be difficult to teach only with verbal explanations, as well as improves understanding of social cues, body language, and emotional expressions related to relationships and personal safety. Moreover, video modeling can be easily implemented in various settings, including homes and schools, and ensures a secure and structured learning environment, where levels of stress and anxiety are reduced (Miltenberger & Charlop, 2015). Despite its advantages, implementing video modeling interventions in health education also poses challenges. There may be questions about whether the material is acceptable or not, and whether parental participation is required in reinforcing the concepts taught (Solomon et al., 2019).

The main purpose of this study was to determine the effects of a video modeling health education program for school-aged children diagnosed with ASD and the extent to which children are able to acquire a better knowledge of the human body and to be informed about issues related to personal safety through video modeling. A four-week and eight-session health education intervention program was implemented in four children with ASD focusing on body awareness and privacy. Each session included four short videos about body parts that are male/female or common to both genders, as well as privacy issues and desired behaviors of exposing or not exposing body parts in order for a child to feel safe. Then, based on videos, all children proceeded to related assessment exercises.

Results showed that all participants responded positively to the process. Furthermore, the degree and quality of their engagement and joint attention skills appeared to improve through the video modeling intervention sessions. The use of video modeling techniques and their combination with joint attention skills is consistent with the research of Rudy et al. (2014), who used and endorsed the effect of video modeling in combination with joint attention skills in children with autism.

The performance of all children seems to be connected with intellectual disability severity level, because the child with the higher intellectual anility and fewer deficits in functional behavior had better scores in all phases of the program. Contrary, the student with the most severe degree of cognitive disability and the largest functional level deficits recorded the lowest performance. Yet, all participants showed significant intrapersonal improvement during the interventions irrespective of the severity of the intellectual disability.

Current results are aligned with the study of Acar et al., (2016), which showed that video modeling interventions were effective in teaching social skills to children with ASD and children could maintain and generalize their acquired skills. Furthermore, Godish et al. (2017) designed a video modeling intervention program to teach abduction prevention skills to children with autism, such as saying no, walking away from a stranger and heading to a trusted person and was found to be effective and important in developing safety skills, so that could reduce exploitation and abduction rates. Piccin et al. (2018), also, demonstrated that video modeling is a useful tool in learning self-care skills. Meta-analysis by Hong et al. (2016) examined the effects of video modeling on teaching functional living skills, which could include aspects of health education and their results indicate that video modeling interventions are overall moderately effective. Respectively, meta-analysis of Bellini & Akullian (2007) examined the effectiveness of video modeling interventions for children and adolescents with ASD and their findings imply that video modeling is an effective intervention strategy for teaching social communication and behavioral functioning skills that are maintained over time.

CONCLUSION

Current study's originality lies in the implementation of a video modeling program to teach both body awareness and privacy as dimensions of health education, as well as permissible social engagement in children with ASD. Understanding body differences according to gender and adopting appropriate behaviors in private and public places is crucial for children with ASD. This video modeling intervention had positive outcomes, with all participants showing significant improvement in body awareness and privacy issues. Notably, despite differences in intellectual disability severity, all participants demonstrated significant intra-individual progress.

However, the current study had some limitations to take into consideration. Firstly, this was a preliminary study as a part of a general health education program for teaching skills to children diagnosed with ASD through video modeling. Since there were only four participants, additional replication is required to determine the robustness of our findings. Second, follow-up data to evaluate the maintenance of these skills were not obtained. Thus, future research should evaluate the maintenance of body awareness and safety skills across extended time periods and across other participants.

In the future, researchers may investigate whether teaching children with ASD other safety skills through video modeling might be also beneficial. Considering that video modeling was effective in teaching all four participants body awareness and safety skills, video modeling may be effective in teaching other safety skills as well. Moreover, future studies may focus on the implementation of similar interventions in children with ASD of different ages (e.g. preschoolers, adolescents). Parent and caregiver involvement to an intervention health education program could also be a future research direction. Parents of children with ASD play a pivotal role in the process of their education and their involvement to a similar video modeling health education program may reinforce the concepts at home.

In conclusion, the aim of this study was to create an educational program that aims to expand knowledge about the human body and how to manage it in the best possible way towards others. Understanding body differences according to gender and adopting appropriate ways of behaving in a public or private place is essential for children with ASD of all ages. Teaching health education to school-aged children with ASD using video modeling seemed to be a promising intervention approach. Educators can create an engaging and effective learning environment that addresses the specific needs of children with autism. Additionally, better knowledge and understanding of health education can empower children with ASD to get involved in social situations with greater confidence and safety. As society continues to recognize the importance of inclusive education, the integration of innovative strategies such as video modeling has the potential to promote and transform the educational experiences of children with ASD.

REFERENCES

Acar, C., Tekin Iftar, E., & Yıkmış, A. (2016). Effects of mother-delivered social stories and video modeling in teaching social skills to shildren with Autism Spectrum Disorders. *The Journal of Special Education.* Advance online publication. DOI: 10.1177/0022466916649

Alhuzimi, T. (2022). Efficacy of video modeling (VM) in developing social skills in children with autism spectrum disorder (ASD) at school in Saudi Arabia. *International Journal of Disability Development and Education*, *69*(2), 550–564. DOI: 10.1080/1034912X.2020.1716962

Alpaydın, B. (2020). The effectiveness of video modeling on social and communication skills: A systematic review. *International Journal of Scholars in Education*, *3*(2), 363–373. https://dergipark.org.tr/en/pub/ueader/issue/59308/827006

American Psychiatric Association. (2013). *Diagnostic and statistical manual of mental disorders* (5th ed.).

American Psychiatric Association. (2022). *Diagnostic and statistical manual of mental disorders* (5th ed., text rev.).

Ballan, M. S., & Freyer, M. B. (2017). Autism spectrum disorder, adolescence, and sexuality education: Suggested interventions for mental health professionals. *Sexuality and Disability*, *35*(2), 261–273. DOI: 10.1007/s11195-017-9477-9

Bellini, S., & Akullian, J. (2007). A Meta-Analysis of Video Modeling and Video Self-Modeling Interventions for Children and Adolescents with Autism Spectrum Disorders. *Exceptional Children*, *73*(3), 264–287. DOI: 10.1177/001440290707300301

Besler, F., & Kurt, O. (2016). Effectiveness of video modeling provided by mothers in teaching play skills to children with autism. *Educational Sciences: Theory & Practice*, *16*(1), 209–230. DOI: 10.12738/estp.2016.1.0273

Brignell, A., Chenausky, K. V., Song, H., Zhu, J., Suo, C., & Morgan, A. T. (2018). Communication interventions for autism spectrum disorder in minimally verbal children. *Cochrane Database of Systematic Reviews*, *2018*(11). Advance online publication. DOI: 10.1002/14651858.CD012324.pub2 PMID: 30395694

Chen, C. H., Lee, I. J., & Lin, L. Y. (2016). Augmented reality-based video-modeling storybook of nonverbal facial cues for children with autism spectrum disorder to improve their perceptions and judgments of facial expressions and emotions. *Computers in Human Behavior*, *55*, 477–485. Advance online publication. DOI: 10.1016/j.chb.2015.09.033

Chianese, A. A., Jackson, S. Z., & Souders, M. C. (2021). Psychosexual knowledge and education in autism spectrum disorder individuals. *Journal of the American Association of Nurse Practitioners, 33*(10), 776–784. DOI: 10.1097/JXX.0000000000000508 PMID: 33273264

Davis, R., & Crompton, C. J. (2021). What do new findings about social interaction in autistic adults mean for neurodevelopmental research? *Perspectives on Psychological Science, 16*(3), 649–653. DOI: 10.1177/1745691620958010 PMID: 33560175

Dekker, L. P., Van Der Vegt, E. J., Visser, K., Tick, N., Boudesteijn, F., Verhulst, F. C., Maras, A., & Greaves-Lord, K. (2015). Improving psychosexual knowledge in adolescents with autism spectrum disorder: Pilot of the tackling teenage training program. *Journal of Autism and Developmental Disorders, 45*(6), 1532–1540. DOI: 10.1007/s10803-014-2301-9 PMID: 25399394

Delano, M. E. (2007). Video modeling interventions for individuals with autism. *Remedial and Special Education, 28*(1), 33–42. DOI: 10.1177/07419325070280010401

Dueñas, A. D., Plavnick, J. B., & Bak, M. Y. S. (2019). Effects of Joint Video Modeling on Unscripted Play Behavior of Children with Autism Spectrum Disorder. *Journal of Autism and Developmental Disorders, 49*(1), 236–247. DOI: 10.1007/s10803-018-3719-2 PMID: 30136112

Georgiadi, M. (2022). Definition and modern diagnostic issues. In Georgiadi, M. (Ed.), *Children and Adolescents with Autism Spectrum Disorder. Contemporary Research Data and Therapeutic Interventions*. Papazisi.

Georgiadi, M., Tombrou, D. M., Plexousakis, S., & Loizidou-Ieridoy, N. (2022). Strengthening Sexual Education of Students with Autism Spectrum DisorderIn Children and Adolescents with Autism Spectrum Disorder. In Georgiadi, M. (Ed.), *Children and Adolescents with Autism Spectrum Disorde:Contemporary Research Data and Therapeutic Interventions*. Papazisi.

Godish, D., Miltenberger, R., & Sanchez, S. (2017). Evaluation of Video Modeling for Teaching Abduction Prevention Skills to Children with Autism Spectrum Disorder. *Advances in Neurodevelopmental Disorders, 1*(3), 168–175. Advance online publication. DOI: 10.1007/s41252-017-0026-4

Greek Ministry of Education-Pedagogical Institute. (2009). *Learning Readiness Activities. Oral Speech, Psychomotricity, Mental abilities, Emotional Organization. Book for the teacher of Special Education and training and students* (Drossinou, M., Ed.). Pedagogical Institute, Organization for the Publication of Teaching Books., http://www.pi-schools.gr/download/lessons/drast_math_etoimotitas/vivlio_ekp/vivlio.pdf

Halle, S., Ninness, C., Ninness, S. K., & Lawson, D. (2016). Teaching social skills to students with autism: A video modeling social stories approach. *Behavior and Social Issues*, *25*(1), 42–54. DOI: 10.5210/bsi.v25i0.6190

Ho, T. Q., Gadke, D. L., Henington, C., Evans-McCleon, T. N., & Justice, C. A. (2019). The effects of animated video modeling on joint attention and social engagement in children with autism spectrum disorder. *Research in Autism Spectrum Disorders*, *58*, 83–95. DOI: 10.1016/j.rasd.2018.09.004

Holmes, L. G., Himle, M. B., & Strassberg, D. S. (2016). Parental sexuality-related concerns for adolescents with autism spectrum disorders and average or above IQ. *Research in Autism Spectrum Disorders*, *21*, 84–93. DOI: 10.1016/j.rasd.2015.10.001

Holopainen, A., de Veld, D. M., Hoddenbach, E., & Begeer, S. (2019). Does theory of mind training enhance empathy in autism? *Journal of Autism and Developmental Disorders*, *49*(10), 3965–3972. DOI: 10.1007/s10803-018-3671-1 PMID: 30074122

Kaestle, C. E., & Halpern, C. T. (2005). Sexual intercourse precedes partner violence in adolescent romantic relationships. *The Journal of Adolescent Health*, *36*(5), 386–392. DOI: 10.1016/j.jadohealth.2004.02.030 PMID: 15837342

Kirk, S., Gallagher, J., & Coleman, M. R. (2021). *Educating Exceptional children* (Georgiadi, M., Plexousakis, S., & Tomprou, D. M., Eds.). Utopia Publishing.

Littner, L., Littner, M., & Bae, Y. S. (2017). Sexuality Education for Students with Autism Spectrum Disorder. *Curricula for Teaching Students with Autism Spectrum Disorder*, 251-271. DOI: 10.1007/978-3-319-69983-7_11

Lord, C., & Tager-Flusberga, H. Does Gestural Communication Influence Later Spoken Language Ability in Minimally Verbal Autistic Children?. *Journal of Speech, Language, and Hearing Research, 1*, 14. DOI: 10.1044/2024_JSLHR-23-00433

MacKenzie, A. (2018). Prejudicial stereotypes and testimonial injustice: Autism, sexuality and sex education. *International Journal of Educational Research*, *89*, 110–118. DOI: 10.1016/j.ijer.2017.10.007

McCoy, K., & Hermansen, E. (2007). Video modeling for individuals with autism: A review of model types and effects. *Education & Treatment of Children*, *30*(4), 183–213. https://www.jstor.org/stable/42899952. DOI: 10.1353/etc.2007.0029

Meister, C., & Salls, J. (2015). Video modeling for teaching daily living skills to children with autism spectrum disorder: A pilot study. *Journal of Occupational Therapy, Schools & Early Intervention*, *8*(4), 307–318. DOI: 10.1080/19411243.2015.1107005

Miltenberger, C. A., & Charlop, M. H. (2015). The comparative effectiveness of portable video modeling vs. traditional video modeling interventions with children with autism spectrum disorders. *Journal of Developmental and Physical Disabilities, 27*(3), 341–358. DOI: 10.1007/s10882-014-9416-y

Mitsch, M. K., Riggleman, S., & Buchter, J. M. (2021). Responding to young children's social-emotional needs through video modeling. *Young Exceptional Children, 24*(1), 16–27. DOI: 10.1177/1096250620910708

Noel, J. P., & Angelaki, D. E. (2023). A theory of autism bridging across levels of description. *Trends in Cognitive Sciences, 27*(7), 631–641. DOI: 10.1016/j.tics.2023.04.010 PMID: 37183143

Pain, O., Pocklington, A. J., Holmans, P. A., Bray, N. J., O'Brien, H. E., Hall, L. S., Pardiñas, A. F., O'Donovan, M. C., Owen, M. J., & Anney, R. (2019). Novel insight into the etiology of autism spectrum disorder gained by integrating expression data with genome-wide association statistics. *Biological Psychiatry, 86*(4), 265–273. DOI: 10.1016/j.biopsych.2019.04.034 PMID: 31230729

Piccin, S., Crippa, A., Nobile, M., Hardan, A. Y., & Brambilla, P. (2018). Video modeling for the development of personal hygiene skills in youth with autism spectrum disorder. *Epidemiology and Psychiatric Sciences, 27*(2), 127–132. DOI: 10.1017/S2045796017000610 PMID: 29122040

Plexousakis, S., Georgiadi, M., & Kourkoutas, E. (2011). Asperger syndrome and Sexuality: Intervention issues in a case of an Adolescent with Asperger syndrome in a context of a Special Educational Setting. *Procedia: Social and Behavioral Sciences, 15*, 490–495. DOI: 10.1016/j.sbspro.2011.03.128

Pugliese, C. E., Ratto, A. B., Granader, Y., Dudley, K. M., Bowen, A., Baker, C., & Anthony, L. G. (2020). Feasibility and preliminary efficacy of a parent-mediated sexual education curriculum for youth with autism spectrum disorders. *Autism, 24*(1), 64–79. DOI: 10.1177/1362361319842978 PMID: 31096780

Qi, C. H., Barton, E. E., Collier, M., & Lin, Y.-L. (2018). A Systematic Review of Single-Case Research Studies on Using Video Modeling Interventions to Improve Social Communication Skills for Individuals with Autism Spectrum Disorder. *Focus on Autism and Other Developmental Disabilities, 33*(4), 249–257. DOI: 10.1177/1088357617741282

Rosenberg, A., Patterson, J. S., & Angelaki, D. E. (2015). A computational perspective on autism. *Proceedings of the National Academy of Sciences of the United States of America, 112*(30), 9158–9165. DOI: 10.1073/pnas.1510583112 PMID: 26170299

Rudy, N. A., Betz, A. M., Malone, E., Henry, J. E., & Chong, I. M. (2014). Effects of video modeling on teaching bids for joint attention to children with autism. *Behavioral Interventions, 29*(4), 269–285. DOI: 10.1002/bin.1398

Schilbach, L. (2022). Autism and other disorders of social interaction: Where we are and where to go from here. *European Archives of Psychiatry and Clinical Neuroscience, 272*(2), 173–175. DOI: 10.1007/s00406-022-01391-y PMID: 35141808

Schöttle, D., Briken, P., Tüscher, O., & Turner, D. (2017). Sexuality in autism: Hypersexual and paraphilic behavior in women and men with high-functioning autism spectrum disorder. *Dialogues in Clinical Neuroscience, 19*(4), 381–393. DOI: 10.31887/DCNS.2017.19.4/dschoettle PMID: 29398933

Schreibman, L., Dawson, G., Stahmer, A. C., Landa, R., Rogers, S. J., McGee, G. G., Kasari, C., Ingersoll, B., Kaiser, A. P., Bruinsma, Y., McNerney, E., Wetherby, A., & Halladay, A. (2015). Naturalistic developmental behavioral interventions: Empirically validated treatments for autism spectrum disorder. *Journal of Autism and Developmental Disorders, 45*(8), 2411–2428. DOI: 10.1007/s10803-015-2407-8 PMID: 25737021

Shaw, C. A., Sheth, S., Li, D., & Tomljenovic, L. J. O. A. (2014). Etiology of autism spectrum disorders: Genes, environment, or both. *OA Autism, 2*(2), 11. https://www.vaccinssansaluminium.org/wp-content/uploads/2015/11/Etiology-of-autism-spectrum-disorders-Tomljenovic-Shaw.pdf

Solomon, D., Pantalone, D. W., & Faja, S. (2019). Autism and adult sex education: A literature review using the information–motivation–behavioral skills framework. *Sexuality and Disability, 37*(3), 339–351. DOI: 10.1007/s11195-019-09591-6 PMID: 33311815

Taheri-Torbati, H., & Sotoodeh, M. S. (2019). Using video and live modeling to teach motor skill to children with autism spectrum disorder. *International Journal of Inclusive Education, 23*(4), 405–418. DOI: 10.1080/13603116.2018.1441335

Tissot, C., & Evans, R. (2003). Visual teaching strategies for children with autism. *Early Child Development and Care, 173*(4), 425–433. DOI: 10.1080/0300443032000079104

Tomprou, D. M. (2022). The etiological background of Autism Spectrum Disorder. In Georgiadi, M. (Ed.), *Children and Adolescents with Autism Spectrum Disorder. Contemporary Research Data and Therapeutic Interventions* (pp. 37–58). Papazisi.

Tomprou, D. M., Georgiadi, M., Anagnopoulou, N. A., Maragkou, E., Stefanaki, M., & Chatzaki, E. M. (2022). Educational and therapeutic approaches for students with Autism Spectrum Disorder. In Georgiadi, M. (Ed.), *Children and Adolescents with Autism Spectrum Disorder. Contemporary Research Data and Therapeutic Interventions* (pp. 61–92). Papazisi.

Turner, A. (2017). *Teaching social skills to children with special needs using video modeling* (Doctoral dissertation, University of Waikato). https://hdl.handle.net/10289/11126

Walsh, K., Zwi, K., Woolfenden, S., & Shlonsky, A. (2015). School-based education programmes for the prevention of child sexual abuse. *Cochrane Database of Systematic Reviews, 2015*(4). Advance online publication. DOI: 10.1002/14651858.CD004380.pub3 PMID: 25876919

Wang, S. Y., Cui, Y., & Parrila, R. (2011). Examining the effectiveness of peer-mediated and video-modeling social skills interventions for children with autism spectrum disorders: A meta-analysis in single-case research using HLM. *Research in Autism Spectrum Disorders, 5*(1), 562–569. DOI: 10.1016/j.rasd.2010.06.023

White, P. J., O'Reilly, M., Streusand, W., Levine, A., Sigafoos, J., Lancioni, G., Fragale, C., Pierce, N., & Aguilar, J. (2011). Best practices for teaching joint attention: A systematic review of the intervention literature. *Research in Autism Spectrum Disorders, 5*(4), 1283–1295. DOI: 10.1016/j.rasd.2011.02.003

Wilson, K. P. (2013). Incorporating video modeling into a school-based intervention for students with autism spectrum disorders. https://doi.org/DOI: 10.1044/0161-1461(2012/11-0098)

Wood-Downie, H., Wong, B., Kovshoff, H., Mandy, W., Hull, L., & Hadwin, J. A. (2021). Sex/gender differences in camouflaging in children and adolescents with autism. *Journal of Autism and Developmental Disorders, 51*(4), 1353–1364. DOI: 10.1007/s10803-020-04615-z PMID: 32691191

Xiong, J., Chen, S., Pang, N., Deng, X., Yang, L., He, F., Wu, L., Chen, C., Yin, F., & Peng, J. (2019). Neurological diseases with autism spectrum disorder: Role of ASD risk genes. *Frontiers in Neuroscience, 13*, 349. DOI: 10.3389/fnins.2019.00349 PMID: 31031587

Zhao, J., Gao, Z., Lai, J., & Joshi, R. M. (2021). The relationship between autism traits and listening comprehension among Chinese preschool children with autism spectrum disorder. *Reading and Writing*, •••, 1–19. DOI: 10.1007/s11145-021-10216-8

Chapter 2
The Role of AI in Children's Mental Health and Well-Being Empowerment

Louiza Ioannidou
https://orcid.org/0000-0002-5320-1581
European University, Cyprus

Agathi Argyriadi
https://orcid.org/0000-0003-3935-0414
Frederick University, Cyprus

Alexandros Argyriadis
https://orcid.org/0000-0001-5754-4787
Hellenic Mediterranean University, Greece

ABSTRACT

The integration of artificial intelligence (AI) into mental health intervention programs for children has emerged as a promising avenue for enhancing emotional well-being. AI technologies can facilitate early detection of mental health issues. AI-driven applications can analyze behavioral data from various sources, including social media and mobile devices, to identify patterns indicative of anxiety or depression. By utilizing machine learning algorithms, AI programs can adapt therapeutic approaches based on individual responses, preferences, and progress. This personalized approach increases engagement in children, empowering them to take an active role in their mental health management. AI-powered tools, such as chatbots and virtual therapists provide 24/7 support, enabling children to seek help

DOI: 10.4018/979-8-3373-5072-1.ch002

without the barriers often associated with traditional therapy settings. Moreover, gamification elements in these programs can make mental health management more engaging for children. Incorporating AI into mental health programs also allows for enhanced parental involvement.

INTRODUCTION

The mental health of children has emerged as an increasing public health issue, with around one in five children facing mental health difficulties, including anxiety, depression, or other behavioral disorders during their developmental stages (Kessler et al., 2005; Polanczyk et al., 2015). Prompt identification and intervention are crucial, since neglected mental health issues can result in significant long-term repercussions, such as scholastic failure, social seclusion, and a heightened likelihood of chronic mental health disorders (Patel et al., 2018). Traditional mental health care systems frequently fail to provide accessible, personalized, and timely support, especially for younger children. The incorporation of artificial intelligence technologies presents significant potential to transform the field, particularly regarding children's emotional well-being (Kazdin & Blase, 2011; Li et al., 2023; Vial & Almon). In this context, artificial intelligence (AI) has emerged as a transformative instrument in mental health prevention and intervention programs, providing creative methods to rectify these deficiencies (Fiske et al., 2019; Shatte et al., 2019).

AI-driven solutions can enhance the early identification of mental health disorders, deliver tailored interventions, and substantially increase access to mental health resources for young populations (Fiske et al., 2019; Olawade et al., 2024). The extensive utilization of digital technologies by children and adolescents, alongside the COVID-19 pandemic's effects on mental health, has intensified the demand for novel, technology-based solutions in this area (Holmes et al., 2020; Ornell et al., 2020). AI-driven solutions are currently employed for the prediction, detection, and treatment of mental health disorders. These advances, including machine learning, natural language processing (NLP), and chatbots, possess the capacity to improve diagnosis and treatment while tackling global mental health issues (D'Alfonso et al., 2017; Patel et al., 2023; Yeh et al., 2025).

AI technologies utilize data-driven insights to improve early detection, individualized care, and accessibility in mental health management. AI algorithms can examine behavioral and environmental data from sources, including social media, mobile applications, and clinical records, to detect early indicators of mental health disorders, such as anxiety and depression (Imran, Hashmi, & Imran, 2023). These technologies facilitate the creation of predictive models that track mental health trajectories, similar to growth charts, assuring proactive interventions. Additionally, AI-driven platforms, such as virtual therapists and gamified applications, offer round-the-clock access to mental health resources, diminishing stigma and enhancing engagement among youngsters (Karam et al., 2019). The personalization of mental health care represents a substantial benefit of AI. Machine learning algorithms adjust therapeutic tactics in real-time, tailoring interventions to accommodate individual needs and preferences. This customized technique improves the efficacy of mental health efforts and empowers youth to take an active role in managing their well-being (Torous et al., 2021). Furthermore, AI solutions facilitate parental engagement by delivering insights into children's emotional conditions and offering recommendations for appropriate caregiving, therefore enhancing family dynamics (Luxton, 2016).

Although the prospective advantages of AI in children's mental health are considerable, ethical issues, including data privacy, algorithmic bias, and equitable access, must be resolved to guarantee the responsible implementation of these technologies (Mittelstadt et al., 2016). This chapter analyzes the influence of AI on the evolution of mental health prevention and intervention programs for children, highlighting its uses, constraints, and future advancements. Furthermore, the chapter aims to clarify AI's ability to enhance emotional well-being and empower youngsters through the incorporation of modern advancements.

EARLY DETECTION OF MENTAL HEALTH ISSUES IN CHILDREN AND DIAGNOSIS

Mental health issues are prevalent among children and adolescents, influencing approximately 10–20% of young individuals worldwide each year (Kessler et al., 2005; Polanczyk et al., 2015). Anxiety, depression, and attention deficit hyperactivity disorder (ADHD) are common disorders that appear throughout early developmental stages (Patel et al., 2007). Despite its substantial prevalence, a significant number of cases go undiagnosed or untreated due to the insidious nature of early symptoms, restricted access to mental health care, and societal stigma (Merikangas et al., 2010). Studies have shown that prompt identification is essential, as expeditious management significantly reduces the likelihood of developing enduring mental health disorders and improves long-term outcomes (McGorry et al., 2018). Artificial intelligence technologies have demonstrated substantial potential in addressing the challenges associated with early mental health diagnosis. AI systems can identify subtle patterns that indicate the onset of mental health issues by analyzing a vast amount of clinical, environmental, and behavioral data (Torous et al., 2021). AI algorithms provide data-driven insights, which enhance diagnostic precision and objectivity, in contrast to conventional procedures that rely on subjective evaluations. Early indicators of mental health disorders are identified through the evaluation of multiple data sources by artificial intelligence algorithms. Behavioral data from social media platforms, such as language usage, sentiment trends, and interaction frequency, have been shown to be effective in detecting symptoms of anxiety, despair, and loneliness in adolescents (Guntuku et al., 2017; Reece & Danforth, 2017).

Mobile devices and wearable technologies improve data collection by monitoring physical activity, sleep patterns, and physiological responses, such as heart rate variability, which are associated with emotional well-being (Guntuku et al., 2017). The use of multimodal data facilitates thorough evaluations that consider multiple dimensions of children's mental health. AI-driven screening instruments are transforming early detection through automated, real-time evaluations of mental health disorders (Torous et al., 2021). Natural language processing (NLP) algorithms examine text and speech to identify indicators of emotional discomfort, including negative sentiment or alterations in communication style (Coppersmith et al., 2015; Doe & Wilson, 2025; Mikolov et al., 2013). Chatbots utilizing conversational AI, like Woebot and Replika, interact with children to evaluate their emotional condition and identify potential issues for further assessment (Miner et al., 2016).

Benefits of Early Detection of Mental Health Issues in Children

Timely identification of mental health disorders provides multiple advantages for children, families, and healthcare systems. Initially, it facilitates prompt interventions that avert the advancement of mental health disorders, thereby diminishing the treatment load in subsequent phases (McGorry et al., 2018). Recent comparative studies have confirmed the effectiveness of AI in mental health prediction. For example, Kheterpal and Gill (2024) demonstrated that AI-driven models, such as Boosting algorithms, achieved an accuracy of 81.75%, outperforming traditional statistical models like logistic regression (79.63%). Their findings emphasize the potential of AI not only for early detection but also for building clinically interpretable tools that assist mental health professionals in tailoring interventions based on individual lifestyle and demographic factors. Similarly, Garg and Patil (2021) reported that computer vision-based models achieved a 96% accuracy rate in detecting ADHD and ASD. These findings support the growing consensus that AI technologies can significantly enhance early detection efforts compared to conventional diagnostic approaches.

Furthermore, AI-facilitated early detection minimizes diagnostic delays by recognizing at-risk individuals prior to the onset of severe or disruptive symptoms (Torous et al., 2021). This proactive strategy enhances resilience and emotional stability, hence improving academic achievement, social relationships, and general quality of life. Furthermore, AI technologies facilitate equitable access to mental health care by providing affordable, scalable solutions. Automated screening techniques can approach underserved populations, including children in rural or low-income regions, who may otherwise be deprived of professional mental health services (Guntuku et al., 2017). AI technologies enhance accessibility, fostering fair mental health care delivery and guaranteeing that all children can grow emotionally and socially.

PERSONALIZED INTERVENTIONS THROUGH AI

One of the most notable breakthroughs that AI contributes to mental health care is its capacity to provide highly individualized interventions. In contrast to conventional methods that typically employ broad strategies for varied populations, AI facilitates customized assistance by examining individual data and dynamically adjusting interventions to meet the specific requirements of each child (Torous et al., 2021). Machine learning algorithms could be implemented to enable AI-driven personalization. These algorithms use data from a range of sources to discover trends and forecast outcomes, including health records, behavioral surveillance, and self-reported surveys (Li et al., 2023; Shatte et al., 2019). Machine learning algorithms can evaluate children's responses to various therapeutic modalities, allowing systems to make real-time adjustments to improve efficacy. Additionally, reinforcement learning, a subdivision of machine learning, enables systems to improve their recommendations by incorporating user feedback and interactions, thereby preserving the efficacy and relevance of therapeutic interventions over time (Torous et al., 2021). By incorporating data on children's interests, cultural contexts, and emotional states, AI can customize therapeutic approaches. AI algorithms can detect stress or anxiety patterns, which can then be used to customize the content and duration of exercises in individualized mindfulness programs (Coppersmith et al., 2015). Similarly, the cognitive-behavioral treatment (CBT) processes utilized by AI apps can be customized to target specific cognitive distortions or emotional triggers discovered during assessments (Reece & Danforth, 2017). As children become more actively involved in interventions that are specifically tailored to their needs, this individualized approach promotes a sense of agency.

Examples of AI-Driven Applications

Numerous AI-powered applications are advancing tailored mental health care for children:

Woebot

Woebot (https://woebothealth.com) is an AI-driven chatbot. It can provide evidence-based therapeutic techniques, such as Cognitive Behavioral Therapy (CBT), in a conversational format. Woebot enhances emotional resilience by providing tailored reactions, motivation, and coping mechanisms based on the study of user input (Fitzpatrick et al., 2017). Woebot is particularly effective in alleviating symptoms of anxiety and depression, particularly among young individuals and those who are hesitant to pursue conventional therapy, according to research. In contrast to human clinicians, Woebot is accessible 24 hours a day, providing consumers with immediate psychological support at any given moment.

The chatbot's responses are customized and responsive to the mental health needs of users through the use of machine learning algorithms. Recent research has shown that Woebot's ability to provide immediate and non-judgmental assistance enhances user engagement and conformance with therapeutic methods (Fitzpatrick et al., 2017; Yeh, Kuo & Tsai, 2024). Moreover, its organized dialogues enable the implementation of CBT-based methods, such as recognizing negative thought patterns and cultivating effective coping mechanisms. Woebot is an economical and easily available tool that complements conventional mental health therapy, especially for children and teenagers adept in digital communication, while it does not substitute for human therapists.

Replika: AI-Powered Conversational Companion

Replika utilizes natural language processing (NLP) to produce customizable dialogues that simulate human interaction with empathy. This AI companion adjusts its tone and responses in accordance with the user's emotional state, thereby fostering a sense of recognition and respect in both children and adults. In contrast to conventional chatbot engagements, Replika cultivates an ongoing relationship with users by incorporating their remarks and modifying its conversational strategy over time. Replika employs natural language processing (NLP) to generate customized dialogues that mimic empathetic human contact. This AI companion modifies its tone and responses according to the user's emotional state, assisting both youngsters and adults in feeling acknowledged and esteemed. In contrast to conventional chatbot engagements, Replika fosters an ongoing relationship with users by incorporating their comments and evolving its conversational strategy over time. The chatbot employs attentive listening, sympathetic replies, and organized writing methods to improve emotional well-being. Although Replika offers substantial psychological support, issues around data protection, ethical AI interactions, and its efficacy compared to human therapy persist as contested subjects. Nevertheless, it functions as a pioneering instrument in digital mental health, providing non-judgmental and readily accessible assistance for children, adolescents, and adults with emotional difficulties.

Mental Health Trajectories Program: AI for Personalized Pediatric Mental Health

The Mental Health Trajectories Program (https://www.cincinnatichildrens.org), created by researchers at Cincinnati Children's Hospital, is an AI-driven system intended to longitudinally assess children's mental health through the analysis of clinical and environmental data. This application combines machine learning algorithms with electronic health records (EHR), academic performance data, and behavioral evaluations to monitor mental health trends and forecast probable psychological concerns. A principal strength of the program is its capacity to furnish clinicians with customized intervention recommendations that correspond to the child's developmental requirements and socio-environmental context. AI-driven risk stratification models facilitate the identification of children at elevated risk for mental health disorders, hence enabling early intervention measures. Furthermore, predictive analytics enable healthcare providers to personalize treatment programs by evaluating the efficacy of previous therapies and modifying recommendations as required.

The program employs AI-enhanced sentiment analysis to identify linguistic indicators of distress, anxiety, or despair in the speech and social media interactions of children. The Mental Health Trajectories Program has made substantial strides in the field of pediatric mental healthcare. However, further research is required to address concerns regarding data privacy, ethical AI utilization, and algorithmic biases. This AI-driven initiative represents a significant stride forward in the application of technology to create mental health care that is adaptive, responsive, and personalized for children. Further investigation is required to tackle issues related to algorithmic biases, ethical AI use, and data protection. This AI-driven effort greatly enhances the development of adaptable, responsive, and individualized mental health treatment for children through the application of technology.

WYSA: AI for Personalized Emotional Well-being

WYSA (https://www.wysa.com) is a mental health chatbot powered by AI that offers personalized emotional support. It is founded on the principles of cognitive behavioral therapy (CBT) and mindfulness techniques. WISA facilitates meaningful dialogues with users by employing sentiment analysis and natural language processing (NLP) to provide interactive self-help activities that aid in managing stress, anxiety, and depression. In contrast to conventional mental health interventions, WISA is especially advantageous for individuals who are hesitant to participate in professional therapy, as it is accessible 24 hours a day and offers immediate, non-judgmental support. Furthermore, WYSA implements structured mindfulness techniques and AI-based mood monitoring, which allows users to evaluate their pemotional well-being over time and receive personalized self-care recommendations. WYSA is not a replacement for professional therapy; however, it serves as a beneficial adjunct for individuals who require immediate psychological support and self-improvement strategies.

GAMIFICATION IN MENTAL HEALTH MANAGEMENT

AI-driven customization markedly improves engagement and enables youngsters to actively participate in controlling their mental health. Studies indicate that interventions customized to individual preferences are more likely to be regarded as significant and pleasurable, hence enhancing compliance with therapy programs (Lukka & Palva, 2023). Gamification components, like incentives for task completion and interactive narratives, enhance participation by transforming mental health management from a burdensome obligation into an empowering experience. Gamification has become an effective instrument for increasing children's involvement in mental health interventions. By integrating gamified aspects, AI applications enhance the attraction and interactivity of mental health management, hence augmenting children's propensity to engage consistently in these programs (Blohm et al., 2013; Morris et al., 2013). Gamified mental health applications utilize tactics including rewards, progress tracking, and challenges to maintain children's attention and promote ongoing participation. Some applications encourage regular mindfulness practices for children or enable mood tracking via interesting, interactive games. These strategies foster a sense of accomplishment and normalcy regarding mental health care, incorporating it into their daily routines. These tools not only enhance engagement but also reinforce advantageous behavioral habits over time (Cheng et al., 2023).

Gamification enhances emotional resilience by promoting regular and enjoyable interaction with mental health services. Research demonstrates that youngsters participating in gamified mental health programs exhibit greater adherence to therapeutic activities, including mindfulness and relaxation exercises, than those utilizing conventional methods (Pestian et al., 2022). Furthermore, gamified elements may reduce anxiety and depression regarding mental health management by framing it as a pleasant and rewarding activity instead of a burdensome obligation (Abd-Alrazaq et al., 2022). Furthermore, gamification may augment social connectedness (McGonigal, 2011). Some systems offer multiplayer features or collaborative progress tracking, allowing youth to interact with peers facing similar challenges. This sense of community can further alleviate feelings of isolation and loneliness, enhancing their general well-being.

IMPORTANCE OF PARENTAL INVOLVEMENT IN CHILDREN'S MENTAL HEALTH

Parents have an important role in their children's emotional and psychological development. Their aid is critical in spotting potential mental health issues and creating a supportive environment in which children feel safe expressing their emotions (Cong et al., 2020; Pine et al., 2024). According to research, active parental involvement in mental health therapies improves program efficacy by boosting emotional support, communication, and therapeutic practice (Haine-Schlagel et al., 2015). AI-powered tools are transforming parental engagement in their children's mental health by giving actionable insights and practical advice. AI tools, such as Companion and WYSA, can provide parents with insights into their child's emotional state and offer guidance on supporting them effectively. These instruments use data from children's interactions with digital platforms, wearable technologies, and behavioral assessments to provide immediate insights into their emotional state (Garg & Patil, 2021). Applications that use mood tracking or speech analysis can detect signs of stress, anxiety, or depression, allowing parents to intervene quickly. Unlike conventional approaches that rely heavily on subjective observations and periodic clinical assessments, AI tools provide continuous monitoring, offering parents a dynamic understanding of their child's mental state. Alerts generated by predictive models allow caregivers to intervene early, adapting strategies based on data-driven recommendations. Comparative studies have demonstrated that integrating AI-driven parental feedback mechanisms leads to improved treatment adherence, stronger emotional bonds, and better therapeutic outcome (Kheterpal & Gill, 2024).

CONTINUOUS SUPPORT VIA AI TECHNOLOGIES AND MITIGATION OF STIGMA

Artificial intelligence (AI) has considerably enhanced access to mental health care by removing the barriers that were previously associated with mental health services, including geographical restrictions, financial constraints, and stigma. AI-driven solutions enable children to access mental health resources around the clock, enabling them to seek assistance at any time and in any location (Adesina et al., 2024)

Chatbots and virtual therapists that are propelled by AI provide adolescents with immediate, on-demand support. Natural language processing (NLP) is employed by applications like Woebot and Replika to simulate empathic and engaging discussions, which is regarded as conversational therapy. For children who may experience feelings of intimidation or apprehension regarding requesting assistance from human therapists, these tools offer evidence-based guidance, coping strategies, and emotional support, thereby enhancing their access to mental health resources (Yulia et al., 2024). Moreover, AI solutions of this kind are scalable and cost-effective, making them especially beneficial in underserved or remote communities with limited access to mental health professionals.

AI technologies substantially reduce the stigma around mental health. Traditional therapeutic settings can be intimidating for adolescents, particularly those who fear judgment or feel shame when discussing personal issues (Batool, 2024). AI systems provide a confidential and impartial setting in which children can freely explore their emotions and seek help without the fear of stigma. This anonymity cultivates a sense of security and confidence, prompting youngsters to interact more freely with mental health providers.

ETHICAL CONSIDERATIONS AND CHALLENGES

AI-based mental health tools usually rely on sensitive personal data, such as behavioral patterns, emotional states, and communication records, raising serious privacy concerns. Children's data is particularly vulnerable since they may lack a thorough grasp of how their information is used. It is critical to adhere to data protection requirements such as the General Data Protection Regulation (GDPR) and the Children's Online Privacy Protection Act (COPPA). Developers should prioritize transparency by providing comprehensive descriptions of data collection methods, obtaining informed consent, and using strict encryption mechanisms to prevent unauthorized access.

Despite high reported accuracies, AI models are not infallible. Misdiagnoses can occur, leading to inappropriate labelling of children with disorders they may not have, causing potential stigmatization or unwarranted medical interventions. False negatives are equally harmful, delaying necessary treatments. Furthermore, while AI can enhance early detection and treatment personalization, it cannot replace the empathetic relationship and contextual understanding that human therapists provide (Garg & Patil, 2021). Over-reliance on algorithmic outputs risks oversimplifying complex emotional states into binary classifications.

The efficacy of AI in children's mental health care can be completely actualized only if these tools are universally available. Socioeconomic inequalities and inadequate internet infrastructure can obstruct access to AI-driven mental health interventions, especially in rural or low-income areas. Policymakers and stakeholders must confront these difficulties by investing in digital inclusion initiatives and subsidizing AI technology to guarantee equal access. Moreover, interventions must be crafted with cultural sensitivity, integrating varied viewpoints to ensure their relevance across all demographics.

Bias in AI systems may result in erroneous evaluations or actions, disproportionately affecting specific groups of children. Models trained on non-representative datasets may neglect cultural, linguistic, or socioeconomic variation, leading to biased results. Conducting regular audits, developing inclusive datasets, and collaborating with experts from many disciplines are essential for reducing prejudice and enhancing algorithmic fairness. Developers must embrace ethical AI frameworks to guarantee that the tools are transparent, accountable, and aligned with the best interests of children.

FUTURE DIRECTIONS AND RESEARCH OPPORTUNITIES

Progress in artificial intelligence technology persistently broadens the domain of mental health care. Innovations like generative AI, deep learning, and multimodal data analysis provide more advanced evaluations and tailored treatments. Wearable gadgets equipped with AI systems can track physiological indicators such as heart rate and sleep patterns, offering immediate insights into emotional health (Pestian et al., 2022). Furthermore, AI-driven immersive experiences utilizing virtual reality (VR) are being investigated to provide interactive and captivating therapeutic settings.

Multiple domains require additional scrutiny to enhance AI's contribution to pediatric mental health care:

Long-Term Efficacy: Investigation is required to assess the sustained effectiveness of AI-driven therapies across varied populations.

Hybrid Models: Research should investigate the integration of AI with conventional treatment methods, including cognitive-behavioral therapy (CBT) and family counseling.

Ethical Safeguards: Examining strategies to improve privacy, mitigate prejudice, and foster openness in AI systems is an essential objective.

Impact on Specific Groups: Additional study is necessary to evaluate how AI technologies might be customized to assist vulnerable populations, such as children with autism spectrum disorder (ASD) or histories of trauma. Many

AI models are developed with datasets lacking sufficient cultural, ethnic, and socioeconomic diversity. Culturally adaptive AI frameworks are urgently needed.

As AI-driven virtual companions advance, future innovations should emphasize their integration into comprehensive therapeutic frameworks. Through collaboration with mental health specialists, developers can devise hybrid solutions that integrate digital interventions with conventional therapy, thereby augmenting the overall effect on children's social and emotional well-being. AI technologies possess the capacity to augment, rather than supplant, conventional therapeutic approaches. AI solutions can serve as mediators between therapy sessions, offering continuous assistance and monitoring of progress. Virtual therapists assist clinicians in remotely tracking patient progress, facilitating prompt modifications to therapy methods. Integrating AI into current frameworks enables mental health care professionals to develop more comprehensive and adaptive care models.

CONCLUSION

The use of AI into children's mental health treatment could transform prevention and intervention methodologies. AI provides novel answers to critical difficulties in mental health care by enabling early identification, offering individualized interventions, improving accessibility, and fostering parental participation. These technologies enable youngsters to actively participate in controlling their well-being, enhancing resilience, and cultivating emotional development.

In order to fully realize the potential of AI, it is imperative that academics, practitioners, and policymakers work together to address critical issues and ensure responsible application. Researchers are interested in focusing on the development of culturally inclusive instruments, the improvement of AI algorithms, and the conduct of comprehensive efficacy assessments. The potential of AI technologies to enhance traditional methods must be leveraged by practitioners in therapeutic techniques. Policymakers must prioritize the provision of financing for digital inclusion initiatives and establish robust ethical frameworks to ensure fair access and protect the privacy of minors. Stakeholders may create a supportive ecosystem that prioritizes the emotional well-being of children and fosters favorable developmental outcomes by combining sophisticated technology with human expertise. AI has the potential to revolutionize the field of mental health treatment, ensuring that no child is overlooked in their pursuit of emotional resilience and well-being as it continues to develop.

REFERENCES

Abd-Alrazaq, A., Al-Jafar, E., Alajlani, M., Toro, C., Alhuwail, D., Ahmed, A., Reagu, S. M., Al-Shorbaji, N., & Househ, M. (2022). The effectiveness of serious games for alleviating depression: Systematic review and meta-analysis. *JMIR Serious Games*, *10*(1), e32331. DOI: 10.2196/32331 PMID: 35029530

Abd-Alrazaq, A., Alajlani, M., Alhuwail, D., Schneider, J., Akhu-Zaheya, L., Ahmed, A., & Househ, M. (2022). The effectiveness of serious games in alleviating anxiety: Systematic review and meta-analysis. *JMIR Serious Games*, *10*(1), e29137. DOI: 10.2196/29137 PMID: 35156932

Adesina, A., Abuka, O., & Adesiyan, J. (2024). Enhancing adolescent mental health outcomes through integrated technology (AI) innovations in the United States. *International Journal of Advanced Psychitric Nursing*, *6*(2), 22–30. DOI: 10.33545/26641348.2024.v6.i2a.170

Batool, S. F., Fazal, A., Sajid, U., & Alam, R. (2024). AI-Driven Mental Health Tools: Their Potential in Reducing Stigma in Pakistan. *Pakistan Journal of Medical and Health Education*, *4*(2), 107–112.

Blohm, I., & Leimeister, J. M. (2013). Gamification. Design of IT-Based Enhancing Services for Motivational Support and Behavioral Change. *Business & Information Systems Engineering*, *5*(4), 275–278. DOI: 10.1007/s12599-013-0273-5

Cheng, V. W., Davenport, T., Johnson, D., Vella, K., & Hickie, I. B. (2019). Gamification in apps and technologies for improving mental health and well-being: Systematic review. *JMIR Mental Health*, *6*(6), e13717. DOI: 10.2196/13717 PMID: 31244479

Cong, X., Hosler, A. S., Tracy, M., & Appleton, A. A. (2020). The relationship between parental involvement in childhood and depression in early adulthood. *Journal of Affective Disorders*, *1*(273), 173–182. DOI: 10.1016/j.jad.2020.03.108 PMID: 32421599

Coppersmith, G., Dredze, M., & Harman, C. (2015). Quantifying mental health signals in Twitter. *Proceedings of the Workshop on Computational Linguistics and Clinical Psychology: From Keyboard to Clinic,* 51–60.

D'Alfonso, S., Santesteban-Echarri, O., Rice, S., Wadley, G., Lederman, R., Miles, C., Gleeson, J., & Alvarez-Jimenez, M. (2017). Artificial intelligence-assisted online social therapy for youth mental health. *Frontiers in Psychology*, *8*, 796. DOI: 10.3389/fpsyg.2017.00796 PMID: 28626431

Doe, S., & Wilson, L. (2025). Understanding the role of artificial intelligence in reducing mental health stigma and improving public awareness. *Advances and Challenges in Artificial Intelligence and Cybersecurity*, *1*(2), 1–25.

Fiske, A., Henningsen, P., & Buyx, A. (2019). Your robot therapist will see you now: Ethical implications of embodied artificial intelligence in psychiatry, psychology, and psychotherapy. *Journal of Medical Internet Research, 21*(5), e13216. DOI: 10.2196/13216 PMID: 31094356

Fitzpatrick, K. K., Darcy, A., & Vierhile, M. (2017). Delivering Cognitive Behavioral Therapy to young adults with depression and anxiety via a smartphone app: A randomized controlled trial of Woebot. *JMIR Mental Health*, *4*(3), e7679.

Garg, M. & Patil, H. (2021). Comparative study on AI in mental health and wellbeing – Current applications and trends. *International Research Journal of Engineering and Technology, 8(6).*

Guntuku, S. C., Yaden, D. B., Kern, M. L., Ungar, L. H., & Eichstaedt, J. C. (2017). Detecting depression and mental illness on social media: An integrative review. *Current Opinion in Behavioral Sciences*, *18*, 43–49. DOI: 10.1016/j.cobeha.2017.07.005

Haine-Schlagel, R., & Walsh, N. E. (2015). A review of parent participation engagement in child and family mental health treatment. *Clinical Child and Family Psychology Review*, *18*(2), 133–150. DOI: 10.1007/s10567-015-0182-x PMID: 25726421

Holmes, E. A., O'Connor, R. C., Perry, V. H., Tracey, I., Wessely, S., Arseneault, L., Ballard, C., Christensen, H., Cohen Silver, R., Everall, I., Ford, T., John, A., Kabir, T., King, K., Madan, I., Michie, S., Przybylski, A. K., Shafran, R., Sweeney, A., & Bullmore, E. (2020). Multidisciplinary research priorities for the COVID-19 pandemic: A call for action for mental health science. *The Lancet. Psychiatry*, *7*(6), 547–560. DOI: 10.1016/S2215-0366(20)30168-1 PMID: 32304649

Imran, N., Hashmi, A., & Imran, A. (2023). Chat-GPT: Opportunities and Challenges in Child Mental Healthcare. *Pakistan Journal of Medical Sciences*, *39*(4), 1191–1193. DOI: 10.12669/pjms.39.4.8118 PMID: 37492313

Karam, Z. N., Provost, E. M., Singh, S., Montgomery, J., Archer, C., Harrington, G., & McInnis, M. G. (2019). Ecologically valid long-term mood monitoring of individuals with bipolar disorder using speech. *Journal of Affective Disorders*, *273*, 386–393.

Kazdin, A. E., & Blase, S. L. (2011). Rebooting psychotherapy research and practice to reduce the burden of mental illness. *Perspectives on Psychological Science*, *6*(1), 21–37. DOI: 10.1177/1745691610393527 PMID: 26162113

Kessler, R. C., Berglund, P., Demler, O., Jin, R., Merikangas, K. R., & Walters, E. E. (2005). Lifetime prevalence and age-of-onset distributions of DSM-IV disorders in the National Comorbidity Survey Replication. *Archives of General Psychiatry*, *62*(6), 593–602. DOI: 10.1001/archpsyc.62.6.593 PMID: 15939837

Kheterpal, A., & Singh Gill, K. (2024). Therapeutic tech: A comparative study of AI-drive mental health interventions. *4th International Conference on Advancement in Electronics & Communication Engineering,* 1187-1190, GHAZIABAD, India. DOI: 10.1109/AECE62803.2024.10911418

Li, H., Zhang, R., Lee, Y.C., Kraut, R.E., & Mohr, D.C. (2023). Systematic review and meta-analysis of AI-based conversational agents for promoting mental health and well-being. *NPJ Digit Med.,* 9, 6(1):236.

Lukka, L., & Palva, J. (2023). The Development of Game-Based Digital Mental Health Interventions: Bridging the Paradigms of Health Care and Entertainment. *JMIR Serious Games, 11*, e42173. DOI: 10.2196/42173 PMID: 37665624

Luxton, D. D. (2016). *An introduction to artificial intelligence in behavioral and mental health care.* Academic Press. DOI: 10.1016/B978-0-12-420248-1.00001-5

McGonigal, J. (2011). *Reality Is Broken: Why Games Make Us Better and How They Can Change the World.* Penguin Press.

McGorry, P. D., Hartmann, J. A., Spooner, R., & Nelson, B. (2018). Beyond the "at risk mental state" concept: Transitioning to transdiagnostic psychiatry. *World Psychiatry; Official Journal of the World Psychiatric Association (WPA)*, *17*(2), 133–142. DOI: 10.1002/wps.20514 PMID: 29856558

Merikangas, K. R., He, J. P., Burstein, M., Swanson, S. A., Avenevoli, S., Cui, L., Benjet, C., Georgiades, K., & Swendsen, J. (2010). Lifetime prevalence of mental disorders in US adolescents: Results from the National Comorbidity Survey Replication–Adolescent Supplement (NCS-A). *Journal of the American Academy of Child and Adolescent Psychiatry*, *49*(10), 980–989. DOI: 10.1016/j.jaac.2010.05.017 PMID: 20855043

Mikolov, T., Sutskever, I., Chen, K., Corrado, G., & Dean, J. (2013). Distributed representations of words and phrases and their compositionality. *Proceedings of Neural Information Processing Systems (NeurIPS), 3111-3119.*

Miner, A. S., Milstein, A., Schueller, S. M., & Brown, S. (2016). Smartphone-based conversational agents and artificial intelligence for mental health care. *JAMA Psychiatry*, *73*(8), 827–828.

Mittelstadt, B. D., Allo, P., Taddeo, M., Wachter, S., & Floridi, L. (2016). The ethics of algorithms: Mapping the debate. *Big Data & Society*, *3*(2), 2053951716679679. DOI: 10.1177/2053951716679679

Morris, B. J., Croker, S., Zimmerman, C., Gill, D., & Romig, C. (2013). Gaming science: The "Gamification" of scientific thinking. *Frontiers in Psychology*, *4*, 607. DOI: 10.3389/fpsyg.2013.00607 PMID: 24058354

Olawade, D., Wada, O., Odetayo, A., David-Olawade, A., Asaolu, F., & Eberhardt, J. (2024). Enhancing mental health with Artificial Intelligence: Current trends and future prospects. *Journal of Medicine, Surgery, and Public Health*, *3*, 3. DOI: 10.1016/j.glmedi.2024.100099

Ornell, F., Schuch, J. B., Sordi, A. O., & Kessler, F. H. (2020). "Pandemic fear" and COVID-19: Mental health burden and strategies. *The British Journal of Psychiatry*, *42*(3), 232–235. DOI: 10.1590/1516-4446-2020-0008 PMID: 32267343

Patel, V., Flisher, A. J., Hetrick, S., & McGorry, P. (2007). Mental health of young people: A global public-health challenge. *Lancet*, *369*(9569), 1302–1313. DOI: 10.1016/S0140-6736(07)60368-7 PMID: 17434406

Patel, V., Saxena, S., Lund, C., Thornicroft, G., Baingana, F., Bolton, P., & Unützer, J. (2018). The Lancet Commission on global mental health and sustainable development. *Lancet*, *392*(10157), 1553–1598. DOI: 10.1016/S0140-6736(18)31612-X PMID: 30314863

Patel, V., Saxena, S., Lund, C., Thornicroft, G., Baingana, F., Bolton, P., & Unützer, J. (2023). The role of digital technology in mental health care: Opportunities and challenges. *The Lancet. Digital Health*, *5*(1), e15–e25.

Pine, A., Baumann, M., Modugno, G., & Compas, B. (2024). Parental Involvement in Adolescent Psychological Interventions: A Meta-analysis. *Clinical Child and Family Psychology Review*, *27*(3), 1–20. DOI: 10.1007/s10567-024-00481-8 PMID: 38748300

Polanczyk, G. V., Salum, G. A., Sugaya, L. S., Caye, A., & Rohde, L. A. (2015). Annual research review: A meta-analysis of the worldwide prevalence of mental disorders in children and adolescents. *Journal of Child Psychology and Psychiatry, and Allied Disciplines*, *56*(3), 345–365. DOI: 10.1111/jcpp.12381 PMID: 25649325

Reece, A. G., & Danforth, C. M. (2017). Instagram photos reveal predictive markers of depression. *EPJ Data Science*, *6*(1), 15. DOI: 10.1140/epjds/s13688-017-0110-z

Shatte, A. B., Hutchinson, D. M., & Teague, S. J. (2019). Machine learning in mental health: A scoping review of methods and applications. *Psychological Medicine*, *49*(9), 1426–1448. DOI: 10.1017/S0033291719000151 PMID: 30744717

Torous, J., Andersson, G., Bertagnoli, A., Christensen, H., Cuijpers, P., Firth, J., & Haim, A. (2021). Towards a consensus around standards for digital mental health research. *npj. Digital Medicine*, *4*, 13.

Vial, T., & Almon, A. (2023). Artificial Intelligence in Mental Health Therapy for Children and Adolescents. *JAMA Pediatrics*, *177*(12), 1251–1252. DOI: 10.1001/jamapediatrics.2023.4212 PMID: 37843842

Yeh, P. L., Kuo, W. C., & Tsai, C. J. (2024). Counseling students' first impressions of using Woebot: A mental health chatbot. *Bulletin of Educational Psychology*, *56*(1), 45–72.

Yeh, P. L., Kuo, W. C., Tseng, B. L., & Sung, Y.-H. (2025). Does the AI-driven Chatbot Work? Effectiveness of the Woebot app in reducing anxiety and depression in group counseling courses and student acceptance of technological aids. *Current Psychology (New Brunswick, N.J.)*, *44*(9), 8133–8145. Advance online publication. DOI: 10.1007/s12144-025-07359-0

Yulia, S., Serge, N., & Samuel, F. (2023). Combating Loneliness with Artificial Intelligence: An AI-Based Emotional Support Model, *Proceedings of the 56th Hawaii International Conference on System Sciences.*

Chapter 3
Artificial Intelligence Approaches to Autism Spectrum Disorder Screening and Diagnosis

Eleana Charalambous
https://orcid.org/0009-0009-9674-3020
United Arab Emirates University, UAE

Maria Efstratopoulou
https://orcid.org/0000-0002-5162-2104
United Arab Emirates University, UAE

ABSTRACT

Autism Spectrum Disorder (ASD) is a neurodevelopmental condition with rising global prevalence, driven by improved awareness and diagnostic practices. Early diagnosis and intervention are crucial for better outcomes, yet delays persist due to systemic inefficiencies and sociocultural disparities. Artificial Intelligence (AI), including machine learning (ML) and deep learning (DL), offers promising tools for accurate and efficient ASD detection, reducing diagnostic delays and human error. AI-driven tools like Canvas Dx and EarliPoint System show high accuracy, while hybrid models and explainable AI (XAI) enhance precision and interpretability. However, ethical concerns and equitable access remain challenges. AI integration can improve early diagnosis, personalized care, and long-term outcomes for individuals with ASD.

DOI: 10.4018/979-8-3373-5072-1.ch003

DEFINITION OF AUTISM SPECTRUM DISORDER (ASD)

According to the diagnostic and statistical manual of mental health, 5th edition (DSM-5), Autism Spectrum Disorder (ASD) is characterized by persistent challenges in social communication and interaction, alongside restricted, repetitive patterns of behavior, interests, or activities (American Psychiatric Association [APA], 2013). Although ASD can be diagnosed at any age, it is described as a "developmental disorder" because symptoms generally appear in the first two years of life (National Institute of Mental Health, n.d.). Social difficulties include deficits in social-emotional reciprocity, nonverbal communication, and relationship-building, such as struggles with conversation, eye contact, or adapting behavior to different social contexts (APA, 2013). Repetitive behaviors may include motor movements, rigid adherence to routines, fixated interests, or unusual sensory responses, such as hypersensitivity to sounds or fascination with textures (APA, 2013). These challenges must significantly impair daily functioning, and the condition cannot be better explained by intellectual disability or developmental delay, though it may co-occur with these conditions (APA, 2013).

PUBLIC HEALTH SIGNIFICANCE OF ASD

Globally, approximately 1 in 100 children is estimated to have ASD, though this figure is an average and varies widely across studies, depending on design, region, and income level (Talantseva et al., 2023; World Health Organization [WHO], 2023). Some rigorous studies suggest even higher prevalence rates (WHO, 2023). Specifically, a three -level meta-analysis by Talantseva et al. (2023) showed that studies using record-review methods reported higher prevalence, with North America and high-income countries showing greater rates compared to other regions. The highest prevalence was recorded in the U.S. (1.12%), while the lowest was in Taiwan (0.11%) (Talantseva et al., 2023). Similarly, a systematic review by Salari et al. (2022) reported prevalence rates of 1% in America, 0.5% in Europe, and 0.4% in Asia, with limited data for Oceania and Africa. However, data on autism prevalence in many low- and middle-income countries remains scarce (WHO, 2023).

ASD diagnoses have risen significantly in recent years, with this global upward trend starting in the early 1990s (World Population Review, 2024). The Centres for Disease Control and Prevention (CDC) reports that as of 2024, 1 in 36 children in the U.S. is diagnosed with ASD (Centers for Disease Control and Prevention [CDC], 2024). This reflects a steady increase from previous rates of 1 in 44 in 2018, 1 in 68 in 2016, 1 in 88 in 2008, and 1 in 150 in 2000 (World Population Review, 2024). A UK study analysing ASD diagnosis trends from 1998 to 2018 found a 787%

increase in recorded cases (Russell et al., 2022). This rise was more pronounced in adults, older children, and females, with the average age of diagnosis increasing from 9.6 to 14.5 years (Russell et al., 2022).

Similarly, ASD prevalence in Asia has increased, despite prevalence rates being lower in comparison with Western countries (Qiu et al., 2020). In a meta-analysis conducted by Qiu et al. (2020) the pooled prevalence in Asian countries was 0.36%, a rate higher than the 0.15% reported in a 2010 meta-analysis (Qiu et al., 2020). Prevalence was higher in males (0.45%) than females (0.18%), likely due to differences in diagnostic rates, as girls often exhibit less overt atypical behavior (Qiu et al., 2020). Geographically, prevalence was highest in East Asia (0.51%), followed by West Asia (0.35%) and South Asia (0.31%), possibly influenced by cultural perceptions of autism (Qiu et al., 2020). Experts attribute much of this increase to heightened awareness and improved diagnostic practices rather than a surge in actual cases (World Population Review, 2024). Additionally, factors like older parental age and higher survival rates of premature infants, both more common in modern times, may also contribute to the rise (World Population Review, 2024).

IMPORTANCE OF EARLY DIAGNOSIS AND INTERVENTION

Early diagnosis of ASD offers significant advantages, including access to early interventions (Clark et al., 2017; Okoye et al., 2023). Research has consistently shown that the earlier children with ASD begin intervention, the greater their progress will be across various skill areas (Fuller & Kaiser, 2020; Gabbay-Dizdar et al., 2022; Godel et al., 2022; Shi et al., 2021; Vietze & Lax, 2020). Specifically, early intervention programs have been particularly effective in enhancing social and communication skills (Fuller & Kaiser, 2020; Gabbay-Dizdar et al., 2022; Milbourn et al., 2017; Vietze & Lax, 2020), with maximum benefits occurring at age 3.81 years (Fuller & Kaiser, 2020). Additionally, these programs significantly improve cognitive abilities (Godel et al., 2022; Shi et al., 2021; Vietze & Lax, 2020) and foster substantial gains in verbal and language skills (Godel et al., 2022; Milbourn et al., 2017; Shi et al., 2021). Finally, early intervention also promotes meaningful improvements in adaptive behaviour (Okoye et al., 2023; Vietze & Lax, 2020).

Furthermore, it allows for personalized strategies to address autism-specific needs, such as social communication, language development, and behavioural challenges (Milbourn et al., 2017; Okoye et al., 2023). The cultivation of these skills has been shown to reduce stress and enhance family dynamics (Milbourn et al., 2017). Parents are better equipped to understand and address their child's unique needs, thereby fostering a more supportive and nurturing home environment (Milbourn et al., 2017). Additionally, they are more prepared to manage challenging situations and actively contribute to their child's developmental progress (Milbourn et al., 2017). Finally, it connects families to essential support services, educational tools, and community programs (Jacobs et al., 2020; Okoye et al., 2023).

Overall, even though prevalence increased over time, it was significantly higher among children aged six to twelve compared to those under five or over thirteen (Efstratopoulou et al., 2012; Talantseva et al., 2023). Misdiagnosing or missing autism in childhood can deprive individuals and families of essential support, including early intervention critical for development (Kaufman, 2022). Symptoms like social impairments, challenging behaviours, and language loss are often overlooked, misattributed, or normalised by caregivers and professionals, delaying diagnosis (Lupindo et al., 2023). This disparity may impact children's developmental progress, as emotional, behavioral, and social difficulties are closely linked to the timing of an autism diagnosis (Mandy et al., 2022). Children diagnosed later often face significant mental health and social challenges that may worsen during adolescence (Mandy et al., 2022) Furthermore, a lack of early diagnosis and support can lead to long-term psychological effects, including isolation, bullying, and distress, which persist into adulthood (Lupindo et al., 2023). Late diagnosis affects academic achievement, career opportunities, and independence, with individuals often adopting maladaptive coping strategies like masking, substance use, and withdrawal to manage challenges (Lupindo et al., 2023).

The Traditional Process of Identifying and Diagnosing ASD

Diagnosing ASD typically involves a two-step process: first, a developmental screening that identifies at risk children, followed by a comprehensive diagnostic evaluation if the screening indicates potential concerns (Gordon-Lipkin et al., 2016). To optimize outcomes for all children with ASD, the American Academy of Paediatrics (AAP) recommends universal ASD screening, in addition to broadband developmental screening, at the 18- and 24-month well-child paediatric visits (Johnson et al., 2007; Zwaigenbaum et al., 2015). The Modified Checklist for Autism in Toddlers (M-CHAT) and its updates are widely used and extensively studied tools for ASD screening in children aged 16–30 months (Jullien, 2021). They evaluate communication, joint attention, repetitive movements, and pretend play through a parent-rated scale, often followed by an interview. Positive screenings result in referrals for a confirmatory diagnosis (Jullien, 2021).

The Golden Standards for ASD Diagnosis

Toddlers and children should undergo diagnostic evaluation if screening or surveillance indicates an elevated risk of developmental disorders, including ASD (American Academy of Pediatrics, 2023). The most used diagnostic tools for ASD are the autism diagnostic observation schedule, second edition (ADOS-2) and the autism diagnostic interview, revised (ADI-R) (Santos et al., 2024). The combined administration of these two diagnostic tools is considered to be the golden standard for diagnosing ASD (Gray et al., 2008; Vargason et al., 2020). The ADOS-2 is a semi-structured assessment that consists of observed interactions and a series of activities conducted between the referred individual and a trained evaluator (Lord et al., 2012). ADI-R is a structured interview conducted with caregivers to assess communication, social interaction, and repetitive behaviors in individuals suspected of having autism (Rutter et al., 2003).

The Challenges of Early ASD Diagnosis

Significant delays persist between initial parental concern and ASD diagnosis, with an average delay of a minimum of two years (Y. H. Chen et al., 2023; Wong et al., 2017). Specifically, the diagnostic delay averages 26.9 months from the first developmental screening and 21.0 months from the latest screening (Y. H. Chen et al., 2023). Interestingly, no significant difference in delay times was found between children who had single or multiple screenings, suggesting repeated screenings do not necessarily lead to earlier diagnoses (Y. H. Chen et al., 2023). Additionally, the time from a parent's initial concern to an ASD diagnosis varies significantly, averaging 8 months for children diagnosed early (under 3 years old) and 28 months for those diagnosed later (3 years or older) (Becerra-Culqui et al., 2018). Furthermore, the average time between parents first suspecting a problem and receiving a diagnosis was nearly 29 months (Wong et al., 2017). Finally, the average age of diagnosis was 3.26 years and the average delay between the first professional visit and the final diagnosis was 1.20 years (MacKenzie et al., 2023).

Parents often report long waits between referral, diagnosis, and intervention, with up to 88% experiencing referral delays and 70% facing challenges accessing special education programs (Yi et al., 2020). Navigating the diagnostic process often involves attending multiple appointments, assessments, and consultations, which can be emotionally and physically exhausting for families (Milbourn et al., 2017). In Australia, parents reported an average of eight consultations and a one-year delay before receiving a diagnosis, underscoring systemic inefficiencies (Bent et al., 2020). These persistent barriers reflect systemic healthcare issues that delay timely ASD diagnosis and intervention, highlighting the urgent need for streamlined processes and better family support systems.

Delays between a parent's first concern and an ASD diagnosis are often attributed to healthcare providers' tendency to advise a "wait-and-see" approach, which postpones timely diagnoses (Becerra-Culqui et al., 2018; Bent et al., 2020). Some professionals are reluctant to diagnose ASD, often dismissing parental concerns as temporary delays, which frustrates families and hinders early intervention (Milbourn et al., 2017). The "wait-and-see" approach largely stems from the difficulty of distinguishing ASD from other developmental disorders in the early stages, due to overlapping symptoms and the variability of ASD presentations (Garrido et al., 2018; Hus & Segal, 2021). Paediatricians may take a cautious approach, noting that children develop at different rates and early concerns might signal other conditions (Garrido et al., 2018). For example, children with both ASD and attention deficiency/hyperactivity disorder (ADHD) may exhibit difficulties with social interaction, communication, and attention, making it challenging to determine the primary diagnosis (Hus & Segal, 2021).

Research reveals significant gaps in healthcare providers' knowledge and training regarding ASD, which hinder early diagnosis and intervention. Shortcomings in training have been highlighted as a critical issue (Bivarchi et al., 2021). Similarly, insufficient education among healthcare providers has been identified as a key barrier to early diagnosis (Elder et al., 2016). Many parents have reported that medical professionals lack the necessary knowledge or experience to recognize and diagnose ASD, leading to delays and missed opportunities for early intervention (Milbourn et al., 2017). Additionally, barriers to effective screening include limited knowledge, unfamiliarity with screening tools, and a lack of confidence in identifying autism symptoms (Fenikilé et al., 2015; Self et al., 2015). These findings highlight the urgent need for enhanced training and education for healthcare professionals.

The universal screening tools for ASD and the current gold-standard diagnostic tools, such as the Autism Diagnostic Observation Schedule (ADOS) and Autism Diagnostic Interview-Revised (ADI-R), have limitations (McCarty & Frye, 2020). Universal screening has limitations due to the low prevalence of ASD in the general population (Levy et al., 2020; McCarty & Frye, 2020; Sobieski et al., 2022). Even with highly sensitive and specific screening tools like the Modified Checklist for Autism in Toddlers, Revised with Follow-up (M-CHAT-R/F), the positive predictive value is only around 33% (McCarty & Frye, 2020). This means that only 1 in 3 children identified by the M-CHAT-R/F has ASD, leading to a high number of false positives (McCarty & Frye, 2020). Additionally, there is a lack of well-studied screening tools for children older than 30 months (Levy et al., 2020; McCarty & Frye, 2020; Sobieski et al., 2022). These challenges highlight the complexity of diagnosing ASD and underscore the need for improved methods to facilitate early and accurate identification.

Children with a delayed ASD diagnosis are more likely to have received other developmental or psychiatric diagnoses, such as ADHD and language disorders, at baseline than those with early ASD diagnosis (Avlund et al., 2021). Specifically, children and adolescents with a prior ADHD diagnosis were diagnosed with autism an average of 1.8 years later than those without ADHD, regardless of ASD severity or current age (Kentrou et al., 2019). Gender-based differences were observed in the timing of autism diagnoses among children and adolescents with prior ADHD diagnoses (Kentrou et al., 2019). Boys were diagnosed with autism 1.52 years later, and girls 2.64 years later, compared to peers without a preceding ADHD diagnosis (Kentrou et al., 2019). Similarly, children with both ASD and ADHD who were diagnosed with ADHD first received their ASD diagnosis approximately three years later than those diagnosed with ADHD concurrently or after ASD (Miodovnik et al., 2015). These children were nearly 30 times more likely to be diagnosed with ASD after age six, with 39.5% receiving their diagnosis at six years or older, a delay that persisted throughout childhood and was unaffected by ASD severity (Miodovnik et al., 2015).

Early diagnosis of ASD is critical for accessing timely interventions, but certain presentations of the condition can complicate the diagnostic process. Children with milder symptoms or higher verbal abilities often face delays in being diagnosed, as their skills can mask the effects of ASD symptoms and make early identification more challenging (Rattaz et al., 2022). Similarly, children who do not exhibit typical "red flags" for ASD, such as language regression or language delay, are more likely to experience diagnostic delays because these hallmark traits often prompt earlier evaluation and intervention (Brett et al., 2016). Finally, universal screening questions are more skewed towards severe ASD symptoms, while failing to capture and recognize children with more subtle ASD signs (Elder et al., 2016). These findings highlight the need for improved diagnostic strategies that account for subtle or atypical presentations of ASD to ensure timely diagnosis and support.

Sociocultural and socioeconomic disparities significantly contribute to delays in diagnosing ASD, particularly for children from minority and low-income families. Children in these groups face systemic inequities, such as limited access to quality healthcare and resources, resulting in delayed diagnoses (Aylward et al., 2021). Geographic and sociocultural barriers further exacerbate these delays, with African American, Hispanic/Latino children, and those living in rural areas particularly affected (Mazurek et al., 2019). Socioeconomic challenges, including limited healthcare accessibility and lack of continuity of care, also prolong the diagnostic timeline (Malwane et al., 2022). Additionally, children from lower socioeconomic status (SES) families often experience delays due to disparities in access to healthcare and educational resources (Rattaz et al., 2022). In contrast, children from higher SES backgrounds tend to be diagnosed earlier, likely due to increased awareness and better access to healthcare and early intervention resources (Hus & Segal, 2021). These findings emphasize the need for equitable healthcare practices and culturally sensitive approaches to improve early identification and intervention for all children.

Social stigma surrounding ASD significantly impacts the timeliness of diagnosis and access to support services. Fear of judgment and negative societal perceptions often discourage parents from seeking early diagnosis or professional help, further delaying the diagnostic process (Elder et al., 2016). Stigma can also result in isolation and a delayed acceptance of a diagnosis, as families may struggle with societal misconceptions about ASD and its implications (Bivarchi et al., 2021). Additionally, cultural stigma within certain communities can exacerbate delays, as families may hesitate to pursue interventions due to a lack of understanding or fear of being ostracized (Aylward et al., 2021). These findings highlight the importance of education and community outreach to reduce stigma and foster a more supportive environment for individuals with ASD and their families.

THE EMERGENCE OF ARTIFICIAL INTELLIGENCE IN ASD DIAGNOSIS

Artificial Intelligence (AI) refers to computer systems designed to perform tasks that usually require human intelligence (Nguyen & Huang, 2024). A branch of AI, Machine Learning (ML), involves creating algorithms and models that can analyse data, make decisions or predictions, and enhance their performance over time through computational experience, either with or without human guidance (Nguyen & Huang, 2024). Deep Learning (DL), a specialized area within ML, enables computers to mimic human brain functions in data processing (Nguyen & Huang, 2024).

With rapid advancements in data processing and deep learning techniques, AI and ML are poised to revolutionize medical practices, including the growing use of AI, ML, and DL in detecting mental disorders (Helm et al., 2020; Nguyen & Huang, 2024). Specifically, in the field of medical diagnosis, the rise of AI has the potential to transform medical diagnostics by enhancing accuracy, speed, and efficiency (Al-Antari, 2023). AI algorithms can process medical images like X-rays, MRIs, and CT scans, assisting healthcare professionals in detecting diseases with greater precision (Al-Antari, 2023). Additionally, AI can analyze extensive patient data, including imaging, bio-signals (such as ECG and EEG), vital signs, demographics, medical history, and lab results (Al-Antari, 2023). By improving predictive capabilities and decision-making, AI supports healthcare providers in delivering more informed and effective patient care (Al-Antari, 2023).

Recent advancements in neuropsychopharmacology indicate that artificial intelligence (AI) plays a vital role in enhancing the diagnosis of neurodevelopmental disorders, such as ASD, ADHD and more (Song et al., 2022; Uddin et al., 2019; Verma et al., 2021). AI technologies, including machine learning and data analytics, are utilized to process extensive datasets from neuroimaging studies, genetic research, and clinical trials (Azevedo et al., 2023; Skampardoni et al., 2024). These AI applications assist in detecting biomarkers, forecasting treatment responses, and enhancing drug development, potentially resulting in more precise and effective therapies for neurological and psychiatric disorders (Sabbagh et al., 2020).

Benefits of AI in ASD Diagnosis

In the context of ASD, AI holds tremendous potential to revolutionize the diagnosis process (Shahamiri & Thabtah, 2020). Specifically, AI tools, including ML and DL can help improve the accuracy and precision of ASD detection and diagnosis (Ali et al., 2020; Alqaysi et al., 2022; Anagnostopoulou et al., 2020). Specifically, AI algorism can be trained to detect patterns and features in the pre collected data that indicate ASD, allowing them to be used for more accurate and reliable diagnoses (Brueggeman et al., 2020; Radhakrishnan et al., 2021). Additionally, AI-powered tools, such as machine learning algorithms and natural language processing systems, can analyze vast amounts of data—including behavioral patterns, neuroimaging results, genetic indicators, and electronic medical records—to provide meaningful insights into ASD (Anagnostopoulou et al., 2020; Gupta et al., 2022). The combination of the AI's ability to analyze large amount of data (Joudar et al., 2023) and improve accuracy through trials (Jiang et al., 2017), can reduce human error and bias in the diagnostic process (Jiang et al., 2017; Joudar et al., 2023). Finally, AI can minimize the reliance on expensive and lengthy tests while significantly reducing evaluation wait times and assessment costs through its applications (Ali et al., 2020; Anagnostopoulou et al., 2020).

Existing AI Devices for the Screening and Diagnosis of ASD

The Canvas Dx, created by Cognoa Medical Affairs, and the EarliPoint System, developed by EarliTec are two devices developed to aid healthcare providers in ASD in children, both of which received Food and Drug Administration (FDA) Class II clearance (Kleine et al., 2025). Canvas DX was developed using ML techniques. The device analyses historical data to identify predictive ASD behavioral features and integrates inputs from caregivers, clinicians, and trained video analysts through a smartphone app, video uploads, and questionnaires (Megerian et al., 2022a, 2022b). These inputs are processed into a mathematical vector for ML analysis, yielding a diagnostic output of ASD positive, negative, or abstention when insufficient information is available. In a pivotal 2019–2020 validation study involving 425 children aged 18–72 months, Canvas Dx demonstrated strong alignment with specialist diagnoses for determinate cases, with high positive and negative predictive values, sensitivity, and specificity (Megerian et al., 2022a, 2022b). Importantly, the study found no evidence of performance disparities across gender, race/ethnicity, or socioeconomic status, though further research is needed to confirm these findings (Megerian et al., 2022a, 2022b). Canvas Dx serves as an adjunct to clinical judgment, supporting providers in adhering to diagnostic standards while emphasizing the importance of accuracy and equity in AI-driven ASD diagnosis.

The EarliPoint System aids healthcare providers in diagnosing ASD in children aged 16 to 30 months who are at risk for developmental delay (Kleine et al., 2025). Utilizing AI, the system analyzes eye-tracking data collected by measuring a child's visual responses to social information presented in videos (Jones et al., 2023). This approach is supported by evidence showing that eye-tracking-based measurement of social visual engagement is predictive of autism diagnoses, as demonstrated in a study where 475 out of 499 children (95.2%) successfully underwent testing (Jones et al., 2023). The study revealed strong correlations between eye-tracking results and expert clinical assessments of social disability, verbal ability, and non-verbal cognitive ability, with sensitivity and specificity reaching 78.0% and 85.4%, respectively, in children with definitive autism diagnoses (Jones et al., 2023). The EarliPoint WebPortal facilitates the entry and access of patient information and assessment results, delivering a clear positive or negative ASD diagnosis without an indeterminate option (Kleine et al., 2025). These findings highlight the potential of the EarliPoint System as a valuable tool for early autism diagnosis, though further evaluation of its role in routine clinical practice is warranted (Kleine et al., 2025).

Accuracy of AI Tools in the ASD Diagnosis

Machine Learning Methods

Machine learning (ML) has emerged as a powerful tool in the early detection and diagnosis of ASD, offering the potential to improve accuracy, efficiency, and accessibility in clinical settings. Several studies have explored the application of ML models to diverse datasets, including behavioral, linguistic, and neuroimaging data, to identify patterns indicative of ASD. For instance, Shambour et al. (2024) compared six ML models—Support Vector Machine (SVM), Random Forest (RF), k-nearest neighbors (KNN), Logistic Regression (LR), Decision Tree (DT), and Naive Bayes (NB)—for ASD detection in toddlers, They found that more complex models like SVM and RF were particularly effective for non-linearly separable data, suggesting their utility in clinical applications for accurate and efficient ASD diagnosis (Shambour et al., 2024). Similarly, a study Themistocleous et al. (2024) utilized Natural Language Processing (NLP) and ML models such as Hist Gradient Boosting and XGBoost to classify children with ASD based on narrative production and expressive vocabulary. achieving high accuracy rates of 96.75% and 96%, respectively. Building on these findings, Alzakari et al. (2025) employed a two-phase approach using a variety of ML models, including LR, RF, SGD, XGBoost, SVM, KNN, DT, and Extra Trees Classifier (ETC), as well as an LR-SVM ensemble model. Their study achieved a remarkable 99% classification accuracy using the LR-SVM ensemble model with Chi-square (CHI2) feature selection, further validating the effectiveness of combining ML models for ASD detection (Alzakari et al., 2025).

ML techniques have also been applied to neuroimaging data to identify structural abnormalities associated with ASD. Xu et al. (2024) employed six ML models, including SVM and AdaBoost, to analyze brain segmentation data, achieving high prediction accuracy (AUC of 0.91–0.92) and identifying specific brain regions with increased volume in children with ASD. T. Chen et al. (2020) further advanced this approach by developing a Histogram-Based Morphometry (HBM) framework using 3D Histogram of Oriented Gradients (HOG) to distinguish ASD patients from healthy controls based on structural MRI (sMRI) data, achieving 86% accuracy and highlighting the practicality of sMRI over fMRI due to its lower cost and wider clinical availability. These studies underscore the potential of combining ML with neuroimaging for precise and scalable ASD diagnosis

In addition to behavioral and neuroimaging data, ML has been integrated into multi-modular diagnostic systems. Abbas et al. (2020) developed a mobile app with three ML modules—parent questionnaire, clinician questionnaire, and video analysis—using gradient-boosted decision trees, which outperformed conventional autism screeners and provided reliable predictions (positive, negative, or inconclusive). Similarly, Hazim Hammed & Albahri (2023) employed traditional feature selection methods alongside ML models like Gradient Boosting (GB) and Random Forest (RF) to screen ASD, with GB achieving 87% accuracy, demonstrating the effectiveness of combining feature selection with ML for improved diagnostic outcomes [6].

The use of explainable AI (XAI) techniques has further enhanced the interpretability and reliability of ML models in ASD diagnosis. A study by Jeon et al. (2024) utilized XAI methods such as SHAP and LIME to interpret the decision-making processes of models like XGBoost and Neural Networks (NNET), which achieved near-perfect accuracy (1 and 0.9984, respectively), emphasizing the importance of behavioral characteristics in ASD prediction. Similarly, Alzakari et al. (2025) also leveraged SHAP (Shapley Additive Explanations) to understand the importance of features in their model, identifying key contributors such as the A9 and A6 scores, which were crucial for predicting ASD [21]. These advancements highlight the potential of ML to streamline ASD diagnosis, enabling earlier intervention and improving outcomes for children with ASD.

Collectively, these studies demonstrate the versatility and effectiveness of ML in ASD diagnosis, leveraging diverse data types and advanced algorithms to achieve high accuracy and reliability. By integrating ML with clinical tools, such as questionnaires, narrative analysis, and neuroimaging, researchers and clinicians can enhance the diagnostic process, reduce delays, and provide more personalized care for individuals with ASD.

Deep Learning Methods

Deep learning models have shown significant promise in advancing the diagnosis of ASD, leveraging complex architectures to analyze diverse data types such as neuroimaging, facial images, and behavioral patterns. For instance, Parui et al. (2023) utilized a 2D Convolutional Neural Network (2D-CNN) alongside Low Estimated Rank Tensor (LERT) to estimate functional connectivity networks (FCNs) from fMRI data, achieving a maximum accuracy of 70.76% when combining results from multiple brain atlases (CC200, DOS, and AAL) using a majority voting algorithm. Similarly, Ahmad et al. (2024) explored the use of pre-trained CNN models, including ResNet50, VGG16, and MobileNetv2, for ASD detection using facial images, with ResNet50 achieving the highest accuracy of 92% through transfer learning techniques. In a similar vein, Shahamiri & Thabtah (2020) employed CNNs to detect autistic traits based on data provided by individuals, families, or medical professionals. This system, known as AutismAI, revealed higher accuracy, sensitivity, and specificity when compared to conventional screening methods. These studies highlight the effectiveness of deep learning in extracting high-level features from complex datasets, such as brain connectivity and facial characteristics, to improve diagnostic accuracy.

Hybrid deep learning models have also emerged as powerful tools for ASD diagnosis, combining the strengths of multiple architectures to enhance performance. Priyadarshini (2023) proposed two hybrid models—CNN-LSTM with Particle Swarm Optimization (PSO) and GRU-CNN—which achieved remarkable accuracies of 98.89% and 94.02%, respectively, for ASD screening in adults, and an exceptional 99.64% accuracy for toddlers using the CNN-LSTM-PSO model. Colonnese et al. (2024) developed a Gaze-Based Autism Classifier (GBAC) model, which combined three neural networks and utilized eye-tracking data to achieve a test accuracy of 94.35% and an F1-score of 0.9315, outperforming other benchmark models. Additionally, Ulaganathan et al. (2025) introduced a hybrid optimization-enabled DenseNet (JSTO-DenseNet) for classifying ASD using MRI images, which achieved an accuracy of 94.8%. These hybrid approaches demonstrate the potential of integrating optimization techniques and multimodal data to further refine ASD detection.

The application of deep learning in ASD diagnosis is further enhanced by its ability to handle imbalanced datasets and incorporate fairness techniques. Priyadarshini (2023) employed the Synthetic Minority Oversampling Technique (SMOTE) to address data imbalance and used AI fairness methods such as feature engineering and outlier handling to reduce bias. Colonnese et al. (2024) utilized the TracIn method to trace model behavior back to training data, identifying influential samples and improving the interpretability of the GBAC model. These advancements underscore the importance of combining deep learning with ethical AI practices to ensure reliable and unbiased diagnostic outcomes. Collectively, these studies illustrate the transformative potential of deep learning and hybrid models in ASD diagnosis, offering scalable, accurate, and interpretable solutions for early detection and intervention.

ML and DL Integration Approaches

The integration of ML and DL models has shown significant promise in improving the accuracy and reliability of ASD diagnosis across various modalities, including neuroimaging, natural language processing, motion data, eye-tracking, and facial feature analysis. For instance, Jung et al. (2023) proposed the Explainability-guided Region of Interest Selection (EAG-RS) framework, which leverages self-supervised learning and Layer-wise Relevance Propagation (LRP) to identify non-linear high-order functional associations in resting-state functional magnetic resonance imaging (rs-fMRI) data. This framework achieved an Area Under the Curve (AUC) of 0.760 and outperformed several baseline methods, including BrainNetCNN and BrainGNN, on the Autism Brain Imaging Database Exchange (ABIDE) dataset. The study also identified ASD subtypes that align with neuroscientific findings, highlighting the potential of explainable AI in neuroimaging-based ASD diagnosis (Jung et al., 2023).

In the realm of natural language processing, Rubio-Martín et al. (2024) explored the use of ML and DL models to diagnose ASD using text data from Twitter. By analyzing 404,627 tweets from 252 users, the study demonstrated that deep learning models, particularly BERTweet, achieved the highest accuracy (87.7%) compared to traditional ML models like Decision Trees and XGBoost (Rubio-Martín et al., 2024). The authors emphasized the potential of leveraging social media data for ASD detection, though they noted the need for further hyperparameter optimization to enhance model performance (Rubio-Martín et al., 2024). Similarly, Luongo et al. (2024) investigated the use of raw motion data to classify children with ASD, employing an Artificial Neural Network (ANN) to analyze motion trajectories. Their findings revealed that acceleration metrics, such as maximum and minimum acceleration, play a critical role in distinguishing ASD from typically developing children, underscoring the importance of motor pattern analysis in early ASD detection (Luongo et al., 2024).

Eye-tracking data has also been leveraged for ASD diagnosis, with Ahmed et al. (2022) developing a hybrid approach combining machine learning and deep learning techniques. Their study utilized pre-trained CNN models like GoogleNet and ResNet-18, achieving accuracies of up to 99.8% with feedforward neural networks (FFNNs) and artificial neural networks (ANNs) (Ahmed et al., 2022). The hybrid GoogleNet + SVM and ResNet-18 + SVM systems further demonstrated the effectiveness of integrating deep learning with traditional ML classifiers for ASD detection (Alqubati et al., 2023). Additionally, Elangovan et al. (2024) introduced a novel methodology, FTLDA-AASDDC, which fuses transfer learning with the Dandelion Algorithm (DA) for ASD classification using facial features. Their approach achieved a superior accuracy of 97.50%, outperforming standalone models like MobileNetV2 and ResNet50, and highlighted the potential of nature-inspired optimization techniques in enhancing model performance (Elangovan et al., 2024).

Finally, Rony et al. (2024) developed a Data Mining and Logistic Regression model with Shapley Additive exPlanations (DMLRS) for ASD diagnosis, achieving an impressive accuracy of 99%. Their study incorporated explainable AI techniques, such as SHAP, to enhance model interpretability and developed a real-time web application for ASD detection (Rony et al., 2024). This approach underscores the importance of combining advanced ML techniques with user-friendly applications to facilitate early and accurate ASD diagnosis (Rony et al., 2024). Collectively, these studies demonstrate the transformative potential of combining machine and deep learning models with diverse data modalities to improve ASD diagnosis, offering new avenues for early detection and personalized intervention.

AI IN HEALTHCARE POLICIES

The World Health Organization (WHO) and the European Union (EU) have proposed guiding principles and regulations to ensure the ethical, safe, and inclusive use of aAI in healthcare (European Union, 2024; WHO, 2021). WHO's six principles emphasise protecting human autonomy, promoting well-being and public interest, ensuring transparency and explainability, fostering accountability, promoting inclusiveness, and encouraging sustainability and responsiveness in AI design and application (WHO, 2021). Meanwhile, the EU's AI Act, adopted in March 2024, is the first comprehensive legal framework specifically regulating AI in various sectors, including healthcare (Busch et al., 2024; European Union, 2024). It uses a risk-based approach, categorising AI systems by risk level—ranging from prohibited to minimal risk—with high-risk applications like AI-assisted diagnosis requiring strict compliance with safety, transparency, and oversight measures (European Union, 2024; Panel for the Future of Science and Technology, 2022). The AI Act is particularly important for healthcare, as many current and future medical AI applications will be deemed high-risk and must meet specific compliance obligations within 12 months of the Act's enforcement (Busch et al., 2024; European Union, 2024).

Ethical Considerations

Privacy and Data Security is a big concern when it comes to utilizing AI in healthcare general and ASD diagnosis specifically (Elendu et al., 2023; Garg & Chauhan, 2024; Panel for the Future of Science and Technology [STOA], 2022). AI systems in healthcare generate large amounts of sensitive patient data, and ensuring the privacy and security of this data is paramount (Elendu et al., 2023) In the context of ASD diagnosis, the reliance on sensitive health data requires strict compliance with data protection regulations to prevent breaches and maintain confidentiality (Garg & Chauhan, 2024). Data breaches could severely impact patient trust and data integrity (Elendu et al., 2023). Responsible data handling practices, including robust encryption and anonymisation techniques, are needed to protect patient information (Elendu et al., 2023).

Algorithmic bias and fairness is another ethical consideration when using AI in healthcare (Elendu et al., 2023; Li et al., 2023). AI algorithms may unintentionally reinforce biases that exist in past healthcare data (Li et al., 2023). This can lead to disparities in diagnosis and treatment, making it crucial to develop algorithms that mitigate bias and promote fairness (Elendu et al., 2023). Bias can also arise from the use of unrepresentative or incomplete training data (Reddy et al., 2020). Specifically, issues related to discrimination and equality can occur when AI systems lack equality in the training data, or if the target is not appropriately selected (Balthazar et al., 2018). Data-driven AI can lead to discrimination in healthcare, which may result in certain groups being treated unequally (Balthazar et al., 2018).

An additional ethical consideration is transparency and explainability (Carabantes, 2020; STOA, 2022). The "black box" nature of many AI algorithms, especially those using deep learning, can make it difficult to understand their decision-making processes (Currie et al., 2020; D'antonoli, 2020; Panel for the Future of Science and Technology, 2022). This lack of transparency and explainability can reduce trust in AI systems, and it is essential that patients and healthcare providers understand the rationale behind AI-driven recommendations (Elendu et al., 2023). Defining clear accountability for the actions of AI systems and ensuring transparent decision-making processes are essential for fostering trust and promoting ethical use (Elendu et al., 2023).

A final ethical consideration to mention is social gaps and justice (Elendu et al., 2023; Farhud & Zokaei, 2021; Nordling, 2019; STOA, 2022). AI's development may exacerbate existing social inequalities (Farhud & Zokaei, 2021). While AI may improve access to information, it can also worsen social inequality (Farhud & Zokaei, 2021). It is important to ensure that the benefits of AI in healthcare are accessible to all, especially low-income and developing countries, and that the technology does not create further disparities (Farhud & Zokaei, 2021).

CONCLUSION

In summary, the integration of AI tools and models has significantly advanced the accuracy and efficiency of ASD diagnosis. Various approaches, including neuroimaging, natural language processing, motion tracking, and facial feature analysis, have demonstrated promising results in identifying ASD with high precision. Hybrid models that combine multiple AI techniques have further enhanced diagnostic reliability, offering scalable solutions for early intervention. However, while these technological advancements hold great potential, their successful implementation requires careful consideration of ethical factors, such as data privacy, algorithmic bias, and transparency. Ensuring that AI-based ASD diagnostic tools are equitable and interpretable remains crucial in fostering trust among clinicians, caregivers, and individuals with ASD.

Moving forward, continued research and collaboration between data scientists, healthcare professionals, and policymakers will be essential in refining these AI-driven diagnostic models. Addressing challenges such as data imbalance, accessibility disparities, and the need for robust regulatory frameworks will be key to ensuring these technologies benefit all individuals, regardless of socioeconomic background. Furthermore, integrating AI with real-time monitoring and personalized treatment strategies could revolutionize ASD care, providing tailored interventions that adapt to each individual's needs. Ultimately, a balanced approach that combines technological innovation with ethical responsibility will be critical in shaping the future of ASD diagnosis and intervention.

REFERENCES

Abbas, H., Garberson, F., Liu-Mayo, S., Glover, E., & Wall, D. P. (2020). Multi-modular AI approach to streamline autism diagnosis in young children. *Scientific Reports*, *10*(1), 5014. Advance online publication. DOI: 10.1038/s41598-020-61213-w PMID: 32193406

Ahmad, I., Rashid, J., Faheem, M., Akram, A., Khan, N. A., & Amin, R. (2024). Autism spectrum disorder detection using facial images: A performance comparison of pretrained convolutional neural networks. *Healthcare Technology Letters*, *11*(4), 227–239. DOI: 10.1049/htl2.12073 PMID: 39100502

Ahmed, I. A., Senan, E. M., Rassem, T. H., Ali, M. A. H., Shatnawi, H. S. A., Alwazer, S. M., & Alshahrani, M. (2022). Eye tracking-based diagnosis and early detection of autism spectrum disorder using machine learning and deep learning techniques. *Electronics (Basel)*, *11*(4), 530. Advance online publication. DOI: 10.3390/electronics11040530

Al-Antari, M. (2023). Artificial intelligence for medical diagnostics—Existing and future AI technology! *Diagnostics (Basel)*, *13*(4), 688. DOI: 10.3390/diagnostics13040688 PMID: 36832175

Ali, N. A., Syafeeza, A. R., Jaafar, A. S., & Alif, M. K. M. F. (2020). Autism spectrum disorder classification on electroencephalogram signal using deep learning algorithm. *IAES International Journal of Artificial Intelligence*, *9*(1), 91–99. DOI: 10.11591/ijai.v9.i1.pp91-99

Alqaysi, M. E., Albahri, A. S., & Hamid, R. A. (2022). Hybrid diagnosis models for autism patients based on medical and sociodemographic features using machine learning and multicriteria decision-making (MCDM) techniques: An evaluation and benchmarking framework. *Computational and Mathematical Methods in Medicine*, *2022*(1), 9410222. DOI: 10.1155/2022/9410222 PMID: 36439957

Alzakari, S. A., Allinjawi, A., Aldrees, A., Zamzami, N., Umer, M., Innab, N., & Ashraf, I. (2025). Early detection of autism spectrum disorder using explainable AI and optimized teaching strategies. *Journal of Neuroscience Methods*, *413*, 110315. Advance online publication. DOI: 10.1016/j.jneumeth.2024.110315 PMID: 39532186

American Academy of Pediatrics. (2023, May 4). *Autism spectrum disorder*. https://www.aap.org/en/patient-care/autism/?srsltid=AfmBOoqSQJiFO31AyoeWwTT7xYu8205FzS3nN9MkiencGG74ybtMXSyE

American Psychiatric Association. (2013). *The diagnostic and statistical manual of mental disorders* (5th ed.). American Psychiatric Association.

Anagnostopoulou, P., Alexandropoulou, V., Lorentzou, G., Lykothanasi, A., Ntaountaki, P., & Drigas, A. (2020). Artificial intelligence in autism assessment. *International Journal of Emerging Technologies in Learning, 15*(6), 95–107. DOI: 10.3991/ijet.v15i06.11231

Avlund, S. H., Thomsen, P. H., Schendel, D., Jørgensen, M., Carlsen, A. H., & Clausen, L. (2021). Factors associated with a delayed autism spectrum disorder diagnosis in children previously assessed on suspicion of autism. *Journal of Autism and Developmental Disorders, 51*(11), 3843–3856. DOI: 10.1007/s10803-020-04849-x PMID: 33392868

Aylward, B. S., Gal-Szabo, D. E., & Taraman, S. (2021). Racial, ethnic, and socio-demographic disparities in diagnosis of children with autism spectrum disorder. *Journal of Developmental and Behavioral Pediatrics, 45*(8), 682689. https://journals.lww.com/jrnldbp. DOI: 10.1097/DBP.0000000000000996 PMID: 34510108

Azevedo, T., Bethlehem, R. A. I., Whiteside, D. J., Swaddiwudhipong, N., Rowe, J. B., Lió, P., Rittman, T., Li, G., Petrie, E. C., Peskind, E. R., Villena, T., Martinez, W., Sadowsky, C., Lee, A., Ravdin, L., Lin, M., Chiang, G., Relkin, N., Santulli, R. B., … Silbert, L. C. (2023). Identifying healthy individuals with Alzheimer's disease neuroimaging phenotypes in the UK Biobank. *Communications Medicine 2023 3:1, 3*(1), 1–15. DOI: 10.1038/s43856-023-00313-w

Balthazar, P., Harri, P., Prater, A., & Safdar, N. M. (2018). Protecting your patients' interests in the era of big data, artificial intelligence, and predictive analytics. *Journal of the American College of Radiology, 15*(3), 580–586. DOI: 10.1016/j.jacr.2017.11.035 PMID: 29402532

Becerra-Culqui, T. A., Lynch, F. L., Owen-Smith, A. A., Spitzer, J., & Croen, L. A. (2018). Parental first concerns and timing of autism spectrum disorder Diagnosis. *Journal of Autism and Developmental Disorders, 48*(10), 3367–3376. DOI: 10.1007/s10803-018-3598-6 PMID: 29754290

Bent, C. A., Barbaro, J., & Dissanayake, C. (2020). Parents' experiences of the service pathway to an autism diagnosis for their child: What predicts an early diagnosis in Australia? *Research in Developmental Disabilities, 103*, 103689. Advance online publication. DOI: 10.1016/j.ridd.2020.103689 PMID: 32434123

Bivarchi, F. A., Kehyayan, V., & Al-Kohji, S. M. (2021). Barriers to the early detection and intervention of children with autism spectrum disorders: A literature review. *Journal of Nursing Education and Practice, 11*(11), 72. DOI: 10.5430/jnep.v11n11p72

Brett, D., Warnell, F., McConachie, H., & Parr, J. R. (2016). Factors affecting age at ASD diagnosis in UK: No evidence that diagnosis Age has decreased between 2004 and 2014. *Journal of Autism and Developmental Disorders, 46*(6), 1974–1984. DOI: 10.1007/s10803-016-2716-6 PMID: 27032954

Brueggeman, L., Koomar, T., & Michaelson, J. J. (2020). Forecasting risk gene discovery in autism with machine learning and genome-scale data. *Scientific Reports 2020 10:1, 10*(1), 1–11. DOI: 10.1038/s41598-020-61288-5

Busch, F., Kather, J. N., Johner, C., Moser, M., Truhn, D., Adams, L. C., & Bressem, K. K. (2024). Navigating the European Union Artificial Intelligence Act for Healthcare. *Npj Digital Medicine 2024 7:1, 7*(1), 1–6. DOI: 10.1038/s41746-024-01213-6

Carabantes, M. (2020). Black-box artificial intelligence: An epistemological and critical analysis. *AI and Society, 35*(2), 309–317. https://doi.org/ Centers for Disease Control and Prevention. (2024). *Data and statistics on autism spectrum disorder.* https://www.cdc.gov/autism/data-research/index.htmlDOI: 10.1007/S00146-019-00888-W/METRICS

Chen, T., Chen, Y., Yuan, M., Gerstein, M., Li, T., Liang, H., Froehlich, T., & Lu, L. (2020). The development of a practical artificial intelligence tool for diagnosing and evaluating autism spectrum disorder: Multicenter study. *JMIR Medical Informatics, 8*(5), e15767. Advance online publication. DOI: 10.2196/15767 PMID: 32041690

Chen, Y. H., Drye, M., Chen, Q., Fecher, M., Liu, G., & Guthrie, W. (2023). Delay from screening to diagnosis in autism spectrum disorder: Results from a large national health research network. *The Journal of Pediatrics, 260*, 113514. Advance online publication. DOI: 10.1016/j.jpeds.2023.113514 PMID: 37244580

Clark, M. L. E., Vinen, Z., Barbaro, J., & Dissanayake, C. (2017). School age outcomes of children diagnosed early and later with autism spectrum disorder. *Journal of Autism and Developmental Disorders 2017 48:1, 48*(1), 92–102. DOI: 10.1007/s10803-017-3279-x

Colonnese, F., Di Luzio, F., Rosato, A., & Panella, M. (2024). Enhancing autism detection through gaze analysis using eye tracking sensors and data attribution with distillation in deep neural networks. *Sensors (Basel), 24*(23), 7792. Advance online publication. DOI: 10.3390/s24237792 PMID: 39686328

Currie, G., Hawk, K. E., & Rohren, E. M. (2020). Ethical principles for the application of artificial intelligence (AI) in nuclear medicine. *European Journal of Nuclear Medicine and Molecular Imaging, 47*(4), 748–752. DOI: 10.1007/s00259-020-04678-1 PMID: 31927637

D'antonoli, T. A. (2020). Ethical considerations for artificial intelligence: An overview of the current radiology landscape. *Diagnostic and Interventional Radiology (Ankara, Turkey)*, *26*(5), 504–511. DOI: 10.5152/dir.2020.19279 PMID: 32755879

dos Santos, C. L., Barreto, I. I., Floriano, I., Tristão, L. S., Silvinato, A., & Bernardo, W. M. (2024). Screening and diagnostic tools for autism spectrum disorder: Systematic review and meta-analysis. *Clinics (São Paulo)*, *79*, 100323. DOI: 10.1016/j.clinsp.2023.100323 PMID: 38484581

Efstratopoulou, M., Janssen, R., & Simons, J. (2012). Agreement among physical educators, teachers and parents on children's behaviors: A multitrait–multimethod design approach. *Research in Developmental Disabilities*, *33*(5), 1343–1351. DOI: 10.1016/j.ridd.2012.03.015

Elder, J. H., Brasher, S., & Alexander, B. (2016). Identifying the barriers to early diagnosis and treatment in underserved individuals with autism spectrum disorders (ASD) and their families: A Qualitative study. *Issues in Mental Health Nursing*, *37*(6), 412–420. DOI: 10.3109/01612840.2016.1153174 PMID: 27070190

Elendu, C., Amaechi, D. C., Elendu, T. C., Jingwa, K. A., Okoye, O. K., John Okah, M., Ladele, J. A., Farah, A. H., & Alimi, H. A. (2023). Ethical implications of AI and robotics in healthcare: A review. In *Medicine (United States)* (Vol. 102, Issue 50, p. E36671). Lippincott Williams and Wilkins. DOI: 10.1097/MD.0000000000036671

Farhud, D. D., & Zokaei, S. (2021). Ethical issues of artificial intelligence in medicine and healthcare. In *Iran J Public Health* (Vol. 50, Issue 11). https://creativecommons.org/licenses/by-nc/4.0/

Fenikilé, T. S., Ellerbeck, K., Filippi, M. K., & Daley, C. M. (2015). Barriers to autism screening in family medicine practice: A qualitative study. *Primary Health Care Research and Development*, *16*(4), 356–366. DOI: 10.1017/S1463423614000449 PMID: 25367194

Fuller, E. A., & Kaiser, A. P. (2020). The effects of early intervention on social communication outcomes for children with autism spectrum disorder: A meta-analysis. *Journal of Autism and Developmental Disorders*, *50*(5), 1683–1700. DOI: 10.1007/s10803-019-03927-z PMID: 30805766

Gabbay-Dizdar, N., Ilan, M., Meiri, G., Faroy, M., Michaelovski, A., Flusser, H., Menashe, I., Koller, J., Zachor, D. A., & Dinstein, I. (2022). Early diagnosis of autism in the community is associated with marked improvement in social symptoms within 1–2 years. *Autism*, *26*(6), 1353–1363. DOI: 10.1177/13623613211049011 PMID: 34623179

Garg, S., & Chauhan, A. (2024). Insights into the potential benefits and challenges of AI-driven large language models/ChatGPT-4 for predicting Autism Spectrum Disorder. In *Archives of Psychiatric Nursing* (Vol. 53, pp. 85–87). W.B. Saunders., DOI: 10.1016/j.apnu.2024.10.009

Garrido, D., Carballo, G., Artis, J., & Garcia-Retamero, R. (2018). Timing of parents' concerns related to autism spectrum disorder and its diagnosis: A mediation analysis. *The Spanish Journal of Psychology*, *21*, E59. Advance online publication. DOI: 10.1017/sjp.2018.64 PMID: 30477592

Godel, M., Robain, F., Kojovic, N., Franchini, M., Wood de Wilde, H., & Schaer, M. (2022). Distinct patterns of cognitive outcome in young children with autism spectrum disorder receiving the early start Denver model. *Frontiers in Psychiatry*, *13*, 835580. Advance online publication. DOI: 10.3389/fpsyt.2022.835580 PMID: 35815035

Gordon-Lipkin, E., Foster, J., & Peacock, G. (2016). Whittling down the wait time: Exploring models to minimize the delay from initial concern to diagnosis and treatment of autism spectrum disorder. *Pediatric Clinics of North America*, *63*(5), 851–859. DOI: 10.1016/j.pcl.2016.06.007 PMID: 27565363

Gray, K. M., Tonge, B. J., & Sweeney, D. J. (2008). Using the autism diagnostic interview-revised and the autism diagnostic observation schedule with young children with developmental delay: Evaluating diagnostic validity. *Journal of Autism and Developmental Disorders*, *38*(4), 657–667. DOI: 10.1007/s10803-007-0432-y PMID: 17690967

Gupta, C., Chandrashekar, P., Jin, T., He, C., Khullar, S., Chang, Q., & Wang, D. (2022). Bringing machine learning to research on intellectual and developmental disabilities: taking inspiration from neurological diseases. *Journal of Neurodevelopmental Disorders 2022 14:1, 14*(1), 1–22. DOI: 10.1186/s11689-022-09438-w

Hazim Hammed, S., & Albahri, A. S. (2023). Unlocking the potential of autism detection: Integrating traditional feature selection and machine learning techniques. *Applied Data Science and Analysis*, 42–58. DOI: 10.58496/ADSA/2023/003

Helm, J. M., Swiergosz, A. M., Haeberle, H. S., Karnuta, J. M., Schaffer, J. L., Krebs, V. E., Spitzer, A. I., & Ramkumar, P. N. (2020). Machine learning and artificial intelligence: Definitions, applications, and future directions. *Current Reviews in Musculoskeletal Medicine*, *13*(1), 69–76. DOI: 10.1007/s12178-020-09600-8 PMID: 31983042

Hus, Y., & Segal, O. (2021). Challenges surrounding the diagnosis of autism in children. *Neuropsychiatric Disease and Treatment*, *17*, 3509–3529. DOI: 10.2147/NDT.S282569 PMID: 34898983

Jacobs, D., Steyaert, J., Dierickx, K., & Hens, K. (2020). Parents' views and experiences of the autism spectrum disorder diagnosis of their young child: A longitudinal interview study. *European Child & Adolescent Psychiatry*, *29*(8), 1143–1154. DOI: 10.1007/s00787-019-01431-4 PMID: 31686239

Jeon, I., Kim, M., So, D., Kim, E. Y., Nam, Y., Kim, S., Shim, S., Kim, J., & Moon, J. (2024). Reliable autism spectrum disorder diagnosis for pediatrics using machine learning and explainable AI. *Diagnostics (Basel)*, *14*(22), 2504. Advance online publication. DOI: 10.3390/diagnostics14222504 PMID: 39594170

Jiang, F., Jiang, Y., Zhi, H., Dong, Y., Li, H., Ma, S., Wang, Y., Dong, Q., Shen, H., & Wang, Y. (2017). Artificial intelligence in healthcare: Past, present and future. *Stroke and Vascular Neurology*, *2*(4), 230–243. DOI: 10.1136/svn-2017-000101 PMID: 29507784

Johnson, C. P., Myers, S. M., Lipkin, P. H., Cartwright, J. D., Desch, L. W., Duby, J. C., Elias, E. R., Levey, E. B., Liptak, G. S., Murphy, N. A., Tilton, A. H., Lollar, D., Macias, M., McPherson, M., Olson, D. G., Strickland, B., Skipper, S. M., Ackermann, J., Del Monte, M., & Yeargin-Allsopp, M. (2007). Identification and evaluation of children with autism spectrum disorders. *Pediatrics*, *120*(5), 1183–1215. DOI: 10.1542/peds.2007-2361 PMID: 17967920

Jones, W., Klaiman, C., Richardson, S., Aoki, C., Smith, C., Minjarez, M., Bernier, R., Pedapati, E., Bishop, S., Ence, W., Wainer, A., Moriuchi, J., Tay, S. W., & Klin, A. (2023). Eye-tracking–based measurement of social visual engagement compared with expert clinical diagnosis of autism. *Journal of the American Medical Association*, *330*(9), 854–865. DOI: 10.1001/jama.2023.13295 PMID: 37668621

Joudar, S. S., Albahri, A. S., Hamid, R. A., Zahid, I. A., Alqaysi, M. E., Albahri, O. S., & Alamoodi, A. H. (2023). Artificial intelligence-based approaches for improving the diagnosis, triage, and prioritization of autism spectrum disorder: A systematic review of current trends and open issues. *Artificial Intelligence Review*, *56*(S1), 53–117. DOI: 10.1007/s10462-023-10536-x

Jullien, S. (2021). Screening for autistic spectrum disorder in early childhood. *BMC Pediatrics*, *21*(1), 1–9. DOI: 10.1186/s12887-021-02700-5 PMID: 34496788

Jung, W., Jeon, E., Kang, E., & Suk, H.-I. (2023). *EAG-RS: A novel explainability-guided ROI-selection framework for ASD diagnosis via inter-regional relation learning*. http://arxiv.org/abs/2310.03404

Kaufman, N. K. (2022). Rethinking "gold standards" and "best practices" in the assessment of autism. *Applied Neuropsychology. Child, 11*(3), 529–540. DOI: 10.1080/21622965.2020.1809414 PMID: 32847428

Kentrou, V., de Veld, D. M. J., Mataw, K. J. K., & Begeer, S. (2019). Delayed autism spectrum disorder recognition in children and adolescents previously diagnosed with attention-deficit/hyperactivity disorder. *Autism, 23*(4), 1065–1072. DOI: 10.1177/1362361318785171 PMID: 30244604

Kleine, A. K., Kokje, E., Hummelsberger, P., Lermer, E., Schaffernak, I., & Gaube, S. (2025). AI-enabled clinical decision support tools for mental healthcare: A product review. In *Artificial Intelligence in Medicine* (Vol. 160). Elsevier B.V., DOI: 10.1016/j.artmed.2024.103052

Levy, S. E., Wolfe, A., Coury, D., Duby, J., Farmer, J., Schor, E., van Cleave, J., & Warren, Z. (2020). Screening tools for autism spectrum disorder in primary care: A systematic evidence review. *Pediatrics, 145*(Supplement_1), 47–59. DOI: 10.1542/peds.2019-1895H PMID: 32238531

Li, F., Ruijs, N., & Lu, Y. (2023). Ethics & AI: A systematic review on ethical concerns and related strategies for designing with AI in healthcare. In *AI (Switzerland)* (Vol. 4, Issue 1, pp. 28–53). Multidisciplinary Digital Publishing Institute (MDPI). DOI: 10.3390/ai4010003

Lord, C., Rutter, M., DiLavore, P. C., Risi, S., Gotham, K., & Bishop, S. L. (2012). *Autism diagnostic observation schedule* (2nd ed.). Western Psychological Services., ADOS-2.

Luongo, M., Simeoli, R., Marocco, D., Milano, N., & Ponticorvo, M. (2024). Enhancing early autism diagnosis through machine learning: Exploring raw motion data for classification. *PLoS ONE, 19*(4 April). DOI: 10.1371/journal.pone.0302238

Lupindo, B. M., Maw, A., & Shabalala, N. (2023). Late diagnosis of autism: Exploring experiences of males diagnosed with autism in adulthood. *Current Psychology (New Brunswick, N.J.), 42*(28), 24181–24197. DOI: 10.1007/s12144-022-03514-z PMID: 35967496

MacKenzie, K. T., Mazefsky, C. A., & Eack, S. M. (2023). Obtaining a first diagnosis of autism spectrum disorder: Descriptions of the diagnostic process and correlates of parent satisfaction from a national sample. *Journal of Autism and Developmental Disorders, 53*(10), 3799–3812. DOI: 10.1007/s10803-022-05673-1 PMID: 35896863

Malwane, M. I., Nguyen, E. B., Trejo, S., Kim, E. Y., & Cucalón-Calderón, J. R. (2022). A delayed diagnosis of autism spectrum disorder in the setting of complex attention deficit hyperactivity disorder. *Cureus*. Advance online publication. DOI: 10.7759/cureus.25825 PMID: 35836458

Mandy, W., Midouhas, E., Hosozawa, M., Cable, N., Sacker, A., & Flouri, E. (2022). Mental health and social difficulties of late-diagnosed autistic children, across childhood and adolescence. *Journal of Child Psychology and Psychiatry, and Allied Disciplines*, *63*(11), 1405–1414. DOI: 10.1111/jcpp.13587 PMID: 35174492

Mazurek, M. O., Curran, A., Burnette, C., & Sohl, K. (2019). ECHO autism STAT: Accelerating early access to autism diagnosis. *Journal of Autism and Developmental Disorders*, *49*(1), 127–137. DOI: 10.1007/s10803-018-3696-5 PMID: 30043354

McCarty, P., & Frye, R. E. (2020). Early detection and diagnosis of autism spectrum disorder: Why is it so difficult? In *Seminars in Pediatric Neurology* (Vol. 35). W.B. Saunders., DOI: 10.1016/j.spen.2020.100831

Megerian, J. T., Dey, S., Melmed, R. D., Coury, D. L., Lerner, M., Nicholls, C., Sohl, K., Rouhbakhsh, R., Narasimhan, A., Romain, J., Golla, S., Shareef, S., Ostrovsky, A., Shannon, J., Kraft, C., Liu-Mayo, S., Abbas, H., Gal-Szabo, D. E., Wall, D. P., & Taraman, S. (2022b). Performance of Canvas Dx, a novel software-based autism spectrum disorder diagnosis aid for use in a primary care setting (P13-5.001). *Neurology*, *98*(18, supplement), 1025. Advance online publication. DOI: 10.1212/WNL.98.18_supplement.1025

Megerian, J. T., Dey, S., Melmed, R. D., Coury, D. L., Lerner, M., Nicholls, C. J., Sohl, K., Rouhbakhsh, R., Narasimhan, A., Romain, J., Golla, S., Shareef, S., Ostrovsky, A., Shannon, J., Kraft, C., Liu-Mayo, S., Abbas, H., Gal-Szabo, D. E., Wall, D. P., & Taraman, S. (2022a). Evaluation of an artificial intelligence-based medical device for diagnosis of autism spectrum disorder. *NPJ Digital Medicine*, *5*(1), 57. Advance online publication. DOI: 10.1038/s41746-022-00598-6 PMID: 35513550

Milbourn, B., Falkmer, M., Black, M. H., Girdler, S., Falkmer, T., & Horlin, C. (2017). An exploration of the experience of parents with children with autism spectrum disorder after diagnosis and intervention. *Scandinavian Journal of Child and Adolescent Psychiatry and Psychology*, *5*(3), 104–110. DOI: 10.21307/sjcapp-2017-014

Miodovnik, A., Harstad, E., Sideridis, G., & Huntington, N. (2015). Timing of the diagnosis of attention-deficit/hyperactivity disorder and autism spectrum disorder. *Pediatrics*, *136*(4), e830–e837. DOI: 10.1542/peds.2015-1502 PMID: 26371198

National Institute of Mental Health. (n.d.). *Autism spectrum disorder*. Retrieved January 5, 2025, from https://www.nimh.nih.gov/health/topics/autism-spectrum-disorders-asd#hts-intro

Nguyen, K., & Huang, Y. (2024). Applying artificial intelligence in diagnosis and treatment of autism spectrum disorder in children. *Journal of Student Research, 13*(2). Advance online publication. www.JSR.org/hs. DOI: 10.47611/jsrhs.v13i2.6803

Nordling, L. (2019). A fairer way forward for AI in health care. *Nature, 573*(7775), S103–S105. DOI: 10.1038/d41586-019-02872-2 PMID: 31554993

Okoye, C., Obialo-Ibeawuchi, C. M., Obajeun, O. A., Sarwar, S., Tawfik, C., Waleed, M. S., Wasim, A. U., Mohamoud, I., Afolayan, A. Y., & Mbaezue, R. N. (2023). Early diagnosis of autism spectrum disorder: A review and analysis of the risks and benefits. *Cureus, 15*(8), e43226. DOI: 10.7759/cureus.43226 PMID: 37692637

Panel for the Future of Science and Technology. (2022). *Artificial intelligence in healthcare*. DOI: 10.2861/568473

Parui, S., Samanta, D., Chakravorty, N., Ghosh, U., & Rodrigues, J. J. P. C. (2023). Artificial intelligence and sensor-based autism spectrum disorder diagnosis using brain connectivity analysis. *Computers & Electrical Engineering, 108*, 108720. Advance online publication. DOI: 10.1016/j.compeleceng.2023.108720

Priyadarshini, I. (2023). Autism screening in toddlers and adults Using deep learning and fair AI techniques. *Future Internet, 15*(9), 292. Advance online publication. DOI: 10.3390/fi15090292

Qiu, S., Lu, Y., Li, Y., Shi, J., Cui, H., Gu, Y., Li, Y., Zhong, W., Zhu, X., Liu, Y., Cheng, Y., Liu, Y., & Qiao, Y. (2020). Prevalence of autism spectrum disorder in Asia: A systematic review and meta-analysis. *Psychiatry Research, 284*, 112679. Advance online publication. DOI: 10.1016/j.psychres.2019.112679 PMID: 31735373

Radhakrishnan, M., Ramamurthy, K., Choudhury, K. K., Won, D., & Manoharan, T. A. (2021). Performance analysis of deep learning models for detection of Autism Spectrum Disorder from EEG signals. *TS. Traitement du Signal, 38*(3), 853–863. DOI: 10.18280/ts.380332

Rattaz, C., Loubersac, J., Michelon, C., Geoffray, M. M., Picot, M. C., Munir, K., & Baghdadli, A. (2022). Factors associated with age of diagnosis in children with autism spectrum disorders: Report from a French cohort. *Autism, 26*(8), 2108–2116. DOI: 10.1177/13623613221077724 PMID: 35257591

Reddy, S., Allan, S., Coghlan, S., & Cooper, P. (2020). A governance model for the application of AI in health care. *Journal of the American Medical Informatics Association : JAMIA*, *27*(3), 491–497. DOI: 10.1093/jamia/ocz192 PMID: 31682262

Rony, M. A. T., Johora, F. T., Thalji, N., Raza, A., Fitriyani, N. L., Syafrudin, M., & Lee, S. W. (2024). Innovative approach to detecting autism spectrum disorder using explainable features and smart web application. *Mathematics*, *12*(22), 3515. Advance online publication. DOI: 10.3390/math12223515

Rubio-Martín, S., García-Ordás, M. T., Bayón-Gutiérrez, M., Prieto-Fernández, N., & Benítez-Andrades, J. A. (2024). Enhancing ASD detection accuracy: A combined approach of machine learning and deep learning models with natural language processing. *Health Information Science and Systems*, *12*(1), 20. Advance online publication. DOI: 10.1007/s13755-024-00281-y PMID: 38455725

Russell, G., Stapley, S., Newlove-Delgado, T., Salmon, A., White, R., Warren, F., Pearson, A., & Ford, T. (2022). Time trends in autism diagnosis over 20 years: A UK population-based cohort study. *Journal of Child Psychology and Psychiatry, and Allied Disciplines*, *63*(6), 674–682. DOI: 10.1111/jcpp.13505 PMID: 34414570

Rutter, M., LeCouteur, A., & Lord, C. (2003). *Autism diagnostic interview-Revised*. Western Psychological Services.

Sabbagh, M. N., Boada, M., Borson, S., Chilukuri, M., Dubois, B., Ingram, J., Iwata, A., Porsteinsson, A. P., Possin, K. L., Rabinovici, G. D., Vellas, B., Chao, S., Vergallo, A., & Hampel, H. (2020). Early detection of mild cognitive impairment (MCI) in primary care. *The Journal of Prevention of Alzheimer's Disease*, *7*(3), 165–170. DOI: 10.14283/jpad.2020.21 PMID: 32463069

Salari, N., Rasoulpoor, S., Rasoulpoor, S., Shohaimi, S., Jafarpour, S., Abdoli, N., Khaledi-Paveh, B., & Mohammadi, M. (2022). The global prevalence of autism spectrum disorder: A comprehensive systematic review and meta-analysis. *Italian Journal of Pediatrics*, *48*(1), 112. Advance online publication. DOI: 10.1186/s13052-022-01310-w PMID: 35804408

Self, T. L., Parham, D. F., & Rajagopalan, J. (2015). Autism spectrum disorder early screening practices: A survey of physicians. *Communication Disorders Quarterly*, *36*(4), 195–207. DOI: 10.1177/1525740114560060

Shahamiri, S. R., & Thabtah, F. (2020). Autism AI: A New autism screening system based on artificial intelligence. *Cognitive Computation*, *12*(4), 766–777. Advance online publication. DOI: 10.1007/s12559-020-09743-3

Shambour, Q. Y., Qandeel, N., Alraba'nah, Y., Abumariam, A., & Shambour, M. K. (2024). Artificial intelligence techniques for early autism detection in toddlers: A comparative analysis. *Journal of Applied Data Sciences*, *5*(4), 1754–1764. DOI: 10.47738/jads.v5i4.353

Shi, B., Wu, W., Dai, M., Zeng, J., Luo, J., Cai, L., Wan, B., & Jing, J. (2021). Cognitive, language, and behavioral outcomes in children with autism spectrum disorders exposed to early comprehensive treatment models: A meta-analysis and meta-regression. In *Frontiers in Psychiatry* (Vol. 12). Frontiers Media S.A., DOI: 10.3389/fpsyt.2021.691148

Skampardoni, I., Nasrallah, I. M., Abdulkadir, A., Wen, J., Melhem, R., Mamourian, E., Erus, G., Doshi, J., Singh, A., Yang, Z., Cui, Y., Hwang, G., Ren, Z., Pomponio, R., Srinivasan, D., Govindarajan, S. T., Parmpi, P., Wittfeld, K., Grabe, H. J., & Davatzikos, C. (2024). Genetic and clinical correlates of AI-based brain aging patterns in cognitively unimpaired individuals. *JAMA Psychiatry*, *81*(5), 456–467. DOI: 10.1001/jamapsychiatry.2023.5599 PMID: 38353984

Sobieski, M., Sobieska, A., Sekułowicz, M., & Bujnowska-Fedak, M. M. (2022). Tools for early screening of autism spectrum disorders in primary health care – a scoping review. *BMC Primary Care*, *23*(1), 1–26. DOI: 10.1186/s12875-022-01645-7 PMID: 35291950

Song, C., Jiang, Z. Q., Liu, D., & Wu, L. L. (2022). Application and research progress of machine learning in the diagnosis and treatment of neurodevelopmental disorders in children. *Frontiers in Psychiatry*, *13*, 960672. DOI: 10.3389/fpsyt.2022.960672 PMID: 36090350

Talantseva, O. I., Romanova, R. S., Shurdova, E. M., Dolgorukova, T. A., Sologub, P. S., Titova, O. S., Kleeva, D. F., & Grigorenko, E. L. (2023). The global prevalence of autism spectrum disorder: A three-level meta-analysis. *Frontiers in Psychiatry*, *14*, 1071181. Advance online publication. DOI: 10.3389/fpsyt.2023.1071181 PMID: 36846240

Themistocleous, C. K., Andreou, M., & Peristeri, E. (2024). Autism detection in children: Integrating machine learning and natural language processing in narrative analysis. *Behavioral Sciences (Basel, Switzerland)*, *14*(6), 459. Advance online publication. DOI: 10.3390/bs14060459 PMID: 38920791

Uddin, M., Wang, Y., & Woodbury-Smith, M. (2019). Artificial intelligence for precision medicine in neurodevelopmental disorders. *Npj Digital Medicine 2019 2:1*, *2*(1), 1–10. DOI: 10.1038/s41746-019-0191-0

Ulaganathan, S., Harshavardhanan, P., Ganapathi Raju, N. V., & Parthasarathy, G. (2025). Hybrid optimization enabled DenseNet for autism spectrum disorders using MRI image. *Computational Biology and Chemistry*, *115*, 108335. Advance online publication. DOI: 10.1016/j.compbiolchem.2024.108335 PMID: 39793514

Vargason, T., Grivas, G., Hollowood-Jones, K. L., & Hahn, J. (2020). Towards a multivariate biomarker-based diagnosis of autism spectrum disorder: Review and discussion of recent advancements. *Seminars in Pediatric Neurology*, *34*, 100803. DOI: 10.1016/j.spen.2020.100803 PMID: 32446437

Verma, R. K., Pandey, M., Chawla, P., Choudhury, H., Mayuren, J., Bhattamisra, S. K., Gorain, B., Raja, M. A. G., Amjad, M. W., & Obaidur Rahman, S. (2021). An insight into the role of artificial intelligence in the early diagnosis of Alzheimer's disease. *CNS & Neurological Disorders - Drug Targets*, *21*(10), 901–912. DOI: 10 .2174/1871527320666210512014505 PMID: 33982657

Vietze, P., & Lax, L. E. (2020). Early intervention ABA for toddlers with ASD: Effect of age and amount. *Current Psychology (New Brunswick, N.J.)*, *39*(4), 1234–1244. DOI: 10.1007/s12144-018-9812-z

Wong, V., Yu, Y., Keyes, M. L., & McGrew, J. H. (2017). Pre-diagnostic and diagnostic stages of autism spectrum disorder: A parent perspective. *Child Care in Practice*, *23*(2), 195–217. DOI: 10.1080/13575279.2016.1199537

World Health Organization. (2021). *WHO issues first global report on Artificial Intelligence (AI) in health and six guiding principles for its design and use*. https://www.who.int/news/item/28-06-2021-who-issues-first-global-report-on-ai-in-health-and-six-guiding-principles-for-its-design-and-use

World Health Organization. (2023, November 15). *Autism*. https://www.who.int/news-room/fact-sheets/detail/autism-spectrum-disorders

World Population Review. (2024). *Autism rates by country 2024*. https://worldpopulationreview.com/country-rankings/autism-rates-by-country

Xu, X., Li, Y., Ding, N., Zang, Y., Sun, S., Shen, G., & Song, X. (2024). Quantitative assessment of brain structural abnormalities in children with autism spectrum disorder based on artificial intelligence automatic brain segmentation technology and machine learning methods. *Psychiatry Research: Neuroimaging*, *345*, 111901. Advance online publication. DOI: 10.1016/j.pscychresns.2024.111901 PMID: 39307122

Yi, H., Siu, Q. K. Y., Ngan, O. M. Y., & Chan, D. F. Y. (2020). Parents' experiences of screening, diagnosis, and intervention for children with autism spectrum disorder. *The American Journal of Orthopsychiatry*, *90*(3), 297–311. DOI: 10.1037/ort0000433 PMID: 31829647

Zwaigenbaum, L., Bauman, M. L., Fein, D., Pierce, K., Buie, T., Davis, P. A., Newschaffer, C., Robins, D. L., Wetherby, A., Choueiri, R., Kasari, C., Stone, W. L., Yirmiya, N., Estes, A., Hansen, R. L., McPartland, J. C., Natowicz, M. R., Carter, A., Granpeesheh, D., & Wagner, S. (2015). Early screening of autism spectrum disorder: Recommendations for practice and research. *Pediatrics*, *136*(Supplement_1), S41–S59. DOI: 10.1542/peds.2014-3667D PMID: 26430169

Chapter 4
The Intersection of Occupational Therapy, Speech Therapy, and Artificial Intelligence in Mental Health and Education

Dimitra V. Katsarou
https://orcid.org/0000-0001-8690-0314
University of the Aegean, Greece

ABSTRACT

The integration of artificial intelligence nto occupational therapy and speech therapy marks a significant advancement in making therapeutic interventions more accessible, effective, and tailored to individual needs. Particularly in the realms of education and mental health, AI has demonstrated its potential to transform the delivery of care for individuals with disabilities, speech and motor impairments, and mental health challenges. In educational settings, AI-based tools have revolutionized the approach to personalized learning. For students with special needs, including speech and motor impairments or developmental delays, Ethical concerns and the risk of dehumanizing care must be addressed. Importantly, AI serves as a complementary tool, enhancing human expertise rather than replacing the critical empathetic role of therapists. Looking forward, AI's potential in OT and speech therapy is vast. From early diagnosis and intervention to cognitive rehabilitation and social-emotional development, AI's evolving capabilities promise to further enhance therapy outcomes.

DOI: 10.4018/979-8-3373-5072-1.ch004

INTRODUCTION

The integration of artificial intelligence (AI) into occupational therapy (OT) and speech therapy has opened new frontiers in enhancing the accessibility, effectiveness, and personalization of therapeutic interventions, particularly in education and mental health. AI has the potential to bridge gaps in service delivery, provide tailored interventions, and improve outcomes for patients and students who may otherwise face challenges accessing or benefiting from traditional therapy. In educational settings, AI-based tools have revolutionized the approach to individualized learning, particularly for students with special needs. AI allows for personalized therapeutic interventions by adapting exercises and activities to meet the unique abilities and pace of each learner. This ensures that students with speech or motor impairments, learning disabilities, or developmental delays receive targeted support that aligns with their learning goals. AI technologies, such as speech recognition and adaptive motor skills training, not only make therapy more accessible but also create more inclusive classroom environments. These tools enable students to progress independently and at their own pace, increasing engagement, motivation, and confidence. Moreover, AI plays a crucial role in addressing mental health needs within OT and speech therapy by offering enhanced support for emotional regulation, cognitive skills, and communication. By providing personalized feedback, AI-driven systems empower individuals to work on therapeutic goals in a private, low-stress environment. These technologies also help reduce anxiety and stigma often associated with seeking therapy, making mental health support more approachable for those who may otherwise avoid traditional services. Additionally, AI enables real-time tracking of patient progress, allowing for immediate adjustments to interventions, which is crucial for addressing mental health concerns such as depression, anxiety, and PTSD. AI tools also offer the advantage of continuous monitoring, helping therapists keep track of symptoms and make timely interventions. However, the integration of AI into therapy and education is not without its challenges. Ethical considerations surrounding data privacy, bias in AI algorithms, and the potential for dehumanization of care must be addressed. AI cannot replace the empathetic human connection that is integral to therapeutic practices. The role of therapists remains essential, with AI serving as a complementary tool rather than a substitute. Despite these limitations, AI has proven to be a valuable asset in enhancing therapy outcomes, particularly when combined with human expertise. Looking ahead, the future of AI in OT and speech therapy holds great promise, particularly in areas such as early diagnosis and intervention, cognitive rehabilitation, and social-emotional development. As AI systems become increasingly sophisticated, their ability to tailor therapy to specific patient needs will improve, offering more effective and efficient therapeutic interventions. With careful ethical implementation and a balanced approach, AI has the potential to significantly enhance access to high-quality therapy services, ultimately fostering a more inclusive, accessible, and effective model of care in education and mental health. This intersection of AI, OT, and speech therapy represents an exciting evolution in the fields of education and healthcare, offering opportunities for improved outcomes and quality of life for individuals facing challenges related to speech, motor skills, and mental health.

The integration of Artificial Intelligence (AI) into healthcare is revolutionizing many fields, with Occupational Therapy (OT) and Speech Therapy (ST) among the most promising areas for innovation. These two therapeutic disciplines are focused on improving individuals' functional abilities and communication skills, respectively, but both face challenges in delivering personalized and efficient care. AI's ability to process large volumes of data and recognize patterns has created opportunities to enhance both the practice and outcomes of these therapies. By incorporating AI tools, healthcare providers can offer more individualized treatment plans, improve diagnostic accuracy, and track patient progress in real-time, ultimately promoting more effective interventions (Mousavi Baigi et al., 2024).

In Occupational Therapy, AI technologies are being utilized to develop innovative solutions for patient rehabilitation. The implementation of AI-driven wearable devices, such as sensors and motion trackers, enables therapists to monitor patients' physical movements and functional progress with greater precision. AI algorithms can analyze data from these devices to assess motor skills, range of motion, balance, and other functional abilities, offering clinicians valuable insights into a patient's physical and cognitive development (Râdulescu, 2023). These tools enable clinicians to tailor interventions more accurately to the needs of individual patients, which is especially beneficial for those with complex conditions such as neurodevelopmental disorders, physical disabilities, or cognitive impairments. Furthermore, AI-powered rehabilitation devices can adapt to the patient's abilities over time, making therapy more dynamic and responsive. As a result, patients benefit from activities that are both challenging and achievable, promoting faster recovery and enhancing overall therapy effectiveness (Pineda-Alpizar et al., 2024).

Similarly, AI in Speech Therapy is advancing the diagnosis and treatment of communication disorders by offering precise, data-driven insights into speech patterns. AI technologies such as natural language processing (NLP) and speech recognition software are transforming how speech disorders are identified and addressed. For instance, these tools can detect subtle issues such as articulation problems, stuttering, or voice irregularities, which might not be easily identifiable through traditional assessment methods (Zhang et al., 2024). By analyzing voice recordings, AI systems can provide in-depth reports on speech fluency, rhythm, pitch, and intonation, assisting clinicians in diagnosing conditions more accurately. In addition to diagnostic improvements, AI can also enhance treatment delivery. For example, AI-enabled applications can simulate real-time conversations, allowing patients to practice their communication skills in various scenarios while receiving instant feedback (Wong et al., 2018). These applications can be particularly helpful for individuals with aphasia, voice disorders, or developmental language delays, as they offer a safe environment for practicing speech outside of the clinical setting.

One of the key advantages of integrating AI into OT and ST is its potential to bridge gaps in access to care, especially for underserved populations. Telehealth platforms powered by AI enable therapists to provide remote care, allowing patients to receive therapy without the need for frequent in-person visits. This has been particularly valuable during the COVID-19 pandemic, where many healthcare facilities faced restrictions or capacity challenges. AI-driven remote monitoring tools allow clinicians to observe patients' progress and adjust treatment plans accordingly, even from a distance (Olawade et al., 2025). In addition, AI-based systems can provide caregivers with guidelines and resources to support patients at home, helping to extend the benefits of therapy between clinical sessions. This is especially important for patients with chronic conditions or long-term therapy needs, as it ensures continuous care and reduces treatment gaps.

While AI holds immense promise in both OT and ST, it also raises important ethical and practical considerations. One major concern is ensuring the privacy and security of patient data. AI applications in healthcare rely on the collection and analysis of sensitive patient information, which necessitates robust data protection measures. Without these safeguards, there is a risk of breaches of confidentiality and potential misuse of personal health data (Martinez, 2023). Additionally, the implementation of AI tools in therapy must be approached carefully to ensure that they complement rather than replace human interaction. While AI can enhance the efficiency of diagnosis and treatment, the therapeutic relationship between patient and clinician remains crucial in fostering trust and empathy. AI should be viewed as a tool to augment clinical expertise, not as a substitute for the essential human element in therapy (Al Kuwaiti et al., 2023). Furthermore, the development of AI technologies should be guided by principles of equity to ensure that these tools are accessible to diverse populations and that they do not inadvertently exacerbate existing health disparities.

As AI continues to evolve, there is also the potential for expanding its application within OT and ST to include predictive modeling. For instance, AI could analyze patient data to predict future outcomes, enabling clinicians to identify potential complications early and adjust interventions proactively. Predictive analytics could be particularly valuable in areas such as early intervention for children with developmental delays or in post-stroke rehabilitation, where early detection of setbacks can significantly impact recovery (Pineda-Alpizar et al., 2024). The ability to provide personalized, anticipatory care based on predictive models would mark a significant shift from reactive to proactive healthcare, enhancing both the efficiency and effectiveness of therapy delivery.

In conclusion, the intersection of Occupational Therapy, Speech Therapy, and Artificial Intelligence offers transformative potential for improving the delivery of care. AI technologies are enhancing the precision, accessibility, and personalization of therapy, creating new opportunities for both patients and healthcare providers. However, as the use of AI in therapy grows, it is essential to address ethical challenges, including data security, equity, and the preservation of the human touch in therapeutic relationships. With thoughtful implementation, AI can be a powerful tool that complements the work of therapists, leading to more effective, individualized, and accessible care for people with a range of functional and communication challenges.

AI TECHNOLOGY IN OCCUPATIONAL AND SPEECH THERAPY

Advantages of Occupational Therapy With AI Technology

One of the primary advantages of integrating Artificial Intelligence (AI) in Occupational Therapy (OT) is the ability to personalize treatment plans more effectively. AI algorithms can analyze a patient's unique functional abilities, progress, and therapy needs, allowing for tailored interventions. By continuously monitoring data from wearable devices and sensors, AI can adjust therapy activities in real-time to ensure that they are appropriately challenging and aligned with the patient's current capabilities (Râdulescu, 2023). This level of customization increases the likelihood of positive outcomes, as each treatment plan is specifically designed to meet the individual needs of the patient.

AI in OT provides clinicians with objective, data-driven insights into patient progress. Wearable devices and motion sensors can collect detailed information about a patient's range of motion, movement patterns, and functional abilities. AI algorithms then process this data, offering therapists objective measurements of progress over time (Mousavi Baigi et al., 2024). This helps to minimize the reliance on subjective observations and allows for more precise tracking of improvements, ensuring that the therapy remains aligned with the patient's goals.

AI-driven tools can streamline the assessment and treatment process, leading to greater efficiency in therapy sessions. AI technologies can automate routine tasks, such as data entry, progress tracking, and initial assessments, freeing up more time for therapists to focus on direct patient interaction and complex interventions. For instance, AI can quickly analyze data from sensors to determine a patient's progress and suggest adjustments, reducing the time required for manual evaluations

(Pineda-Alpizar et al., 2024). This not only optimizes time during therapy but also accelerates the overall rehabilitation process.

AI allows for continuous monitoring of a patient's progress, even outside of scheduled therapy sessions. Wearable devices equipped with AI can track movement, posture, and other functional abilities throughout the day. This data is then sent to therapists, enabling them to provide real-time feedback on performance and offer immediate adjustments when necessary (Râdulescu, 2023). Such constant feedback ensures that patients stay engaged in their rehabilitation process and helps to correct issues before they become larger problems.

AI technologies can also support the early detection of functional decline in patients, which is particularly valuable for individuals with chronic conditions or those recovering from surgeries. By analyzing data over time, AI can identify patterns that suggest a deterioration in a patient's abilities. Early identification of functional setbacks allows for quicker interventions, which can prevent further decline and potentially improve long-term outcomes (Olawade et al., 2025). This predictive capability ensures that OT professionals can act swiftly and adjust therapeutic strategies before problems become more significant.

The use of AI in OT has the potential to increase access to therapy, particularly for individuals in remote or underserved areas. Telehealth platforms integrated with AI enable patients to receive therapy remotely, allowing for continued treatment without the need for frequent in-person visits. This is especially beneficial for individuals who live in rural areas or those with mobility challenges. AI tools can provide therapists with the data they need to assess progress and suggest interventions remotely, ensuring that therapy can be maintained even without physical presence (Martinez, 2023).

The integration of AI in OT can also contribute to cost savings by improving the efficiency of treatment and reducing the need for extended therapy sessions. With AI-powered tools, therapists can optimize treatment plans to focus on the most effective interventions, potentially reducing the total number of therapy sessions required. Furthermore, remote monitoring and telehealth platforms help to lower healthcare costs by reducing travel expenses and making therapy more accessible to a wider range of patients (Pineda-Alpizar et al., 2024). This can be especially beneficial for healthcare systems with limited resources.

AI technologies are also playing a significant role in cognitive rehabilitation within OT. AI-driven tools can help patients with cognitive impairments, such as those recovering from brain injuries or stroke, by providing adaptive and personalized cognitive training exercises. These tools can monitor a patient's cognitive performance and adjust exercises to match their abilities, gradually increasing in complexity as the patient improves. This enables a more efficient rehabilitation process, as cognitive training is tailored to the specific needs of the individual (Mousavi Baigi et al., 2024).

AI technologies empower patients and caregivers by providing them with tools to track and manage rehabilitation progress independently. Through user-friendly interfaces, patients can access their own data and receive reminders to perform therapy exercises at home. This level of autonomy encourages patients to take a more active role in their recovery. For caregivers, AI systems can offer guidance on how to assist patients with exercises and monitor their progress, reducing the burden on family members and improving overall outcomes (Olawade et al., 2025).

AI in OT can also facilitate more coordinated care by integrating with other healthcare disciplines. AI systems can share data across various platforms, allowing occupational therapists to collaborate with physical therapists, speech therapists, and other healthcare providers more effectively. This integrated approach ensures that all aspects of a patient's rehabilitation are considered, promoting holistic care that addresses the patient's physical, cognitive, and emotional needs. Such collaboration can lead to more comprehensive treatment plans and improved patient outcomes (Pineda-Alpizar et al., 2024).

Advantages of Speech Therapy with AI Technology

One of the most significant advantages of integrating Artificial Intelligence (AI) into Speech Therapy (ST) is the improvement in diagnostic accuracy. AI-driven tools, such as speech recognition and natural language processing (NLP), can analyze an individual's speech patterns in great detail, identifying issues such as mispronunciations, irregularities in speech fluency, and language delays. AI systems can detect even subtle speech disorders that may go unnoticed by clinicians in traditional assessments, ensuring early detection and timely intervention (Zhang et al., 2024). This allows for more precise diagnoses and tailored treatment plans based on the specific needs of the patient.

AI technology helps speech therapists create highly personalized treatment plans for individuals. By using machine learning algorithms, AI can track a patient's speech patterns and identify specific areas of difficulty. This data can be used to develop exercises and activities that focus on the patient's particular needs. For example, a patient with a stutter may be provided with targeted exercises that address fluency, while a child with speech delays could be given tasks that enhance their vocabulary or articulation skills (Wong et al., 2018). Personalized approaches ensure that therapy is more effective and aligned with each patient's developmental stage and goals.

AI enables real-time feedback during speech therapy sessions, which is invaluable for patients who are working to improve their speech skills. Through speech recognition tools, AI can analyze a patient's speech and provide immediate feedback on aspects like pronunciation, rhythm, pitch, and tone. This instant feedback helps patients make adjustments on the spot, fostering quicker improvements in their speech abilities. Additionally, AI systems can continuously monitor a patient's progress over time, offering therapists valuable insights into how effectively a patient is responding to treatment (Olawade et al., 2025).

AI-based tools also increase access to speech therapy, particularly for individuals in underserved or rural areas. With telehealth platforms that incorporate AI, patients can receive therapy from the comfort of their homes. Speech therapists can remotely monitor progress, provide feedback, and adjust treatment plans based on the data collected by AI systems. This accessibility ensures that patients who may not have local access to speech therapy services can still receive high-quality care (Martinez, 2023). For children with speech disorders, this is especially beneficial, as parents can facilitate home-based sessions under the guidance of an AI-assisted platform.

The integration of AI in speech therapy can also reduce costs associated with treatment. By automating repetitive tasks such as speech assessments and progress tracking, AI reduces the administrative workload on speech therapists. Additionally, AI can provide remote support, decreasing the need for frequent in-person visits. This not only makes therapy more affordable but also more efficient, as clinicians can focus on delivering targeted interventions rather than spending time on administrative tasks (Pineda-Alpizar et al., 2024). For healthcare systems, AI-powered platforms can serve a larger number of patients without significantly increasing costs.

AI-driven applications, such as virtual assistants and interactive games, are increasingly being used in speech therapy to engage patients, especially children. These applications use speech recognition and NLP to interact with patients, guiding them through exercises and providing instant feedback. For example, a child practicing pronunciation might receive encouragement from a virtual character when they correctly pronounce a word, or be guided through a series of tasks to improve fluency. These gamified and interactive approaches make speech therapy more enjoyable and motivate patients to continue their practice outside of therapy sessions (Zhang et al., 2024).

For patients with more severe speech impairments, AI offers valuable assistive technologies that facilitate communication. AI-driven devices, such as speech-generating devices (SGDs), use text-to-speech technology to help individuals with speech disorders communicate more effectively. These devices can be personalized to the user's voice or preferences, allowing individuals with conditions such as cerebral palsy or ALS to have more fluid communication. AI can also adapt to a patient's needs over time, offering more intuitive interfaces as their abilities or preferences change (Râdulescu, 2023). This empowerment leads to improved quality of life and greater independence for individuals with significant speech impairments.

AI's ability to analyze patterns in speech data allows for the early detection of speech disorders, even before they become clinically evident. By analyzing large datasets of speech samples, AI can identify patterns that indicate early speech or language development issues in children. Early intervention is critical for improving long-term outcomes in speech therapy, and AI can help clinicians identify the need for therapy at a younger age, enabling quicker and more effective treatment (Pineda-Alpizar et al., 2024). This early detection also reduces the likelihood of more severe communication difficulties in the future.

AI can adapt speech therapy interventions for different populations, ensuring that treatment is tailored to the specific needs of various age groups and conditions. For instance, the needs of a child with speech delay differ significantly from those of an adult recovering from a stroke. AI tools can adjust therapy techniques based on the patient's age, cognitive abilities, and speech disorder. For individuals with neurodegenerative diseases, such as Parkinson's disease, AI can track speech changes over time and help modify interventions to address the progressive nature of their condition (Wong et al., 2018). This adaptability makes AI a versatile tool in speech therapy.

AI technology also facilitates better collaboration between speech therapists, patients, and caregivers. With AI-powered apps and platforms, caregivers can access resources and track their loved one's progress in real time. For children, this means that parents can monitor their child's speech exercises at home, ensuring consistency and reinforcing the work done in therapy sessions. Caregivers can also receive reminders to engage in specific activities with the patient, ensuring that therapeutic practices are followed between sessions (Olawade et al., 2025). This enhanced involvement leads to more effective care and improved patient outcomes.

AI technology has the potential to assist in language and accent modification, which is particularly helpful for individuals learning a second language or those working on accent reduction. AI speech recognition systems can help individuals practice pronunciation and intonation in a nonjudgmental, supportive environment. Through consistent practice and feedback, these systems help users modify their speech patterns and enhance their fluency in the desired language. AI also tracks the user's progress, offering suggestions for improvement based on the collected data, making language learning more efficient and focused (Zhang et al., 2024).

AI's predictive analytics capabilities provide speech therapists with the ability to foresee how patients might respond to treatment. By analyzing historical data from patients with similar conditions, AI can predict potential outcomes and help clinicians make more informed decisions about future treatment plans. Predictive modeling helps to identify the most effective interventions for a given patient, leading to better resource utilization and more accurate forecasting of therapy goals

(Râdulescu, 2023). This predictive power allows therapists to take a proactive rather than reactive approach to treatment.

AI tools can also be equipped with multilingual capabilities, making speech therapy more accessible to non-native speakers or individuals who speak multiple languages. This is especially useful in multicultural societies or for individuals who wish to improve their proficiency in multiple languages. AI systems that support multiple languages allow for seamless therapy across linguistic barriers, ensuring that patients receive the same quality of care, regardless of their primary language (Wong et al., 2018). This can enhance inclusivity and support linguistic diversity in therapy.

In large-scale settings, such as hospitals or rehabilitation centers, AI can improve the efficiency of speech therapy services. AI can automate administrative tasks like scheduling, progress tracking, and reporting, allowing therapists to focus more on clinical care. Additionally, AI systems can help manage patient intake and prioritize therapy sessions based on urgency or progress. This ensures that therapists can provide timely care to patients with the greatest need, optimizing the overall effectiveness of speech therapy programs in busy healthcare environments (Martinez 2023).

Even after the formal therapy sessions have concluded, AI systems can continue to monitor a patient's speech and provide ongoing support. These tools allow patients to practice their speech skills independently, and therapists can offer long-term tracking of speech patterns through data collected via AI applications. This continued support ensures that patients maintain the progress they have made during therapy and can address any setbacks early on (Olawade et al., 2025). The ability to continue monitoring and adjusting therapy remotely ensures better long-term outcomes and helps prevent regression in speech abilities.

Disadvantages of AI in Occupational Therapy

One of the main drawbacks of using AI in occupational therapy (OT) is the absence of human empathy and interaction. Occupational therapy is deeply rooted in building trust and rapport between therapists and patients. The therapeutic relationship helps patients feel comfortable and supported, which is crucial for motivating them to engage in exercises, especially those with complex physical or mental health conditions. AI systems, despite their technical capabilities, cannot provide the emotional support and human understanding that therapists offer. As a result, the therapeutic experience may feel more mechanical and less holistic (Li & Aflatoony, 2024).

AI systems, if overly relied upon, may replace critical human judgment and intuition in OT. Occupational therapists assess the needs of patients by considering not only their physical impairments but also their emotional, psychological, and social factors. While AI can assist by tracking progress and providing data, it lacks the capacity to understand a patient's emotional state or the context of their daily life. Over-relying on AI tools might lead to standardized treatments that overlook the complexities and individuality of each patient, which could reduce the overall quality of care (Mousavi Baigi et al., 2024).

AI-based tools in OT may struggle to adapt to patients with complex, multifaceted conditions. For example, individuals with severe cognitive impairments, multi-trauma injuries, or rare conditions may require highly customized therapy plans. While AI can analyze large amounts of data to create generalized solutions, it may not be effective in developing interventions that require a deep understanding of a patient's nuanced needs (Manole et al., 2024). The lack of flexibility in AI systems may hinder their ability to address the dynamic and diverse nature of occupational therapy practices.

AI tools in OT tend to focus on measurable, physical outcomes, such as mobility or task performance, but they often fail to address the psychological and emotional aspects of rehabilitation. Many patients undergoing OT struggle with anxiety, depression, or post-traumatic stress disorder (PTSD) due to their injuries or conditions. AI cannot recognize or address these psychological barriers, which are often key factors in a patient's recovery. A comprehensive OT approach requires a balance of physical and emotional support, which AI technology, at this stage, cannot fully provide (Fulmer et al., 2018).

AI tools in occupational therapy often rely on the collection and analysis of sensitive personal data, such as detailed medical histories, physical assessments, and behavioral data. This raises significant privacy and data security concerns. The risk of data breaches or unauthorized access to patient information is a significant challenge in healthcare technology. In addition, many AI systems operate through cloud-based platforms, which increases the potential for security vulnerabilities. Ensuring that AI tools comply with privacy regulations and that patient data remains confidential is a major challenge that cannot be overlooked (Nebeker et al., 2022).

The implementation of AI in OT may deepen existing healthcare inequities, particularly for underserved populations. Access to AI-based rehabilitation tools often requires reliable internet, smartphones, or specialized equipment, which many low-income individuals or those living in rural areas may not have. Additionally, the digital literacy required to navigate AI tools may pose an additional barrier for older adults or those unfamiliar with technology. As such, AI in OT could inadvertently widen the gap between individuals who have access to advanced therapies and those who do not (Mousavi Baigi et al., 2024).

AI systems are trained on large datasets, and if these datasets are not diverse or representative, the resulting algorithms can be biased. For example, if an AI system in OT is trained primarily on data from a specific demographic, it may not work as effectively for patients from different backgrounds. This could result in unequal treatment and a lack of tailored interventions for individuals from diverse cultural or ethnic groups. Ensuring that AI systems are trained on diverse datasets and undergo regular testing for biases is critical to mitigating these issues (Manole et al., 2024).

Occupational therapy often deals with unstructured and unpredictable problems, particularly when assessing the functional capacity of individuals with severe disabilities. While AI can process and analyze structured data well, such as scores from standardized assessments, it struggles with unstructured data or situations that require creative problem-solving (Li & Aflatoony, 2024). For example, when addressing complex home modifications or adaptive equipment needs, AI may be unable to generate solutions that are appropriate for unique living environments or specific patient preferences.

The cost of integrating AI into occupational therapy practice can be prohibitive for many healthcare providers. While AI tools may eventually save costs in terms of efficiency, the initial financial investment required for purchasing hardware, software, and training clinicians can be significant. Small clinics or independent OT practitioners may not have the resources to invest in these technologies, limiting their access to the potential benefits of AI (Nebeker et al., 2022). This economic barrier could slow the adoption of AI in OT, particularly in underserved areas.

AI tools often require significant changes in how occupational therapy is delivered, which can disrupt established workflows. Integrating AI into a healthcare system requires training therapists, modifying documentation practices, and adjusting patient care routines to accommodate the new technology. These changes can be challenging for clinicians who may not be familiar with AI or who may feel that the technology is a threat to their professional role. Additionally, not all healthcare systems have the infrastructure to support AI-based therapies effectively, which may lead to inconsistent implementation and varying quality of care (Mousavi Baigi et al., 2024).

Disadvantages of AI in Speech Therapy

One of the primary disadvantages of integrating AI into speech therapy is the reduced level of human interaction. While AI can provide real-time feedback and track progress, it cannot replicate the emotional support, empathy, and nuanced understanding that human therapists offer. The therapeutic relationship between a patient and a clinician is crucial for building trust and motivation, particularly for children or individuals with complex speech disorders (Deka et al., 2023). Without the presence of a human therapist, some patients may find it difficult to engage fully in therapy, potentially limiting the effectiveness of AI-driven interventions.

As AI becomes more prevalent in speech therapy, there is a risk of overreliance on technology, which could compromise the quality of care. While AI tools are designed to assist therapists, they cannot replace the intuition and experience that human clinicians bring to the treatment process. Overreliance on AI could lead to therapists relying too heavily on automated feedback, potentially overlooking subtle but important aspects of a patient's progress that require professional judgment (Kumar, 2024). This could lead to a diminished role for speech therapists, undermining the personalized and holistic nature of therapy.

The use of AI in speech therapy often requires the collection and analysis of sensitive patient data, including voice recordings and personal health information. While AI systems are designed to store and process this data securely, there is always a risk of data breaches or misuse. Unauthorized access to private health data can compromise patient confidentiality and trust. As AI technologies become more integrated into healthcare, ensuring the security of patient data becomes increasingly critical (Schönberger, 2019). The potential for privacy violations is a significant concern, particularly in telehealth or remote therapy settings.

Although AI can tailor treatment plans for some speech disorders, it may struggle to fully personalize interventions for patients with complex or rare speech conditions. AI systems typically rely on large datasets and established patterns, which may not account for the unique nuances of individual patients (Bhardwaj et al., 2024). For example, individuals with multiple speech or cognitive impairments may not respond well to standardized AI-driven exercises, requiring the intervention of a clinician who can adjust treatment plans based on a deeper understanding of the patient's specific needs.

Speech therapy often involves addressing emotional and psychological barriers that affect speech development, such as anxiety, low self-esteem, or social challenges. AI lacks the ability to empathize with patients or understand their emotional state during therapy sessions. While AI tools can provide technical feedback, they cannot offer the emotional support that a human therapist can provide, which is particularly important in speech therapy where emotional well-being plays a significant role in the patient's progress (Deka et al., 2023). This limitation means that AI, despite its potential, cannot address all aspects of speech therapy.

AI systems in speech therapy are heavily dependent on high-quality input data, such as clear speech recordings or accurate patient assessments. If the data collected is of low quality, such as distorted speech or background noise in recordings, the AI system may fail to accurately assess the patient's speech patterns or provide useful feedback. This limitation can result in inaccurate diagnoses or ineffective treatment suggestions, which could delay progress or lead to suboptimal therapy outcomes (Kumar, 2024). Ensuring that input data meets high standards is crucial for the effectiveness of AI-driven speech therapy.

Currently, there is limited regulatory oversight regarding the use of AI in speech therapy, which can raise concerns about the safety and efficacy of these technologies. The lack of standardized guidelines means that AI tools may vary significantly in quality, and some may not meet the necessary clinical standards for patient care (Schönberger, 2019). Without proper oversight, patients may be exposed to AI-based therapy tools that have not been thoroughly tested for effectiveness, potentially leading to subpar treatment or harmful outcomes. This calls for the development of more comprehensive regulatory frameworks to ensure the safe and responsible use of AI in healthcare.

For AI-driven speech therapy to be effective, patients need access to the necessary technology, such as smartphones, computers, or specialized devices. This can pose a barrier to certain populations, especially those in lower socioeconomic groups or rural areas who may not have access to the required technology (Bhardwaj et al., 2024). Furthermore, technical issues such as device malfunctions, software glitches, or internet connectivity problems can interfere with therapy sessions and hinder progress. For patients who are not technologically savvy, using AI-based tools may also be challenging and lead to frustration or disengagement.

AI systems are created using data, and if the data used to train these systems is biased, the AI could perpetuate or even amplify existing biases in speech therapy. For instance, if an AI tool is primarily trained on speech samples from a homogeneous group, it may not perform as accurately for individuals from different linguistic or cultural backgrounds (Bhardwaj et al., 2024). This raises ethical concerns about the inclusivity and fairness of AI systems. Additionally, AI systems may unintentionally reinforce stereotypes or provide recommendations that are not culturally sensitive, potentially disadvantaging certain patient groups.

Despite the potential long-term cost savings, the initial investment in AI technology for speech therapy can be prohibitively high. The development and implementation of AI-based tools require significant financial resources, including purchasing hardware, software, and training clinicians to use the technology effectively (Kumar, 2024). Smaller clinics or independent speech therapists may find it challenging to afford such investments, potentially widening the gap between those who can benefit from AI in speech therapy and those who cannot. The high costs associated with AI integration may delay or limit its adoption in some healthcare s

The Effect of AI in Occupational Therapy and Speech Therapy on Mental Health

AI technologies in both occupational therapy (OT) and speech therapy have the potential to increase access to mental health support, particularly for individuals who may face barriers to traditional therapy. AI-driven tools can be utilized remotely, allowing patients in underserved areas or those with mobility limitations to receive therapy without the need for in-person visits (Li & Aflatoony, 2024). By providing patients with tools to engage in self-guided therapy, AI can reduce feelings of isolation, which is particularly beneficial for individuals with mental health conditions like depression or anxiety. The accessibility of these tools ensures that mental health support is more readily available to a wider population, potentially improving the overall mental well-being of patients.

For many individuals with speech and occupational challenges, the thought of undergoing therapy can be intimidating or anxiety-inducing. AI-based tools may help reduce therapy anxiety by providing a less stressful environment for practice. These tools can offer real-time feedback in a nonjudgmental, private space, allowing patients to practice their skills at their own pace and on their own terms (Li, 2023). This reduces the pressure that some individuals feel in face-to-face therapy sessions, which can be a significant barrier to participation in therapy, especially for individuals with social anxiety or fear of judgment.

AI technologies can increase engagement in both OT and speech therapy by introducing gamified elements or interactive tools that make therapy more enjoyable. By incorporating game-like features such as points, levels, or rewards, AI tools encourage patients to actively participate and practice skills that contribute to their mental health recovery. This can be especially helpful for individuals with mental health conditions like depression, who may struggle with motivation or experience low energy levels. The ability to engage with therapy in a fun and low-pressure environment fosters motivation and adherence to treatment plans, which in turn can lead to better mental health outcomes (Mousavi Baigi et al., 2024).

AI's ability to analyze data and tailor treatment plans offers a significant advantage in addressing the specific mental health needs of individuals in OT and speech therapy. For instance, AI algorithms can assess an individual's progress over time, identify patterns, and adjust therapy routines to meet changing needs. This personalized approach can enhance the effectiveness of therapy by ensuring that interventions are relevant and appropriately challenging (Manole et al., 2024). For individuals with mental health conditions such as anxiety, PTSD, or depression, personalized therapy interventions can target specific triggers or coping strategies, leading to more effective treatment outcomes and better mental well-being.

AI tools can be integrated with wearable devices or mobile applications to track mental health symptoms in real-time, providing therapists with valuable data to monitor patient progress. For example, AI-powered tools can assess speech patterns, body language, or emotional states during therapy sessions and provide instant feedback on mental health-related symptoms such as anxiety or stress levels (Fulmer et al., 2018). This data-driven approach enables therapists to adapt interventions accordingly, which can be beneficial in addressing mental health concerns that may be affecting a patient's engagement or progress in therapy.

The use of AI in speech and occupational therapy can also help reduce the stigma often associated with seeking mental health care. Many individuals with mental health conditions feel shame or embarrassment about seeking help, especially when it comes to speech disorders or physical impairments that are visible to others. AI-based therapy tools can be used in private settings, away from the judgment of others, which can encourage individuals to seek help more freely (Li & Aflatoony, 2024). The anonymity provided by AI may help individuals feel more comfortable addressing their challenges, fostering a more positive mental health experience.

AI in speech therapy and OT is particularly beneficial for individuals with cognitive disabilities, such as those with autism or dementia, where traditional therapy may face limitations. AI-powered tools can provide consistent, structured interventions that cater to an individual's cognitive abilities and learning pace, reducing frustration and mental stress (Deka et al., 2023). In speech therapy, AI systems can adapt exercises to accommodate cognitive impairments by using simpler language or visual aids. In OT, AI tools can help with activities of daily living in a way that is cognitively manageable, allowing individuals to achieve a sense of accomplishment and improving their self-esteem and mental well-being.

AI-based systems can provide real-time feedback during therapy sessions, offering patients immediate insight into their performance and progress. This feedback loop can be particularly helpful for individuals who struggle with emotional regulation, such as those with mood disorders or trauma-related conditions. The timely nature of AI feedback allows patients to understand how their behavior affects their therapy, enabling them to regulate their emotional responses more effectively (Nebeker et al., 2022). This continuous feedback fosters greater self-awareness, which is essential for improving emotional regulation, reducing symptoms of mental distress, and enhancing overall well-being.

Both speech therapy and occupational therapy often aim to increase an individual's independence, which can have a profound impact on mental health. By using AI to support the development of skills, individuals with speech or motor impairments can experience a sense of accomplishment as they progress at their own pace. This autonomy fosters increased self-esteem and confidence, which are key factors in mental health recovery (Bhardwaj et al., 2024). As AI-based tools enable patients to perform tasks independently, the positive reinforcement received through successful completion can enhance their psychological well-being.

While AI can offer significant benefits for mental health in therapy, it also has limitations in providing the emotional support that a human therapist can offer. AI lacks the ability to empathize or intuitively respond to a patient's emotional needs, which is a crucial aspect of mental health care. For patients dealing with complex mental health conditions, such as trauma, AI cannot replace the therapeutic value of a counselor or a trained clinician who understands the intricacies of human emotions. In such cases, AI may need to be used as a complementary tool rather than a substitute for human intervention (Deka et al., 2023).

The integration of AI into mental health treatment raises ethical concerns, especially regarding privacy and the potential for bias. AI algorithms used in therapy may inadvertently reinforce stereotypes or fail to account for the emotional and cultural complexities of mental health (Koh et al., 2024). Furthermore, the use of AI to collect and analyze sensitive data about a patient's mental state raises significant privacy issues. Ensuring that AI systems adhere to strict ethical guidelines is critical to safeguarding patient rights and ensuring that these technologies enhance rather than hinder mental health care.

The Effect of AI in Occupational Therapy and Speech Therapy on Education

One of the most significant advantages of AI in occupational and speech therapy is its ability to offer personalized learning experiences for students with special needs. AI systems can adapt therapy sessions and educational content to the individual's learning style, pace, and abilities. In speech therapy, AI tools can provide personalized exercises to target specific speech sounds, language structures, or communication skills. In OT, AI can assist students by tailoring motor tasks or activities of daily living to their specific needs. This level of customization allows students to receive support that is aligned with their unique educational goals, helping them progress at their own pace and improving their educational outcomes (Olawade et al., 2024).

AI technologies in therapy can improve student engagement in both educational and therapeutic contexts. By incorporating gamification, interactive elements, and rewards, AI can make therapeutic exercises feel more like fun activities than tasks. This can be particularly beneficial for children or students with learning disabilities, autism, or speech impairments, who may find traditional therapy sessions or classroom tasks boring or overwhelming. The use of AI-driven games, rewards, or challenges helps maintain motivation, which can have positive spillover effects on the student's academic performance and engagement in school (Mousavi Baigi et al., 2024). The interactive and engaging nature of AI tools also encourages students to actively participate in their therapy, which can enhance both their learning and therapy progress.

In many educational settings, there is a shortage of specialized professionals, such as speech therapists or occupational therapists, who can provide individualized support for students with disabilities. AI tools can help bridge this gap by providing supplemental therapy, especially in remote or under-resourced areas. For instance, AI applications in speech therapy can assist students with speech and language impairments by offering real-time feedback and tailored exercises, even when a therapist is not available. Similarly, AI can help students with fine motor skills in OT by guiding them through exercises or tasks designed to improve their ability to engage with the physical aspects of learning, such as handwriting or using educational tools (Nebeker et al., 2022). In this way, AI enhances access to high-quality therapy services in educational environments where such services may be limited.

AI tools in occupational and speech therapy can play a critical role in the early detection of learning disabilities, communication disorders, or developmental delays. Through continuous monitoring and assessment, AI can help identify patterns in a child's behavior or learning progress that may indicate a need for further evaluation. For example, AI-powered speech recognition tools can detect subtle speech delays or abnormalities in pronunciation that might otherwise go unnoticed. Similarly, AI systems can assess fine motor skills and coordination in students with OT needs. Early detection is crucial for timely intervention, and AI provides an efficient means of monitoring developmental milestones, enabling educators to provide support at the earliest possible stage (Bhardwaj et al., 2024).

AI technology promotes inclusive education by offering students with disabilities a more accessible and tailored learning environment. Students with speech and motor impairments often face significant barriers to accessing traditional education, but AI tools can reduce these obstacles by adapting tasks to meet individual needs. For example, AI can assist students with visual or auditory impairments by providing alternative methods of communication or interactive learning strategies (Onesi-Ozigagun et al., 2024). In speech therapy, AI can use voice-controlled interfaces, real-time captioning, or language translation features, making lessons more inclusive for students with communication challenges (Li & Aflatoony, 2024). The integration of AI in educational settings promotes equity by ensuring that students with a variety of needs have access to the same opportunities for success.

AI-driven tools allow for continuous monitoring of student progress, offering real-time feedback that can be used to adjust educational and therapeutic plans. In both speech and occupational therapy, AI systems can track performance, highlight areas where students are struggling, and adjust the level of difficulty accordingly. This immediate feedback is essential for ensuring that students are constantly engaged and progressing toward their educational goals. For example, speech therapy

AI can track the clarity of pronunciation or language usage, while OT AI systems can assess how well students perform physical tasks. This data helps educators and therapists make timely adjustments, providing the best possible support for each student's unique learning needs (Deka et al., 2023).

AI tools can empower students to take ownership of their learning and therapy. By allowing students to practice at their own pace and in their own time, AI reduces dependency on teachers and therapists for every session. This fosters independence and builds self-confidence, especially for students who struggle in traditional classroom settings (Onesi-Ozigagun et al., 2024). For instance, AI in speech therapy enables students to repeat exercises as many times as they need until they achieve the desired results, promoting self-efficacy. Similarly, in OT, students can independently engage with tasks that improve their motor skills, such as using adaptive technology or practicing functional movements. This autonomy can have a significant positive impact on students' mental health and overall sense of control in their learning journey (Mousavi Baigi et al., 2024).

AI in therapy supports students with physical and cognitive barriers to learning, such as those with mobility issues or cognitive impairments. AI-driven OT tools can help students develop motor skills needed for tasks such as writing, using computers, or engaging in classroom activities (Onesi-Ozigagun et al., 2024). In speech therapy, AI tools can offer interactive exercises that focus on articulation, fluency, or voice modulation, addressing communication barriers that may affect a student's academic success. By addressing these barriers, AI helps students engage more fully in the learning process and reduces frustration, thereby promoting positive mental health and well-being (Nebeker et al., 2022).

AI tools in speech and occupational therapy can also support the development of social-emotional skills, which are essential for success in both academic and life contexts. For example, speech therapy AI can include role-playing exercises, where students practice communication in social scenarios, enhancing both verbal and non-verbal communication skills. OT tools, on the other hand, can support the development of adaptive skills such as managing frustration, interacting with peers, and following routines. These social-emotional skills are essential for students' academic performance and mental health, as they contribute to better relationships with peers and greater confidence in academic settings (Li & Aflatoony, 2024).

AI can enhance collaboration between speech therapists, occupational therapists, and educators. By providing therapists and teachers with detailed data on a student's progress, AI tools allow for more coordinated care and instruction. Teachers and therapists can work together to adjust the student's educational plan based on insights provided by AI systems, ensuring that therapy aligns with classroom learning goals. This collaboration ensures that students receive a consistent and holistic approach to their development, which can have a positive impact on both their academic success and mental well-being (Deka et al., 2023).

AI tools can reduce the financial burden on schools and educational systems, particularly in areas with limited access to specialized services. AI can provide cost-effective alternatives to traditional therapy sessions by automating some of the assessment, feedback, and intervention processes. This enables schools to offer additional support to students with disabilities without requiring significant financial resources. In this way, AI in occupational and speech therapy makes specialized education more affordable, which can be a key factor in improving outcomes for students with diverse needs (Bhardwaj et al., 2024).

THE FUTURE OF AI IN OCCUPATIONAL THERAPY AND SPEECH THERAPY IN EDUCATION AND MENTAL HEALTH

As we look to the future, the integration of artificial intelligence (AI) in occupational therapy (OT) and speech therapy represents a transformative shift in how we approach education and mental health support. AI's ability to provide personalized, data-driven interventions has the potential to revolutionize the way therapy is delivered, ensuring that students and individuals with disabilities or speech and motor impairments receive tailored support that meets their unique needs. The promise of AI lies in its ability to offer solutions that are not only accessible but also scalable, addressing gaps in both educational and therapeutic settings and making critical support available to underserved populations.

In education, AI is poised to break down barriers, providing students with disabilities—whether physical, cognitive, or speech-related—with the tools they need to succeed in a mainstream classroom environment. Personalized learning experiences, real-time feedback, and adaptive technologies all work together to create an inclusive educational experience where every student can thrive. Through AI-driven systems, educators and therapists can collaborate more effectively, ensuring that each child's individual needs are met, fostering both academic achievement and emotional well-being. This collaborative approach could significantly reduce the educational disparity between students with special needs and their peers, helping them reach their full potential.

Similarly, AI in mental health, particularly within the realms of OT and speech therapy, offers significant advantages in reducing stigma and promoting self-efficacy. By offering patients the ability to engage in therapy at their own pace, often in the privacy of their own homes, AI helps alleviate the anxiety and reluctance that many individuals experience when seeking treatment. Furthermore, AI tools can provide consistent, real-time support for emotional regulation, cognitive skills, and physical coordination, all of which are critical components of mental health recovery. In this context, AI is more than just a tool for convenience; it has the potential to be an essential companion in improving mental well-being. However, as with any technological innovation, the integration of AI into these therapeutic practices also presents challenges. Concerns about the ethical use of AI, data privacy, and the potential for bias must be addressed to ensure that these tools are used responsibly. Moreover, AI cannot replace the human touch that is so vital in therapy. The empathetic connection between therapist and patient remains irreplaceable, and AI should be viewed as a complementary tool, not a replacement for human intervention. The future of therapy will likely lie in the synergy between human expertise and AI's capabilities, where technology supports, rather than supplants, the human elements of care.

Looking forward, there is immense potential for AI to continually evolve in ways that enhance therapy outcomes. As AI systems become more sophisticated, their ability to analyze complex data and adjust treatment plans accordingly will likely improve. This could lead to even more precise interventions tailored to individual patients' needs, particularly in the areas of cognitive and speech impairments. Additionally, AI's role in early detection and intervention could lead to faster, more effective treatments, helping to prevent long-term developmental delays or mental health issues from escalating.

In conclusion, the intersection of AI, occupational therapy, and speech therapy offers profound benefits for individuals with disabilities and mental health conditions, as well as for the broader educational landscape. The technology promises to enhance access, improve engagement, and offer personalized, effective interventions that empower patients and students alike. While there are challenges to overcome, the future of AI in these fields holds great promise. As these technologies continue to evolve, they offer the potential for a more inclusive, effective, and accessible approach to therapy and education, paving the way for a brighter, more equitable future for all.

REFERENCES

Al Kuwaiti, A., Nazer, K., Al-Reedy, A., Al-Shehri, S., Al-Muhanna, A., Subbarayalu, A. V., Al Muhanna, D., & Al-Muhanna, F. A. (2023). A review of the role of artificial intelligence in healthcare. *Journal of Personalized Medicine*, *13*(6), 951. DOI: 10.3390/jpm13060951 PMID: 37373940

Bhardwaj, A., Sharma, M., Kumar, S., Sharma, S., & Sharma, P. C. (2024). Transforming pediatric speech and language disorder diagnosis and therapy: The evolving role of artificial intelligence. *Health Sciences Review (Oxford, England)*, *12*, 100188. DOI: 10.1016/j.hsr.2024.100188

Deka, C., Shrivastava, A., Nautiyal, S., & Chauhan, P. (2023, November). Human-centered AI goals for speech therapy tools. In *International Conference on Computer-Human Interaction Research and Applications* (pp. 121–136). Cham: Springer Nature Switzerland. DOI: 10.1007/978-3-031-49368-3_8

Fulmer, R., Joerin, A., Gentile, B., Lakerink, L., & Rauws, M. (2018). Using psychological artificial intelligence (Tess) to relieve symptoms of depression and anxiety: Randomized controlled trial. *JMIR Mental Health*, *5*(4), e9782. DOI: 10.2196/mental.9782 PMID: 30545815

Koh, W. Q., Heins, P., Flynn, A., Mahmoudi Asl, A., Garcia, L., Malinowsky, C., & Brorsson, A. (2024). Bridging gaps in the design and implementation of socially assistive technologies for dementia care: The role of occupational therapy. *Disability and Rehabilitation. Assistive Technology*, *19*(3), 595–603. DOI: 10.1080/17483107.2022.2111610 PMID: 35972877

Kumar, Y. (2024). A comprehensive analysis of speech recognition systems in healthcare: Current research challenges and future prospects. *SN Computer Science*, *5*(1), 137. DOI: 10.1007/s42979-023-02466-w

Li, M., & Aflatoony, L. (2024, October). Exploring the potential of generative AI in DIY assistive technology design by occupational therapists. In *Proceedings of the 26th International ACM SIGACCESS Conference on Computers and Accessibility* (pp. 1–6). DOI: 10.1145/3663548.3688506

Li, X. (2023). Evaluation and analysis of elderly mental health based on artificial intelligence. *Occupational Therapy International*, *2023*(1), 7077568. DOI: 10.1155/2023/7077568 PMID: 36817324

Manole, A., Cârciumaru, R., Brînza , R., & Manole, F. (2024). Harnessing AI in anxiety management: A chatbot-based intervention for personalized mental health support. *Information (Basel)*, *15*(12), 768. DOI: 10.3390/info15120768

Martinez, G. (2023). Ethical considerations in the use of artificial intelligence in healthcare. *Journal of Medical Ethics, 30*(2), 145–160. PMID: 35906018

Mousavi Baigi, S. F., Dahmardeh Kemmak, F., Sarbaz, M., Norouzi Aval, R., & Kimiafar, K. (2024). Application of artificial intelligence in occupational therapy: A systematic review. *Health Education and Health Promotion, 12*(3), 1001–1029.

Nebeker, C., Parrish, E. M., & Graham, S. (2022). The AI-powered digital health sector: Ethical and regulatory considerations when developing digital mental health tools for the older adult demographic. In *Artificial Intelligence in Brain and Mental Health: Philosophical, Ethical & Policy Issues* (pp. 159–176). Springer International Publishing.

Olawade, D. B., Bolarinwa, O. A., Adebisi, Y. A., & Shongwe, S. (2025). The role of artificial intelligence in enhancing healthcare for people with disabilities. *Social Science & Medicine, 364*, 117560. DOI: 10.1016/j.socscimed.2024.117560 PMID: 39612748

Olawade, D. B., Wada, O. Z., Odetayo, A., David-Olawade, A. C., Asaolu, F., & Eberhardt, J. (2024). Enhancing mental health with artificial intelligence: Current trends and future prospects. *Journal of Medicine, Surgery, and Public Health, 3*, 100099. DOI: 10.1016/j.glmedi.2024.100099

Onesi-Ozigagun, O., Ololade, Y. J., Eyo-Udo, N. L., & Ogundipe, D. O. (2024). Revolutionizing education through AI: A comprehensive review of enhancing learning experiences. *International Journal of Applied Research in Social Sciences, 6*(4), 589–607. DOI: 10.51594/ijarss.v6i4.1011

Pineda-Alpizar, A. F., Mourraille-Rojas, J., & Cruz-Alvarenga, A. (2024). Challenges and strategies in AI-enhanced occupational therapy for large-scale dementia rehabilitation. *Clinical Practice and Unmet Challenges in AI-Enhanced Healthcare Systems,* 121–142.

Râdulescu, R. M. (2023). Personalized rehabilitation programs: Tailoring recovery through artificial intelligence. *Applied Medical Informatics, 45*, S11–S11.

Schönberger, D. (2019). Artificial intelligence in healthcare: A critical analysis of the legal and ethical implications. *International Journal of Law and Information Technology, 27*(2), 171–203. DOI: 10.1093/ijlit/eaz004

Wong, A., Plasek, J. M., Montecalvo, S. P., & Zhou, L. (2018). Natural language processing and its implications for the future of medication safety: A narrative review of recent advances and challenges. *Pharmacotherapy, 38*(8), 822–841. DOI: 10.1002/phar.2151 PMID: 29884988

Zhang, M., Tang, E., Ding, H., & Zhang, Y. (2024). Artificial intelligence and the future of communication sciences and disorders: A bibliometric and visualization analysis. *Journal of Speech, Language, and Hearing Research: JSLHR*, *67*(11), 4369–4390. DOI: 10.1044/2024_JSLHR-24-00157 PMID: 39418583

Chapter 5
Of Chatbots and Therapists:
Generative AI as a High School and College Guidance Counselor Support in Philippine Education

Marie Grace Avelino Gomez
https://orcid.org/0000-0003-0180-9875
University of the Philippines, Philippines

ABSTRACT

Mental health issues among Filipino students have escalated since the COVID-19 pandemic, with studies reporting a significant prevalence of anxiety and depression among youth. Filipino schoolchildren face persistent challenges due to poverty, academic pressures, and cultural stigmas surrounding mental health. School guidance counselors play a vital role as mental health therapists, providing emotional support, psychoeducation, and crisis intervention. This chapter explores the potential of generative artificial intelligence (AI) to support mental health services in Philippine schools, particularly for high school and college students. AI-powered tools, such as chatbots, can assist counselors by addressing less complex issues and providing coping strategies.

INTRODUCTION

Mental health issues among Filipinos have increased since the COVID-19 pandemic. There is an estimated 35.89% of the population suffering from anxiety disorder during the pandemic (Mendoza & Dizon, 2022). It is estimated that around

DOI: 10.4018/979-8-3373-5072-1.ch005

35 to 47.2% of students are at risk for depressive and anxiety disorders (Alibudbud, 2021). Filipino children's mental health is continually threatened by typhoons, earthquakes, child labor, and poverty (Malolos et al., 2021).

As the children go back to face-to-face classes after the long and stringent lockdowns in the country, Filipino schoolchildren still suffer from mental health issues (Bollentino et al., 2023). The limited number of guidance counselors has reported an increase in students who have mental health issues since the pandemic and are overburdened by the number of clients (Tangco-Siazon, 2022). This phenomenon created much stress for the counselors who had to address their client's needs while performing other functions given to them by their principals (Tan et al., 2024).

Given the limited number of counselors and their ominous work and caseload, artificial intelligence offers some solutions to the problems that they face (American Counseling Association, 2024). Artificial intelligence (AI) can be viewed as a support for counselors who have too many clients. Chatbots can help clients solve some of their concerns by offering a menu of possible help strategies (Kuhail et al., 2024). AI can also help students identify practical strategies to help them cope with their mental health issues (Maijate et al., 2023).

Despite its wide use, AI has limitations in counseling. It lacks the ability to holistically consider a client's complex personal history, culture, and symptoms associated with their problems (American Counseling Association, June 2024). AI-powered chatbots also have issues with dehumanized and robotic responses, disorganized interaction, and a lack of empathy (Kuhail et al., 2024).

The fifth industrial revolution is characterized by human-machine collaboration (Taj & Jhanjhi, 2022). Therefore, AI permeates almost all areas of our lives. This book chapter explores how generative AI can support mental health services offered by guidance counselors to Filipino high school and college students. It identifies areas of support, limitations, and potential threats to addressing mental health and counseling concerns.

The World Health Organization (WHO) reported that the mental health of children and adolescents rose globally after the COVID-19 pandemic, with an estimated 10 to 20 percent of them having mental health issues. Mental health problems among children and adolescents are increasingly reported amidst the COVID-19 pandemic (Hossain et al., 2022). There is a high prevalence of anxiety, depression, sleep disorders, suicidal behavior, stress-related disorders, attention-deficit/hyperactivity disorder, and other mental health problems among Filipino youth. Mental health has become a pressing concern in the Philippine basic education system. Poverty issues, coupled with increasing academic pressures, societal expectations, and personal struggles, contribute to Filipino students' mental health challenges that impact their overall well-being and academic performance.

The Department of Education (DepEd) also posits that academic stress, family conflicts, bullying, and socio-economic challenges contribute significantly to mental health struggles. The onset of the COVID-19 pandemic exacerbated these issues, leading to increased reports of anxiety, depression, and emotional distress among students. Remote learning, isolation, and technological gaps widened inequalities, creating further barriers to mental well-being.

In basic education, students are often subjected to high academic expectations and rigid performance standards. Filipino parents also prefer that their children perform well in school as education is valued as the only inheritance they can give to their children. Cultural stigmas surrounding mental health add another layer of complexity, as discussing emotions or seeking professional help can remain taboo in many Filipino households. Additionally, bullying, whether in-person or online, continues to be a significant stressor for students, further affecting their mental health.

THE SCHOOL GUIDANCE COUNSELOR AS THE MENTAL HEALTH THERAPIST IN PHILIPPINE EDUCATIONAL INSTITUTIONS

School guidance counselors play a critical role in addressing mental health issues in Philippine educational institutions. As mental health therapists, they provide students with emotional support, crisis intervention, and coping strategies to navigate both personal and academic challenges. Counselors offer individual and group counseling sessions to address concerns such as anxiety, stress, family issues, and peer conflicts. In addition to counseling, school counselors advocate for mental health awareness by conducting psychoeducation programs and workshops. These initiatives aim to reduce stigma, promote emotional well-being, and equip students with the skills necessary to manage their emotions effectively. Counselors also collaborate with teachers, administrators, and parents to create a supportive environment that fosters student growth and resilience.

However, systemic challenges, such as the limited number of counselors in schools, hinder counselors' roles as mental health therapists. Many public schools in the Philippines operate with an insufficient counselor-to-student ratio, making it challenging to provide individualized care. This inadequacy limits counselors' capacity to fully address students' needs and fulfill their role as mental health advocates. Some schools have one registered guidance counselor for every 5,000 students. Worse, some schools have no licensed guidance counselors and rely solely on guidance teachers or guidance advocates. These are teachers who have been assigned guidance roles by their school heads to address the mental health issues of students.

Given this scenario, Filipino school guidance counselors often juggle multiple roles that extend beyond mental health support. In addition to providing counseling services, they are tasked with administrative duties, such as career guidance, student assessment, and records management. Some of them perform administrative tasks such as attendance checking, coordinatorship, and even being the school's discipline officer. Even though having a dual role is shunned, some guidance counselors are left without any choice but to comply with the school administration's demands, as there are no other employees to do the task.

There are also limitations faced by guidance teachers and guidance advocates in the Philippines. These include insufficient training and professional development opportunities in mental health therapy. Many of them are not formally trained to handle complex mental health cases due to a lack of educational background. This puts them at risk of mental health issues.

Aside from inadequate technical resources, another significant constraint is the lack of funding and resources for mental health programs. Schools, particularly in rural and marginalized areas, face budgetary limitations, which affect their ability to hire more counselors or provide adequate mental health services. If guidance counselors are available in these areas, they are left to manage heavy caseloads with minimal institutional support, compromising their effectiveness and well-being.

The mental health crisis in the Philippine basic education system signals the urgent need for comprehensive strategies to support students' emotional well-being. To address these challenges, the Philippine education system must prioritize mental health by increasing the number of trained counselors, reducing counselor-to-student ratios, and promoting mental health awareness across all schools. By empowering counselors and fostering a supportive educational environment, Filipino students can thrive academically, emotionally, and socially in the face of mental health challenges. However, this may not be realistic because of financial constraints and lack of government plantilla. Given this scenario, AI might offer potential solutions.

Purpose of the Chapter

This chapter shows the issues of the use of generative AI in the field of guidance and counseling in Philippine high schools and colleges. It shows the issues of the lack of licensed guidance counselors, deficits in training, and heavy caseloads of Filipino guidance counselors. This chapter shows the areas where generative AI can help Filipino guidance counselors address the counseling needs of their clients. On the other hand, this chapter also presents the potential risks and harm of using generative AI.

Challenges in Traditional Guidance Counseling

While traditional guidance counseling is essential for supporting student well-being and academic success, numerous challenges limit its effectiveness. Among these are the overwhelming counselor-to-student ratios, counselor burnout, the lack or absence of counselors in Philippine public schools, the stigma associated with seeking help, and the pressing need for immediate assistance during emergencies. Each of these issues highlights the gaps in current systems and underscores the urgent need for reform.

One significant challenge in traditional guidance counseling is the disproportionately large counselor-to-student ratios. In many schools, particularly in low-income areas, a single counselor is expected to serve hundreds or even thousands of students. This overwhelming workload makes it nearly impossible for counselors to provide individualized attention, follow-up care, or proactive interventions. The lack of manageable caseloads diminishes the quality of support offered and leaves many students underserved or overlooked entirely.

The workload placed on counselors often leads to burnout. Counselors are tasked with addressing various student needs, including academic advising, mental health support, and career guidance, while navigating bureaucratic demands. Burnout can manifest as emotional exhaustion, reduced efficacy, and even compassion fatigue, which can compromise the counselor's ability to provide adequate care. This issue affects the counselor's well-being and reduces the quality of services available to students.

Another pressing issue is the lack or absence of counselors in public schools, as discussed earlier. In many regions, budget constraints or administrative priorities have led to the exclusion of guidance counselors from school staff. This void is particularly concerning in schools where students face significant socio-economic challenges and heightened risks of mental health issues. Without access to guidance counselors, these students are deprived of critical support systems that could help them navigate academic and personal challenges.

Adding to these structural barriers is the stigma associated with seeking help from a counselor. Many students and their families perceive guidance counseling as a sign of weakness or failure, often due to cultural norms or a lack of awareness about mental health. This stigma discourages students from accessing the available resources, even when in urgent need. As a result, issues that could have been addressed early are left to escalate, sometimes leading to severe consequences.

The need for immediate help in emergencies presents another significant challenge in traditional guidance counseling (Haque & Rubia, 2023). Crises such as bullying, harassment, self-harm, or suicidal ideation require prompt intervention. However, the constraints of traditional systems, such as the limited availability of counselors and procedural delays, can hinder timely responses. In critical moments, delays in assistance can mean the difference between effective intervention and irreversible outcomes.

Moreover, traditional guidance systems often lack the infrastructure to integrate modern technologies that could alleviate some of these challenges. Tools like AI-driven chatbots, virtual counseling platforms, or emergency hotlines could provide additional support layers (Lim et al., 2022). However, the absence of these resources in many schools leaves counselors and students reliant on outdated, insufficient methods for today's fast-paced and complex educational environments.

These challenges are compounded in underserved communities, where resources for education and mental health are already scarce. Students in such environments face additional barriers, such as language differences, cultural sensitivities, and socio-economic stressors, that require specialized approaches. Traditional counseling systems often fail to address these multifaceted needs without adequate training and resources.

Traditionally, systemic changes are essential to address these pressing challenges. These include increasing funding for counseling programs, reducing counselor-to-student ratios, investing in counselor well-being, and integrating innovative technologies into traditional systems. Addressing stigma through awareness campaigns and embedding mental health education into curricula could also foster a culture where seeking help is normalized. Ultimately, reimagining guidance counseling to meet modern demands requires a commitment to holistic, inclusive, and responsive approaches that prioritize the well-being of both students and counselors.

GENERATIVE AI AND ITS ROLE IN MENTAL HEALTH AND GUIDANCE SERVICES

Generative AI is a subset of AI that leverages algorithms, particularly neural networks, to produce new content such as text, images, music, and more. Unlike traditional AI systems, which focus on rule-based outputs, generative AI models simulate human creativity and decision-making. Examples include OpenAI's ChatGPT, Google's Gemini, and similar platforms that generate dynamic responses based on user inputs. These models rely on large-scale datasets and advanced architectures to produce contextually relevant and personalized outputs.

Generative AI and Mental Health

The intersection of generative AI and mental health has opened avenues for scalable, accessible, and personalized mental health support. Tools such as ChatGPT, CiCi, Google Gemini, Woebot, Wysa, and Replika are prime examples of how AI can provide immediate, empathetic, and non-judgmental support to individuals in need.

Singh's (2023) research shows ChatGPT's utility in mental health. ChatGPT, launched by OpenAI on November 30, 2022, is a powerful AI-based chatbot system that quickly became the fastest-growing consumer application, with over 100 million users. It is built on a transformer-based neural network and generates human-like responses. It shows promise in bridging the mental health treatment gap in developing countries, where a lack of professionals and resources creates significant accessibility challenges. By providing companionship, support, and therapy through empathetic and knowledge-based responses, AI chatbots offer convenient and affordable alternatives for those facing barriers due to time, distance, or finances (Tal et al., 2023). However, concerns remain about the reliability of information and potential harm from improperly trained AI, underscoring the need for careful oversight in their application (Singh, 2023).

CiCi or CiCiBot is tailored for therapeutic conversations and specializes in offering empathetic responses. It can address issues such as anxiety, stress, and loneliness. Its interactive design allows users to explore coping mechanisms and develop self-awareness through guided dialogue. CiCi can also help students reduce speaking anxiety when learning a new language (Muthmainnah, 2024).

Alhur's (2024) research on generative AI gives examples of its utility in healthcare. Google Gemini can extend the boundary of AI in healthcare through data analytics, facilitating early disease detection and supporting medical decision-making. On the other hand, co-pilot can seamlessly integrate with healthcare systems, optimize clinical workflows, and encourage a culture of innovation among healthcare professionals (Alhur, 2024)

WoeBot can enable its users to complete assessments of affective and cognitive engagement. It has the capacity to apply therapeutic recommendations in real-world settings and is designed to give cognitive behavior therapy techniques to its users (Hoffmann et al., 2023). On the other hand, Wysa can employ evidence-based therapeutic strategies to address depression (Inkster et al., 2018). Replika acts as a virtual companion, and it focuses on emotional intimacy in order to provide a safe space for its users (Laestadius et al., 2024)

The following is an actual conversation with CiCiBot:

Client: I am sad. I failed a test.

CiciBot: Oh no, I'm so sorry to hear that you're feeling sad about failing a test. That's really tough . It's okay to feel disappointed; it happens to everyone at some point.

CiciBot: Tell me, what can I do to help? Would you like to talk about it? Maybe we can brainstorm ways to approach the next test or chat about something else to take your mind off things? Having someone listen can sometimes make a big difference. Let me know what you need right now.

Client: What should I do?

CiciBot: Okay, let's figure this out together. To best help you, I need more information. What kind of test was it? What do you think went wrong? Was there anything specific you struggled with? Knowing this will help me give you more targeted advice. Don't worry about being perfect; just tell me what's on your mind. We'll work through this step by step.

Failing in tests is a common area of concern for students. CiCiBot can empathize with and validate the client's feelings in the example. It also asks how it can help. It gave suggestions such as brainstorming strategies for the next step or being a companion that can listen. It offered customized support by asking the client what is needed. Emoticons are also given by CiCiBot for further emotional support.

It can be noted that with CiCiBot, the answers are chunked in a way that the client would understand and process the current situation. On the other hand, a conversation with Google Gemini would yield more tips. Here is an example with the same initial prompt.

Client: I am sad. I failed a test.

Google Gemini: Oh, I'm really sorry to hear you're going through such a tough time. It's completely understandable to feel sad when you're facing difficulties with your college classes. You're definitely not alone in experiencing this, and there are absolutely things you can do to navigate this situation.

Let's try to break things down a bit. To get a better handle on what's happening and how to move forward, could you tell me a little more about what you think might be contributing to these difficulties? For example:

- *What specific classes are you finding challenging?*
- *Have you noticed any particular patterns or reasons why you might be struggling (e.g., difficulty with the material, time management, motivation, personal issues)?*
- *Have you reached out to your professors or any support services at your college yet?*

Thinking about these questions can sometimes help clarify the situation. Remember, taking things one step at a time can make a big difference. We can explore some strategies together once we have a clearer picture.

Client: I have noticed that I am failing math and chemistry. I hate calculus. I don't like organic chemistry. I have difficulty with the material and I am de-motivated to study because of my numerous failure. What will do?
Google Gemini: It sounds incredibly frustrating to be struggling with subjects you dislike, especially when those struggles lead to demotivation. It's a tough cycle to be in, but definitely one you can break. Let's focus on some actionable steps you can take:
1. Break Down the Challenge:
• Identify Specific Trouble Spots: Instead of just "Math" and "Chemistry," can you pinpoint specific concepts or types of problems within calculus and organic chemistry that you find most challenging? Knowing the specifics will make it easier to target your efforts. For example, in calculus, is it derivatives, integrals, or a particular application? In organic chemistry, is it nomenclature, reaction mechanisms, or spectroscopy?
• Small, Manageable Tasks: Feeling overwhelmed by the entirety of a subject can be paralyzing. Try breaking down your study sessions into smaller, more manageable tasks. Instead of planning to study calculus for three hours, maybe aim for three 45-minute sessions with breaks in between, focusing on one specific concept each time.
2. Seek Academic Support:
• Talk to Your Professors: This is a crucial step. Schedule a meeting with your math and chemistry professors during their office hours. Explain your difficulties and your feelings of demotivation. They can offer insights into the material, suggest specific resources, and might even adjust their teaching approach slightly if they understand the challenges students are facing. Don't be afraid to ask for clarification on concepts you find confusing.
• Utilize Tutoring Services: Most colleges have tutoring centers staffed by students or professionals who specialize in various subjects. This can provide you with one-on-one help in understanding the material at your own pace. It's a safe space to ask "silly" questions and work through problems step-by-step.
• Form Study Groups: Connecting with classmates can be beneficial. You can explain concepts to each other (which reinforces your own understanding) and work through problems collaboratively. [1] Sometimes, hearing an explanation from a peer can make a concept click in a way a lecture doesn't.
3. Reframe Your Perspective (Even if it's Tough):
• Focus on Progress, Not Just Grades: Instead of solely focusing on the failures, try to acknowledge small improvements you make. Did you understand a concept a little better after a study session? Did you solve one problem correctly that you couldn't before? Celebrating these small wins can help rebuild motivation.

• Connect to Your Goals: Even if you dislike these subjects, try to connect them to your overall academic or career goals. Understanding why these courses are required might provide a slight shift in perspective. Are they foundational for other courses you're more interested in? Do they develop problem-solving skills that are valuable in any field?

• Challenge Negative Self-Talk: It's easy to get caught in a cycle of "I'm bad at this" or "I'll never understand it." Try to consciously challenge these negative thoughts. Replace them with more neutral or even slightly positive statements like, "This is challenging, but I can break it down," or "I haven't understood it yet."

4. Address Demotivation:

• Set Realistic Goals and Reward Yourself: As you start making progress on smaller tasks, reward yourself for your efforts. This could be something small like taking a break to do something you enjoy after a study session, or something bigger once you achieve a more significant milestone.

• Create a Conducive Study Environment: Make sure you have a dedicated study space that is free from distractions. A clean and organized environment can sometimes make studying feel less daunting.

• Prioritize Self-Care: When you're feeling down and demotivated, it's easy to neglect basic self-care. Make sure you're getting enough sleep, eating nutritious meals, and engaging in some form of physical activity. These things can significantly impact your mood and energy levels.

• Seek Emotional Support: Don't hesitate to talk about how you're feeling with friends, family, or a counselor at your college's counseling services. Sometimes, just voicing your frustrations and feeling heard can make a difference. They can also provide strategies for managing stress and improving motivation.

It's important to remember that overcoming academic challenges takes time and effort. Be patient with yourself, celebrate small victories, and don't be afraid to reach out for help. You've already taken a significant first step by acknowledging the problem and asking for guidance. You've got this! Which of these steps feels like something you might be willing to try first? (https://gemini.google.com/app/c4760e0f2f925e5f)

It can be noticed that a lot of information was given for the first and the second prompts. The client would feel that advice coming from websites of how-to-do-it or advice columns are given. The client who feels overwhelmed because of failure might feel more overwhelmed because of the amount of information given.

SUPPORT OF GENERATIVE AI ON GUIDANCE SERVICES

Generative AI has the potential to transform guidance services. By addressing key challenges such as accessibility, scalability, and personalization, these tools enhance the traditional guidance framework. In terms of accessibility and inclusivity, generative AI platforms provide round-the-clock support, ensuring individuals can access mental health resources anytime and anywhere. This is especially critical in underserved areas where professional mental health services are scarce. Generative AI also offers personalization. These AI tools analyze user inputs to deliver tailored interventions. For instance, ChatGPT can adapt its tone and content to suit the user's emotional state, ensuring that the advice resonates with their unique circumstances. Generative AI can also be tapped for skill development. Through interactive exercises and simulated scenarios, generative AI supports the development of coping mechanisms, decision-making skills, and emotional intelligence (Xian et al., 2024).

Generative AI complements human guidance counselors rather than replacing them. It can augment guidance counselor intervention. It can handle routine inquiries, provide preliminary support, and flag critical cases for immediate professional intervention, allowing counselors to focus on complex, high-priority cases (Haber et al., 2024). Generative AI also has the power to collect and analyze anonymized data to identify trends, patterns, and emerging mental health issues (Tortora, 2024). These insights enable educational institutions, organizations, and policymakers to design targeted interventions and improve existing support systems.

Generative AI in Asian Guidance Settings

Recent research shows the growing role of AI in transforming mental health support across diverse Asian contexts. AI technologies, including chatbots and tools like ChatGPT, are reshaping counseling by offering individualized, accessible, and stigma-free alternatives to traditional methods. Increasing acceptance of online and mobile counseling technologies among professionals and users in Asia can be driven by factors such as perceived usefulness, ease of use, and cultural fit.

The research conducted by Ping (2024) investigates the use of AI in counseling, specifically within the Asian context. The study examines user interactions and AI chatbots by employing natural language processing and machine learning to evaluate psychological states and forecast counseling results. The models developed demonstrated an accuracy rate of approximately 89% in assessing psychological conditions, highlighting AI's potential to improve mental health services. This progress points to an increasing acceptance and reliance on AI solutions within Asia's healthcare system, aiming to provide more tailored and effective psychological support. The outcomes suggest a promising future for AI in mental health care, illustrating its growing adoption and trust among Asian communities (Ping, 2024).

Day's (2023) research explores how AI tools like ChatGPT can help address mental health issues in Asian higher education, specifically in Thailand and China. It points out that cultural factors, such as the 'face culture' concept, emphasizing social harmony and hierarchy, affect students' readiness to pursue traditional counseling services. In this scenario, AI-driven interactions provide a more private and less stigmatizing way for students to obtain mental health assistance. The study indicates that human-computer interactions through AI can enhance current university well-being strategies by delivering culturally appropriate support mechanisms. Nonetheless, it also highlights ethical concerns related to AI's application in sensitive contexts, stressing the importance of careful implementation that acknowledges cultural subtleties. The article concludes with a proposed conceptual model that combines cultural dimensions and ethical considerations to improve student well-being through AI technologies in post-COVID-19 Asian higher education. This methodology emphasizes the significant potential of AI tools, like ChatGPT, to transform mental health support within culturally diverse academic settings (Day, 2023).

The research of Srijundaree et al. (2024) explores the determinants affecting the adoption of online counseling technologies by mental health professionals in Thailand. Through a quantitative survey involving 406 Thai counselors, the study employs structural equation modeling to analyze the data. The key findings include that guidance counselors are more inclined to adopt OC technologies if they believe these tools enhance their therapeutic effectiveness and efficiency based on perceived usefulness. The likelihood of technology adoption increases when counselors find the OC platforms user-friendly and easy to navigate based on responses on perceived ease of use. The guidance counselors' positive attitudes and openness to integrating technology into counseling practices significantly influence the acceptance of online counseling tools based on their attitudes toward technology. Their apprehensions regarding confidentiality, data security, and compliance with legal standards hamper the use of online technologies based on ethical and legal concerns responses. The presence of institutional backing and training resources plays a critical role in facilitating the adoption of online counseling modalities (Srijundaree et al., 2024).

Yuduang et al. (2022) explores how Filipinos perceive and accept mobile mental health technologies. Using a hybrid structural equation modeling (SEM) and artificial neural network (ANN) method, the researchers found that voluntariness, convenience, and perceived ease of use are the strongest predictors of whether users find such applications usable. Interestingly, user resistance was not a significant factor, suggesting that many Filipinos are open to adopting digital mental health solutions, including those powered by AI. Other influencing factors include social influence, service awareness, and self-efficacy, which highlight the importance of both personal and community-based enablers. These findings are promising for the integration of AI in counseling, as they reflect a readiness in the population to explore non-traditional mental health tools. The study implies that with proper awareness campaigns and user-friendly designs, AI-based counseling platforms could be widely accepted in the Philippine setting. However, it is critical to address ethical concerns such as data privacy, informed consent, and cultural sensitivity to maintain trust. The findings emphasize that acceptance hinges not only on technological capability but also on how well these tools align with users' values, confidence, and needs. Overall, the Philippine context appears receptive to AI in counseling, especially when designed with the user in mind (Yuduang et al., 2022).

Collectively, these findings underscore AI's potential to enhance psychological services in Asia, while emphasizing the importance of ethical implementation and user-centered design. The use of technology in general in the Philippines is hampered by funding, internet connectivity issues, and a lack of technology use skills among users. Counselors need to learn more about technology and its applications.

Applications of Generative AI in Guidance Counseling

Generative AI is revolutionizing the field of guidance counseling, offering innovative solutions to address longstanding challenges and enhance student support. By leveraging AI-driven tools, counselors can provide timely, effective, and personalized assistance, particularly in contexts with resource constraints or cultural sensitivities. These applications range from initial mental health assessments to culturally responsive interventions, paving the way for more inclusive and efficient counseling systems.

One key application of generative AI in counseling is its ability to conduct initial screenings and assessments for mental health concerns. Traditional methods often rely on time-intensive face-to-face interviews, which can delay support for needy students. AI-powered tools can analyze responses from online surveys, text-based interactions, or spoken inputs to identify early signs of anxiety, depression, or other mental health issues.

The following is another example of AI and Human Interaction:

Client: I have been feeling down for more than two weeks. I feel sad for more than half the day. I don't eat that much and have lost interest in many things. What am I feeling? What is this?

ChatGPT: I'm sorry to hear that you're feeling this way. Based on what you're describing, it might be helpful to consider whether you could be experiencing symptoms of depression. Depression is more than just feeling sad or having a bad day; it's a persistent condition that affects mood, energy, appetite, and interest in daily activities for a prolonged period, often lasting for two weeks or more.

Here are some signs commonly associated with depression which align with what you've shared:

- *Persistent sadness or low mood for most of the day, nearly every day.*
- *Loss of interest or pleasure in activities you used to enjoy.*
- *Changes in appetite or significant weight loss/gain.*
- *Feelings of hopelessness, worthlessness, or guilt.*
- *Fatigue or low energy.*
- *Difficulty concentrating or making decisions.*
- *Changes in sleep patterns (e.g., insomnia or sleeping too much).*
- *Physical symptoms like aches or pains without a clear cause.*
- *Thoughts of self-harm or suicide (if this applies, it's crucial to seek help immediately).*

What Can You Do?

1. Reach Out for Support: Talk to someone you trust, like a friend, family member, or counselor. Sometimes, sharing your feelings can lighten the emotional burden.
2. Seek Professional Help: Consider consulting a mental health professional (psychologist, psychiatrist, or counselor). They can provide a proper assessment and recommend strategies or treatments, such as therapy or medication.
3. Take Small Steps: If it feels overwhelming, try setting small, manageable goals each day, like going for a short walk or eating a meal you enjoy.
4. Practice Self-Care: Engage in activities that help soothe or relax you, even if they feel challenging at first (e.g., listening to music, journaling, or meditating).
5. Emergency Help: If you ever feel like you might harm yourself, please get in touch with a crisis hotline or emergency services in your area right away.

You're not alone, and many people have felt similar emotions. With the proper support and help, things can and do get better. Let me know if you'd like more information or resources.

OpenAI. (2025). ChatGPT [Large language model]. https://chatgpt.com

In the conversation between ChatGPT and the client, the AI suggested depression. The response was quite comprehensive, and it identified characteristics of people who may have depression. Despite the thorough answer, the client can be at risk of self-diagnosis and make the condition worse. On the other hand, therapeutic support might be sought. Further, the response of ChatGPT seems to be overwhelming as too much data was given.

The following is an example of a conversation with CiCiBot:

Client: I have been feeling nervous for the past few weeks. I get tongue-tied. I feel jittery. I feel worried about almost everything. What am I dealing with?

CiciBot: It sounds like you're describing symptoms of anxiety. Feeling nervous, tongue-tied, jittery, and worried about everything are all common signs. It's important to remember that everyone experiences anxiety from time to time, but when it becomes overwhelming and interferes with your daily life, it's a good idea to seek help.

Here are a few things to keep in mind:

- *It's okay to seek help: Anxiety is treatable, and there are many resources available. Talking to a trusted friend, family member, or a mental health professional can make a big difference.*
- *You're not alone: Many people experience anxiety, and it's nothing to be ashamed of.*
- *There are things you can do: There are many strategies to manage anxiety, such as practicing mindfulness, relaxation techniques, and getting regular exercise.*

If you're worried about your anxiety, please don't hesitate to reach out to a mental health professional. They can help you develop a plan to manage your symptoms and live a happier, healthier life.

Remember, you're not alone, and there is help available. Take care of yourself.

In the conversation, it can be noticed that the AI identified that the client might be suffering from anxiety. Reaching out to a mental health professional was identified. There was also empathy present, and the AI can engage in a conversation and wish that the client take care of.

Generative AI also excels in supporting students with emotional regulation and stress management through interactive chatbots. These AI-driven chatbots offer a non-judgmental space for students to express their feelings, practice mindfulness exercises, or receive practical advice for managing stress (Gera, 2024). Unlike traditional systems that require scheduling appointments, chatbots are available 24/7, making them an invaluable resource for students seeking immediate support during crises or after school hours. For instance, a chatbot can guide students through breathing techniques or reframing negative thoughts, providing on-the-spot relief and fostering resilience.

AI's capacity to analyze vast amounts of data makes it instrumental in creating personalized student counseling and wellness plans. By integrating academic performance data, behavioral patterns, and socio-emotional factors, generative AI can offer tailored academic and personal growth recommendations (Licardo & Lipovec, 2023). These plans can include strategies for improving study habits, managing time effectively, or addressing specific emotional needs. Such precision ensures that interventions are relevant to the individual, increasing their likelihood of success and engagement.

The scalability of generative AI makes it particularly useful in addressing the counselor-to-student ratio problem in the Philippines. Many public schools have limited access to counselors, so AI can act as an initial point of contact, addressing basic queries and offering preliminary advice. This reduces the burden on human counselors, allowing them to focus on more complex cases that require in-depth attention. Additionally, AI systems can seamlessly integrate with remote counseling platforms, making mental health services accessible to students in rural or underserved areas. Further, ChatGPT can respond to questions in many Filipino languages, such as Tagalog, Ilokano, Cebuhanon, and Kapampangan, to name a few.

Generative AI also has the potential to reduce the stigma surrounding mental health support. Many students hesitate to approach counselors due to fears of judgment or cultural misconceptions about mental health. AI tools, with their anonymity and impartiality, provide a safe space for students to seek help without fear of stigma. This anonymity is crucial in fostering trust among students who might otherwise avoid seeking assistance.

Moreover, AI systems can assist counselors in their professional development by providing real-time insights and recommendations. For instance, an AI tool could suggest best practices or evidence-based strategies for managing specific student concerns, keeping counselors informed and equipped to handle diverse challenges. These systems can also analyze trends in student interactions, offering valuable data to shape school-wide policies or interventions.

As technology advances, integrating generative AI in guidance counseling holds immense promise for enhancing student well-being and addressing systemic gaps. However, ethical considerations such as data privacy, bias in AI algorithms, and the importance of human oversight must remain at the forefront. By combining AI's strengths with the empathy and expertise of human counselors, schools can create a holistic support system that meets the diverse needs of their student populations.

Generative AI has the potential to transform guidance counseling, offering timely, personalized, and culturally sensitive solutions. From mental health assessments to stress management and personalized guidance plans, AI-driven tools can complement traditional counseling methods, ensuring every student receives the support they need to thrive. The Philippine educational system, in particular, stands to benefit significantly from these advancements, fostering a culture of care and inclusivity for future generations.

COUNSELEE PERSPECTIVES ON AI USE

As AI becomes more prevalent in mental health support, researchers are investigating how users, particularly students, perceive and engage with AI counseling platforms. Studies conducted in diverse settings show a mix of enthusiasm for the accessibility and convenience that AI chatbots provide, alongside worries about their ability to deliver genuine human empathy and maintain confidentiality. This section examines recent research centered on the acceptance of AI in counseling, highlighting counselees' perspectives on its role, effectiveness, and ethical considerations.

Kuhail et al. (2024) examine how college students perceive the use of AI chatbots, specifically one named Pi, in providing emotional support. The study involved 224 participants who interacted with Pi, which was designed to emulate supportive and empathetic human-like conversations. Many students found Pi's responses to be empathic and supportive, appreciating its ability to provide immediate assistance during times of stress or when human counselors were unavailable. They also recognized the convenience of AI counseling, noting its 24/7 availability and the ease of accessing support without the need for appointments. However, despite recognizing the benefits of AI counseling, a significant number of students expressed a preference for human counselors, especially for complex emotional issues. They felt that human interactions offered a deeper understanding and genuine empathy that AI currently lacks. Additionally, students raised concerns about the confidentiality of conversations with AI chatbots. They were uncertain about how their data would be used and whether their privacy would be adequately protected. While AI chatbots like Pi can serve as valuable tools for providing immediate and accessible support, students still value the depth and authenticity of human counseling. The study suggests that AI should complement, rather than replace, human counselors, serving as an initial support mechanism or a bridge when human services are not readily available (Kuhail et al., 2024).

Ajlouni et al. (2023) explore the views of undergraduate Jordanian students on using ChatGPT for mental health support. Students appreciated ChatGPT's immediate availability and its capacity to provide a non-judgmental space for discussing personal issues. However, they also expressed concerns regarding the chatbot's ability to understand complex emotions and its lack of human empathy. Overall, while students recognized the potential of AI tools like ChatGPT as supplementary support, they emphasized the importance of human counselors for deeper emotional understanding and connection (Ajlouni et al., 2023).

Mehmood et al. (2025), explores the integration of AI in mental health therapy of Pakistani startups offering AI-driven mental health solutions. The article provides insights relevant to understanding the broader acceptance and limitations of AI in counseling contexts. Their study found a strong association between the accessibility and scalability of AI applications and positive treatment outcomes. AI tools were recognized for their potential to augment therapeutic services, particularly in enhancing accessibility and efficiency. Despite the benefits, AI was noted to have limitations in addressing complex mental health issues. The lack of human attributes such as empathy and personalized care was highlighted as a significant shortcoming, indicating that AI cannot fully replace human counselors. The study suggests that though counselees benefit from AI-assisted services for accessibility and immediate support, they still value and require human interaction for more complex and nuanced issues (Mehmood et al., 2025).

The study by da Silva and Yamada (2024) investigates the possible role of AI, specifically large language models (LLMs) like ChatGPT, in psychological counseling. The authors highlight that effective counseling fundamentally depends on human connection, empathy, and the therapeutic relationship between the counselor and the client. Their findings do not support the idea of substituting human counselors with AI. Instead, the article proposes that AI could serve as a supportive tool within counseling environments. With strict human oversight and ethical guidelines, AI may assist in specific areas of therapy, such as offering immediate help or managing routine questions. However, the integration of AI into counseling raises concerns regarding ethical issues, reliability, and the trustworthiness of AI-generated responses. The authors emphasize the necessity for rigorous testing and ethical standards to ensure the responsible use of AI tools. Furthermore, they mention that clients may be hesitant to engage with AI counselors unless they trust the system's capacity to handle sensitive information securely and provide accurate, empathetic responses. The human element in counseling is crucial. Clients might question whether AI can genuinely understand and empathize with their experiences (da Silva & Yamada, 2024).

COST AND FEASIBILITY OF AI USE IN SCHOOL COUNSELING

With the increasing interest in AI integration within counseling, critical questions emerge regarding the financial and practical implications of its adoption. Although AI can significantly improve mental health services, substantial investments in infrastructure, training, and ongoing maintenance are necessary. These expenses, combined with the technical and ethical hurdles, underscore the importance of thorough evaluation before implementing AI tools in counseling.

Ganesh and Venkateswaramurthy (2025) examine how AI can be incorporated into counseling practices, identifying four levels of implementation: assistive, augmentative, autonomous, and analytical. Although AI presents potential advantages, the article highlights several associated cost and practical limitations. Notably, these limitations encompass financial costs, technical challenges, ethical and legal issues, as well as training and adaptation needs. In terms of financial costs, the authors acknowledge that adopting AI in counseling involves substantial investments in technological infrastructure, software development, and ongoing maintenance, which can be daunting for institutions, especially those with smaller practices or tighter budgets. Regarding technical challenges, it is noted that AI systems might not fully grasp the complexities of human emotions or the therapeutic relationships fostered by human counselors, which could undermine the quality of care and the success of AI-driven counseling interventions. Ethical and legal issues also arise, as utilizing AI in counseling poses questions about confidentiality, informed consent, and the risk of bias in algorithms. Complying with legal and professional standards adds an extra layer of complexity and potential expenses to the implementation process. Finally, for effective integration, counselors and mental health professionals must receive training to use AI tools appropriately, requiring additional time and financial resources for education and adaptation. In summary, while AI has the potential to enhance counseling services, its implementation involves considerable costs and limitations that must be carefully considered (Ganesh & Venkateswaramurthy, 2025).

Bao et al. (2024) present a cost-effective alternative to conventional motion capture technologies for remote psychological counseling. Traditional motion capture systems involve costly equipment, precise calibration, and labor-intensive setups, which substantially increase operational costs. The Intelligent Control Auxiliary System (ICAS), developed by researchers, offers a user-friendly interface that lessens counselors' mental and physical demands. The study demonstrates that ICAS provides usability and expressiveness comparable to motion capture systems while being simpler and requiring fewer technical resources. Experiment participants valued ICAS for its user-friendliness and efficiency, particularly in situations where time and resources are limited. By minimizing the reliance on expensive hardware and lengthy preparations, ICAS offers a more scalable option for remote counseling services. However, despite its economic benefits, ICAS does not achieve the real-time responsiveness and detailed control of pricier systems, indicating it should be used as a supplementary tool rather than a primary one. Overall, ICAS has the potential to enhance access to counseling services by reducing both technological and financial hurdles (Bao et al., 2024).

SAFEGUARDS AND RESPONSIBLE AI USE

As AI increasingly impacts sectors like counseling and mental health support, there is heightened focus on its ethical, legal, and practical consequences. Experts in the field stress the necessity of developing safeguards and frameworks that guarantee AI systems are both effective and responsible, while aligning with human values. Collectively, their research highlights that for AI to earn trust, it must operate under principles such as human oversight, accountability, transparency, fairness, and a solid foundation in ethical and legal norms.

Díaz-Rodríguez et al. (2023) offers a comprehensive framework for ensuring responsible and trustworthy AI deployment. It emphasizes that AI systems must be lawful, ethical, and robust throughout their lifecycle. Seven key requirements are identified: human agency and oversight; technical robustness and safety; privacy and data governance; transparency; diversity, non-discrimination, and fairness; societal and environmental well-being; and accountability. The authors advocate for a holistic approach that includes ethical principles, philosophical perspectives, risk-based regulation, and practical implementation strategies. They propose the use of auditing processes and regulatory sandboxes to operationalize these safeguards, ensuring that AI systems align with societal values and legal standards. This multidisciplinary perspective underscores the necessity of integrating ethical considerations and human-centric values into AI development and regulation (Díaz-Rodríguez et al., 2023)

Swisher (2022) delves into the ethical, legal, and practical considerations surrounding the deployment of AI in sensitive domains such as counseling and mental health support. It underscores the necessity of implementing robust safeguards to ensure responsible AI usage, emphasizing that while AI can augment human services, it should not supplant the indispensable human elements of empathy and judgment. Key safeguards include human oversight, transparency and accountability, data privacy and security, bias mitigation, and ethical and legal compliance. In human oversight, the author argues that human supervision over AI systems help prevent over-reliance on technology use because critical decisions must be made with human judgment. For transparency and accountability, AI decision-making processes must hold developers and users accountable for AI outcomes. Data privacy and security entail the implementation of stringent data protection measures to safeguard sensitive personal information handled by AI systems. Bias mitigation involves actively identifying and mitigating biases in AI algorithms to prevent discriminatory outcomes. Lastly, aligning AI deployment with existing ethical standards and legal frameworks to uphold individuals' rights and societal values. The author concludes that while AI holds significant promise for enhancing counseling services, its integration must be approached with caution, ensuring that ethical considerations and human-centric values remain at the forefront of technological advancement (Swisher, 2022).

LIMITATIONS AND ETHICAL CONSIDERATIONS

AI technology has risks. Integrating generative AI into guidance counseling offers numerous advantages, but it is not without limitations and ethical challenges. These issues must be carefully addressed to ensure that AI-driven systems are reliable, equitable, and sensitive to students' complex needs of students. Key concerns include the risks of misdiagnosis or inappropriate recommendations, data privacy and confidentiality, lack of emotional depth, and cultural or linguistic biases.

One significant risk is misdiagnosis or inappropriate recommendations. Some reports show that AI can trigger eating disorders (Leamay, 2023). Though machine learning algorithms can recognize patterns that human therapists might overlook, they can also detect inconsistencies and patterns that might lead to pathological conditions (Babu & Joseph, 2024). One of the most pressing limitations of generative AI is the risk of misdiagnosis or inappropriate recommendations.

While AI systems can analyze data and identify patterns efficiently, they lack the nuanced understanding that human counselors bring. An AI tool may misinterpret input data, resulting in recommendations that are either overly simplistic or misaligned with the student's actual needs. For example, an AI might flag a person as at risk for depression based on isolated keywords without considering the broader context of their situation, potentially causing harm.

Data privacy and confidentiality are critical concerns when using AI in counseling. AI systems collect and process vast amounts of personal and sensitive information, such as students' mental health histories, academic records, and behavioral data. Ensuring that this data is stored securely and used responsibly is paramount. Inadequate safeguards could lead to data breaches, exposing students to risks such as identity theft or social stigma. Additionally, questions arise regarding who has access to the data and how it might be used beyond the counseling context. Although AI could help redefine mental illnesses more objectively, identify them at a prodromal stage, personalize treatments, and empower patients in their own care, it must address issues of bias, privacy, transparency, and other ethical concerns (Lee et al., 2021).

Another limitation is the lack of emotional depth in AI-driven interactions. Human counselors are trained to recognize subtle cues such as body language, tone of voice, and emotional undercurrents that are often essential to understanding a student's true feelings. AI, while capable of processing text or voice inputs, cannot fully replicate this depth of perception. As a result, students may feel that AI interactions are impersonal or insufficient in addressing their complex emotional experiences, which could undermine trust in the counseling process.

Cultural or linguistic biases in AI systems further complicate their application in diverse settings. AI algorithms are only as unbiased as the data on which they are trained. The AI may fail to provide culturally appropriate guidance in non-Western contexts if the training data predominantly reflects individualist Western cultural norms. In the collectivist Philippine culture, where cultural values such as *pakikisama* (harmony) and *utang na loob* (debt of gratitude) play significant roles in decision-making, AI tools that do not account for these nuances could offer advice that feels irrelevant or even offensive. Further, the challenges of addressing linguistic diversity are also significant. Many AI tools are primarily developed in English, which may exclude or alienate students more comfortable expressing themselves in their native languages. In multilingual societies like the Philippines, the lack of localized language support could hinder effective communication and limit access to AI-driven counseling for non-English speakers.

Ethical dilemmas also arise concerning the role of AI in decision-making. Can AI make recommendations directly impacting a student's academic path or mental health treatment? Even with safeguards, over-reliance on AI risks reducing students to data points, overlooking the individuality and humanity central to effective counseling. It is essential to balance leveraging AI for efficiency and retaining human oversight to ensure critical decisions are made with empathy and care.

Another concern is the potential for overdependence on AI. Schools or institutions might be tempted to rely too heavily on AI systems to compensate for the lack of human counselors, especially in resource-constrained settings. While AI can complement human efforts, it cannot replace the empathy, intuition, and moral reasoning that professional counselors bring to their roles. Overreliance could lead to a dehumanization of the counseling process, where students are treated as data sets rather than individuals with unique needs and circumstances.

Addressing these limitations requires rigorous ethical guidelines and robust regulatory frameworks. For instance, data privacy laws must be enforced to ensure student information is handled with the utmost care. Clear protocols should also be established for handling AI recommendations, ensuring human counselors review and contextualize them before implementation. Transparency about how AI systems operate and the limitations of their capabilities is equally important in building trust among students and educators.

THREATS OF AI TO COUNSELING

Despite its benefits, the integration of AI poses specific threats to traditional counseling. One of the most significant concerns is the potential for over-reliance on technology, which could dehumanize the counseling process. Students might feel alienated if their concerns are primarily addressed by an AI system rather than a human counselor, reducing the emotional connection critical to effective counseling. Additionally, there is the risk of job displacement, as institutions facing budget constraints might view AI as a cost-effective substitute for human counselors, undermining the profession's value.

Students may also choose not to consult the guidance counselor and rely on AI for help. This can be harmful if faulty intervention is recommended. Though there have been many advances in AI, it must be remembered that this technology is still being refined. Glitches and bugs still need to be addressed.

Despite the risks posed by AI to the field of guidance and counseling, there is a need for the guidance counselor to be educated in this field. To fully harness AI's potential while mitigating its risks, counselors must be trained and upskilled to work effectively with AI tools. Training programs should focus on familiarizing counselors with AI systems' capabilities and limitations, enabling them to interpret AI-generated insights critically. Counselors should also develop skills in data ethics and privacy management, ensuring they responsibly handle sensitive student information. By combining AI literacy with their existing expertise, counselors can use technology to enhance their practice without compromising their professional values.

The most effective integration of AI with traditional counseling lies in fostering a collaborative relationship. AI systems can take over repetitive or technical tasks, while human counselors focus on building trust, providing emotional support, and exercising judgment in complex cases. For example, an AI system might identify early warning signs of stress in a student's behavior, but a human counselor is better equipped to explore the underlying causes and develop a holistic intervention plan.

Preserving the human touch in counseling is essential as AI becomes more prevalent. While AI can analyze data and generate recommendations, it lacks the empathy and intuition to navigate sensitive emotional situations. Students often seek counseling to feel heard and understood, which only a human counselor can fully provide. Institutions must ensure that AI complements, rather than replaces, the relational aspect of counseling central to its effectiveness.

THE ROLE OF EDUCATIONAL INSTITUTIONS

Educational institutions play a pivotal role in integrating AI into counseling practices. They must invest in high-quality AI tools that align with ethical and professional standards while providing adequate resources for training and ongoing professional development for counselors. Additionally, institutions should establish clear guidelines on using AI, emphasizing its role as a supportive tool and ensuring that human counselors remain at the forefront of student support services.

CONCLUSION

As technology evolves, the potential for AI to transform counseling will only grow. Innovations such as real-time language translation, virtual reality counseling environments, and AI-driven emotional analysis could further enhance the profession.

However, the successful integration of these advancements depends on maintaining a balanced approach that leverages the strengths of both AI and human expertise.

Integrating generative AI with traditional counseling offers exciting possibilities for improving student support, but it also requires careful planning and ethical consideration. By viewing AI as a tool to enhance, rather than replace, human counselors, the profession can address systemic challenges while preserving the relational and empathetic core of counseling. With proper training, collaboration, and institutional support, counselors can harness the power of AI to create a more inclusive, effective, and equitable future for guidance services.

REFERENCES

Alhur, A. (2024). Redefining Healthcare With Artificial Intelligence (AI): The Contributions of ChatGPT, Gemini, and Co-pilot. *Cureus*, *16*(4), e57795. DOI: 10.7759/cureus.57795 PMID: 38721180

Alibudbud, R. (2021). Academic experiences as determinants of anxiety and depression of Filipino college students in metro Manila. *Youth Voice Journal.*, *11*, 1–21.

American Counseling Association. (2024). Artificial Intelligence in Counseling. www.counseling.org. https://www.counseling.org/resources/research-reports/artificial-intelligence-counseling

American Counseling Association. (June 2024). AI Can Support — But Not Replace — Human Counselors, According to New Recommendations. https://www.counseling.org/publications/media-center/article/2024/01/25/ai-can-support-not-replace-human-counselors-according-to-new-recommendations

Babu, A., & Joseph, A. P. (2024). Artificial intelligence in mental healthcare: Transformative potential vs. The necessity of human interaction. *Frontiers in Psychology*, *15*, 1378904. DOI: 10.3389/fpsyg.2024.1378904 PMID: 39742049

Bao, Y., Song, Z., Weng, D., Liu, Y., Su, M., & Chen, J. (2024). Intelligent Control of Character for AR-Based Remote Psychological Counseling System. In *Artificial Intelligence and Human-Computer Interaction* (pp. 273–281). IOS Press. DOI: 10.3233/FAIA240162

Bollettino, V., Foo, C. Y. S., Stoddard, H., Daza, M., Sison, A. C., Teng-Calleja, M., & Vinck, P. (2023). COVID-19-related mental health challenges and opportunities perceived by mental health providers in the Philippines. *Asian Journal of Psychiatry*, *84*, 103578. DOI: 10.1016/j.ajp.2023.103578 PMID: 37075675

da Silva, J. T., & Yamada, Y. (2024). Could generative artificial intelligence serve as a psychological counselor? Prospects and limitations. *Central Asian Journal of Medical Hypotheses and Ethics = Central'noaziatskij Zurnal Medicinskich Gipotez i Etiki = Medicinalyk Gipoteza Men Ètikanyn Orta Aziâlyk Zurnaly*, *5*(4), 297–303. DOI: 10.47316/cajmhe.2024.5.4.06

Day, M. J. (2023). Towards ethical Artificial Intelligence in universities: ChatGPT, culture, and mental health stigmas in Asian Higher Education post COVID-19. *Journal of Technology in Counselor Education and Supervision*, *4*(1), 7. DOI: 10.61888/2692-4129.1097

Díaz-Rodríguez, N., Del Ser, J., Coeckelbergh, M., López de Prado, M., Herrera-Viedma, E., & Herrera, F. (2023). Connecting the dots in trustworthy Artificial Intelligence: From AI principles, ethics, and key requirements to responsible AI systems and regulation. *Information Fusion, 99*, 101896. DOI: 10.1016/j.inffus.2023.101896

Ganesh, M. (2025). Artificial Intelligence (AI) Generated Health Counseling For Mental Illness Patients. *Current Psychiatry Research and Reviews, 21*(3), 269–283. DOI: 10.2174/0126660822277500240109050359

Gera, P. (2024). Integrating Mindfulness: Enhancing Art and Design Student Well-being through AI Voice Assistants and Wearable Technology (Doctoral dissertation, OCAD University).

Haber, Y., Levkovich, I., Hadar-Shoval, D., & Elyoseph, Z. (2024). The artificial third: A broad view of the effects of introducing generative artificial intelligence on psychotherapy. *JMIR Mental Health, 11*, e54781. DOI: 10.2196/54781 PMID: 38787297

Haque, M. R., & Rubya, S. (2023). An overview of chatbot-based mobile mental health apps: Insights from app description and user reviews. *JMIR mHealth and uHealth, 11*(1), e44838. DOI: 10.2196/44838 PMID: 37213181

Hoffman, V., Flom, M., Mariano, T. Y., Chiauzzi, E., Williams, A., Kirvin-Quamme, A., Pajarito, S., Durden, E., & Perski, O. (2023). User Engagement Clusters of an 8-Week Digital Mental Health Intervention Guided by a Relational Agent (Woebot): Exploratory Study. *Journal of Medical Internet Research, 25*, e47198. DOI: 10.2196/47198 PMID: 37831490

Hossain, M. M., Nesa, F., Das, J., Aggad, R., Tasnim, S., Bairwa, M., Ma, P., & Ramirez, G. (2022). Global burden of mental health problems among children and adolescents during COVID-19 pandemic: An umbrella review. *Psychiatry Research, 317*, 114814. DOI: 10.1016/j.psychres.2022.114814 PMID: 36055064

Inkster, B., Sarda, S., & Subramanian, V. (2018). An empathy-driven, conversational artificial intelligence agent (Wysa) for digital mental well-being: Real-world data evaluation mixed-methods study. *JMIR mHealth and uHealth, 6*(11), e12106. DOI: 10.2196/12106 PMID: 30470676

Kuhail, M. A., Alturki, N., Thomas, J., & Alkhalifa, A. K. (2024). Human vs. AI Counseling: College Students' Perspectives. *Computers in Human Behavior Reports, 16*, 100534. DOI: 10.1016/j.chbr.2024.100534

Laestadius, L., Bishop, A., Gonzalez, M., Illenčík, D., & Campos-Castillo, C. (2024). Too human and not human enough: A grounded theory analysis of mental health harms from emotional dependence on the social chatbot Replika. *New Media & Society*, *26*(10), 5923–5941. DOI: 10.1177/14614448221142007

Leamey, T. (2023, August 29). Popular AI tools can hurt your mental health, a new study finds. CNET. https://www.cnet.com/health/mental/popular-ai-tools-can-hurt-your-mental-health-new-study-finds/

Lee, E. E., Torous, J., De Choudhury, M., Depp, C. A., Graham, S. A., Kim, H., Paulus, M. P., Krystal, J. H., & Jeste, D. V. (2021). Artificial Intelligence for Mental Health Care: Clinical Applications, Barriers, Facilitators, and Artificial Wisdom. *Biological Psychiatry: Cognitive Neuroscience and Neuroimaging*, *6*(9), 856–864. DOI: 10.1016/j.bpsc.2021.02.001 PMID: 33571718

Licardo, M., & Lipovec, A. (2023). Artificial Intelligence Literacy and Social-Emotional Skills as Transversal Competencies in Education.

Lim, S. M., Shiau, C. W. C., Cheng, L. J., & Lau, Y. (2022). Chatbot-delivered psychotherapy for adults with depressive and anxiety symptoms: A systematic review and meta-regression. *Behavior Therapy*, *53*(2), 334–347. DOI: 10.1016/j.beth.2021.09.007 PMID: 35227408

Majjate, H., Bellarhmouch, Y., Jeghal, A., Yahyaouy, A., Tairi, H., & Zidani, K. A. (2023). AI-powered academic guidance and counseling system based on student profile and interests. *Applied System Innovation*, *7*(1), 6. DOI: 10.3390/asi7010006

Malolos, G. Z. C., Baron, M. B. C., Apat, F. A. J., Sagsagat, H. A. A., Pasco, P. B. M., Aportadera, E. T. C. L., Tan, R. J. D., Gacutno-Evardone, A. J., & Lucero-Prisno Iii, D. E. (2021, August 18). Mental health and well-being of children in the Philippine setting during the COVID-19 pandemic. *Health Promotion Perspectives*, *11*(3), 267–270. DOI: 10.34172/hpp.2021.34 PMID: 34660220

Mehmood, R., Parvez, M. A., Qureshi, M., & Sagheer, Z. (2025). Investigating the Future Role of AI in Therapeutic Settings and whether AI will Eventually Supplement or Replace Human Counselors. *Review of Applied Management and Social Sciences*, *8*(1), 143–156. DOI: 10.47067/ramss.v8i1.442

Mendoza, N. B., & Dizon, J. I. W. T. (2022). Prevalence of severe anxiety in the Philippines amid the COVID-19 outbreak. *Journal of Loss and Trauma*, *27*(8), 1–3. DOI: 10.1080/15325024.2021.2023298

Muthmainnah, M. (2024). AI-CiciBot as Conversational Partners in EFL Education, focusing on Intelligent Technology Adoption (ITA) to Mollify Speaking Anxiety. *Journal of English Language Teaching and Applied Linguistics*, *6*(4), 76–85. DOI: 10.32996/jeltal.2024.6.4.8

Ping, Y. (2024). Experience in psychological counseling supported by artificial intelligence technology. *Technology and Health Care*, *32*(6), 3871–3888. DOI: 10.3233/THC-230809 PMID: 38968060

Singh, O. P. (2023). Artificial intelligence in the era of ChatGPT-Opportunities and challenges in mental health care. *Indian Journal of Psychiatry*, *65*(3), 297–298. DOI: 10.4103/indianjpsychiatry.indianjpsychiatry_112_23 PMID: 37204980

Srijundaree, P., Yurayat, P., & Nipanan, P. (2024). Factors Influencing Acceptance and Use of Online Counseling Technology among Thai Psychologists and Mental Health Counsellors. *Islamic Guidance and Counseling Journal*, *7*(1). Advance online publication. DOI: 10.25217/0020247451200

Swisher, K. (2022). The right to (human) counsel: Real responsibility for artificial intelligence. *South Carolina Law Review*, *74*, 823.

Taj, I., & Jhanjhi, N. Z. (2022). Towards industrial revolution 5.0 and explainable artificial intelligence: Challenges and opportunities. *International Journal of Computing and Digital Systems*, *12*(1), 285–311. DOI: 10.12785/ijcds/120124

Tal, A., Elyoseph, Z., Haber, Y., Angert, T., Gur, T., Simon, T., & Asman, O. (2023). The artificial third: Utilizing ChatGPT in mental health. *The American Journal of Bioethics*, *23*(10), 74–77. DOI: 10.1080/15265161.2023.2250297 PMID: 37812102

Tan, K. A., Villanueva, C., Zhu, X. A., Esguerra, B. J., Agbayani, R. A., & Torralba, M. G. (2024). Examining the Lived Experiences of Guidance Counselors' Self-Care Practices. In FEU Journal of Graduate Students' Research (Vol. 1, Issue 1).

Tangco-Siason, A. (2022). Guiding from the Distance: Counselling Experiences During the Pandemic. *Journal of Positive School Psychology*, •••, 6707–6720.

Tortora, L. (2024). Beyond Discrimination: Generative AI Applications and Ethical Challenges in Forensic Psychiatry. *Frontiers in Psychiatry*, *15*, 1346059. DOI: 10.3389/fpsyt.2024.1346059 PMID: 38525252

Xian, X., Chang, A., Xiang, Y. T., & Liu, M. T. (2024). Debate and Dilemmas Regarding Generative AI in Mental Health Care: Scoping Review. *Interactive Journal of Medical Research*, *13*(1), e53672. DOI: 10.2196/53672 PMID: 39133916

Yuduang, N., Ong, A. K., Vista, N. B., Prasetyo, Y. T., Nadlifatin, R., Persada, S. F., Gumasing, M. J., German, J. D., Robas, K. P., Chuenyindee, T., & Buaphiban, T. (2022, May 31). Utilizing Structural Equation Modeling–Artificial Neural Network Hybrid Approach in Determining Factors Affecting Perceived Usability of Mobile Mental Health Application in the Philippines. *International Journal of Environmental Research and Public Health*, *19*(11), 6732. DOI: 10.3390/ijerph19116732 PMID: 35682313

Chapter 6

Using AI to Support Children With Neurodevelopmental Disorders: A Qualitative Research

Dimitra V. Katsarou
https://orcid.org/0000-0001-8690-0314
University of the Aegean, Greece

Evangelos Mantsos
https://orcid.org/0009-0002-8490-2660
University of Thessaly, Greece

Maria Sofologi
https://orcid.org/0000-0003-0380-2220
University of Ioannina, Greece

Efthymia Efthymiou
https://orcid.org/0000-0003-0411-1720
Zayed University, UAE

Kalliopi Megari
https://orcid.org/0000-0002-5861-7199
City College, University of York, Europe Campus, Greece & University of Western Macedonia, Greece

Soultana Papadopoulou
https://orcid.org/0000-0002-0950-1456
University of Ioannina, Greece

Georgios A. Kougioumtzis
https://orcid.org/0000-0002-2362-2094
National and Kapodistrian University of Athens, Greece

ABSTRACT

Artificial intelligence (AI) can significantly contribute to improving the mental health of children with neurodevelopmental disorders, such as autism and ADHD (Attention Deficit Hyperactivity Disorder), by offering tools to monitor, diagnose and support their emotional state. Through behavioral and voice analysis systems, AI can recognize signs of anxiety, depression or other psychological challenges at

DOI: 10.4018/979-8-3373-5072-1.ch006

an early stage, allowing for early intervention by specialists and caregivers. In addition, personalization-based AI applications can offer interactive exercises and stress management strategies, contributing to children's overall well-being and enhancing their psychological well-being. For this purpose, a semi-structured interview survey was conducted with 30 mental health specialists. Their responses were coded and the following channels emerged from their decoding: AI helps mental health through emotion recognition systems, through personalized stress management applications, and through daily observation and intervention suggestions.

INTRODUCTION

The increasing prevalence of neurodevelopmental disorders, such as autism spectrum disorder (ASD) and Attention Deficit Hyperactivity Disorder (ADHD), has highlighted a pressing need for effective tools to monitor, diagnose, and support the mental health of children affected by these conditions. Children with ASD and ADHD often experience significant emotional and psychological challenges, including anxiety, depression, and difficulties in regulating emotions (Gould et al., 2018; Weiss et al., 2017). These challenges can hinder academic, social, and emotional development, making early intervention and continuous support critical (Hansen et al., 2018). However, traditional methods of assessment and intervention are sometimes limited by time constraints, access to professionals, and the need for ongoing monitoring (Porayska-Pomsta et al., 2018). Artificial intelligence (AI) offers a promising solution to these issues by providing innovative, scalable tools that can enhance early detection, personalize interventions, and offer consistent, real-time support (Pepa et al., 2021).

AI technologies, such as behavioral analysis systems and voice recognition tools, are increasingly being used to detect subtle signs of psychological challenges, including anxiety, depression, and stress, which may not be immediately noticeable to caregivers or professionals (Barua et al., 2022; Bhardwaj et al., 2024). AI's ability to recognize these signs at an early stage allows for quicker intervention, which is crucial for improving long-term outcomes (Rosen et al., 2018). Additionally, AI-based applications can be personalized to offer specific exercises, coping strategies, and stress management techniques tailored to the needs of individual children (Argyriadis et al., 2025; Wankhede et al., 2024). This personalized approach has the potential to enhance emotional regulation and overall well-being for children with neurodevelopmental disorders, providing them with tools to manage their emotions in a more controlled and proactive manner (Sandipa et al., 2023).

To explore the role of AI in improving the mental health of children with neurodevelopmental disorders, a semi-structured interview survey was conducted with 30 mental health specialists who work with children with ASD, ADHD, and other related conditions. The survey aimed to capture expert perspectives on how AI is currently being used or could be integrated into mental health interventions. The responses were analyzed and coded to uncover key themes regarding the potential applications of AI in this field. Three primary channels emerged from the data: emotion recognition systems, personalized stress management applications, and daily observation and intervention suggestions. These findings align with existing research that emphasizes the utility of AI in both the detection and management of psychological issues (do Rego et al, 2024; Song et al., 2022).

Emotion recognition systems, which utilize AI algorithms to analyze facial expressions, voice tone, and physiological signals, have shown promise in identifying emotional states such as anxiety and distress in children with neurodevelopmental disorders (Talaat et al., 2024; Zhang et al., 2019). These systems allow for real-time feedback, enabling caregivers and professionals to intervene promptly when emotional dysregulation occurs (Pepa et al., 2021). Personalized stress management applications, powered by AI, provide tailored coping strategies, including mindfulness exercises, relaxation techniques, and behavioral interventions (Liu et al., 2024). These applications can be used independently by children, fostering autonomy and helping them develop emotional regulation skills at their own pace (Lueken & Hahn, 2020). Finally, daily observation tools powered by AI can monitor children's behavior, emotional states, and interactions, providing caregivers and specialists with valuable insights to inform ongoing intervention strategies (Vistorte et al., 2024).

This paper will delve into the findings of the specialist survey, examining how AI can be used to enhance the mental health support provided to children with neurodevelopmental disorders. By focusing on the themes of emotion recognition, personalized interventions, and continuous monitoring, this paper will explore the transformative potential of AI in supporting children's mental health, offering them the tools they need to manage their emotional and psychological challenges effectively (Lyu et al., 2014; Panagiotakopoulou et al., 2024). The integration of AI into existing therapeutic practices can enable more timely, targeted interventions that can ultimately improve the well-being and development of children with ASD, ADHD, and related disorders (Kasari et al., 2018).

METHODOLOGY

The purpose of this study was to explore the potential role of artificial intelligence (AI) in improving the mental health of children with neurodevelopmental disorders, specifically autism spectrum disorder (ASD) and Attention Deficit Hyperactivity Disorder (ADHD). A semi-structured interview survey was conducted with 30 mental health specialists to gather their perspectives on the applications of AI for emotional recognition, personalized stress management, and intervention suggestions. This section outlines the methodology used, including the demographic characteristics of the sample, data collection procedures, and data analysis techniques.

Participants

A total of 30 mental health specialists participated in this study. Participants were selected based on their experience in working with children diagnosed with neurodevelopmental disorders, including ASD and ADHD, and their familiarity with AI technologies or their potential applications in therapy. The participants represented various professional backgrounds, including clinical psychologists, pediatric psychiatrists, occupational therapists, and speech therapists, ensuring a comprehensive range of perspectives.

The demographic characteristics of the sample are presented in the table below (Table 1):

Table 1. Demographic characteristics

Demographic Characteristic	Category	Frequency (n)	Percentage (%)
Gender	Male	12	40%
	Female	18	60%
Age Range	30-40 years	10	33.3%
	41-50 years	12	40%
	51-60 years	8	26.7%
Profession	Clinical Psychologist	8	26.7%
	Pediatric Psychiatrist	7	23.3%
	Occupational Therapist	10	33.3%
	Speech Therapist	5	16.7%
Years of Experience	5-10 years	5	16.7%
	11-15 years	9	30%
	16-20 years	10	33.3%

continued on following page

Table 1. Continued

Demographic Characteristic	Category	Frequency (n)	Percentage (%)
	21+ years	6	20%
Experience with AI	Extensive experience	6	20%
	Some experience	15	50%
	Minimal experience	9	30%

Data Collection

The data collection process involved conducting semi-structured interviews with the 30 mental health specialists. Each interview lasted approximately 45-60 minutes and was conducted either in person or through an online video conferencing platform, depending on participant availability and preference. The interview consisted of open-ended questions designed to explore participants' views on how AI can support mental health in children with neurodevelopmental disorders. The main topics covered in the interviews included:

1. Emotion Recognition: Participants were asked about their experience and knowledge of AI tools that can detect emotional states in children with neurodevelopmental disorders and how these systems could assist in early diagnosis and intervention.
2. Personalized Stress Management: Questions were posed about the potential for AI applications to offer personalized therapeutic exercises for emotional regulation, anxiety reduction, and other stress management strategies.
3. Daily Observation and Intervention Suggestions: Participants were asked about their views on the use of AI for continuous monitoring of children's behavior and emotions, and how AI could assist in providing real-time intervention recommendations for caregivers and specialists.

In addition to the interview questions, participants were also asked to provide their opinions on the ethical considerations of using AI in mental health treatment for children, including privacy concerns and the need for professional oversight.

Procedure

The data collection process followed a structured approach to ensure thorough and accurate gathering of information. Participants were recruited via professional networks and online platforms targeted at mental health professionals, with an invitation letter outlining the study's purpose and requesting their informed consent. Once recruited, participants were contacted to schedule interviews at their convenience, with the interviews conducted between June and August 2024. The principal investigator (PI) facilitated semi-structured interviews, which were audio-recorded with the participants' consent and subsequently transcribed verbatim. The transcribed data underwent thematic analysis, where responses were systematically coded into themes and categorized into three primary channels: emotion recognition systems, personalized stress management applications, and daily observation and intervention suggestions. This analysis involved identifying patterns and emerging themes from the data to ensure an accurate representation of all participants' perspectives.

Ethical approval for this study was obtained from the institutional review board (IRB) at the researcher's affiliated institution. Informed consent was obtained from all participants, ensuring they were fully aware of the study's objectives, their voluntary participation, and their right to withdraw at any time. Participants were assured that their responses would be confidential and anonymized for the purposes of data analysis and reporting.

The coding and decoding system employed in the thematic analysis followed a systematic approach to categorize and interpret the data derived from the semi-structured interviews. The analysis was carried out in several stages, ensuring that the findings were comprehensive, reliable, and aligned with the participants' views. This process involved coding the interview transcripts and then decoding the identified themes to better understand how mental health specialists perceive the role of artificial intelligence (AI) in supporting children with neurodevelopmental disorders.

Stage 1: Familiarization with Data

The first step in the coding process involved reading through the interview transcripts to familiarize the researcher with the data. This allowed the researcher to get a general sense of the participants' responses and to identify recurring topics, phrases, and ideas.

Stage 2: Initial Coding

The next step involved generating initial codes. The researcher systematically went through the data, identifying meaningful units of text—these could be words, phrases, or entire sentences—reflecting a participant's view on AI's potential applications in mental health. Each unit of text that related to the research questions was assigned a code.

For example, when participants spoke about AI detecting emotional signs such as anxiety or distress, codes such as "emotion detection," "early diagnosis," or "anxiety recognition" were applied. Similarly, when participants discussed AI providing personalized therapeutic exercises, codes like "personalized intervention," "tailored strategies," and "stress management" were used.

Stage 3: Grouping Codes into Themes

Once the initial codes were assigned, the researcher grouped related codes into broader categories or themes. This stage is referred to as the "decoding" process, where the researcher interpreted the connections between the codes and formed meaningful clusters that represented the main ideas emerging from the data.

For example: Emotion Recognition Systems: This theme encompassed codes related to AI's ability to detect emotional states in children, such as "anxiety recognition," "emotion detection," and "behavioral monitoring." It was also linked to discussions about AI detecting early signs of mental health issues, such as "early diagnosis" and "early intervention." Personalized Stress Management Applications: Codes like "personalized strategies," "individualized exercises," and "stress management tools" were grouped together under this theme. This reflected how AI could help develop tailored interventions to manage anxiety or stress based on each child's needs and progress. Daily Observation and Intervention Suggestions: Codes related to AI's continuous monitoring and real-time feedback, such as "behavioral observation," "real-time suggestions," and "continuous tracking," were grouped into this theme. The focus here was on AI offering dynamic support and intervention recommendations based on daily observations of the child's emotional or behavioral state.

Stage 4: Theme Refinement

After the codes were grouped into themes, the researcher revisited the data to ensure that each theme accurately represented the participants' responses. This was done by reviewing the coded data within each theme and ensuring that it was consistent with the meanings and intentions conveyed by the participants. If needed, the researcher further refined or adjusted the themes to better reflect the data.

Stage 5: Interpretation of Findings

Once the final themes were established, the researcher interpreted the data in the context of the research questions. The themes of emotion recognition, personalized stress management, and daily observation and intervention were analyzed to understand how AI can improve mental health care for children with neurodevelopmental disorders.

Each theme was then discussed in relation to how mental health specialists perceive AI's potential applications in therapy, the benefits they see in using such technology, and any concerns they raised. For example, in the theme of Emotion Recognition Systems, the researcher highlighted how AI tools could detect emotional states such as anxiety or stress early on, providing timely interventions and supporting more efficient treatment plans. Similarly, under Personalized Stress Management Applications, the researcher noted the specialists' optimism about AI's ability to provide tailored interventions for children, which could empower children to manage their own mental health. Finally, the Daily Observation and Intervention Suggestions theme was discussed in terms of AI's potential to offer real-time support, which could greatly enhance the ongoing treatment and support that children receive from caregivers and specialists. The finale themes and codes summary are listed in Table 2

Table 2. Final themes and codes summary

Theme	Codes	Description
Emotion Recognition Systems	Emotion detection, anxiety recognition, early diagnosis, early intervention, facial recognition, behavioral monitoring	AI tools designed to detect emotional states such as anxiety or depression in children, enabling early diagnosis and timely interventions.
Personalized Stress Management Applications	Personalized strategies, individualized exercises, stress management tools, coping mechanisms, anxiety management	AI-driven applications offering tailored interventions for emotional regulation, such as relaxation techniques, mindfulness exercises, and coping strategies.
Daily Observation and Intervention Suggestions	Behavioral observation, real-time suggestions, continuous tracking, intervention recommendations, daily monitoring	AI tools that continuously monitor a child's behavior and emotional state, providing real-time intervention suggestions for caregivers and specialists.

Stage 6: Reporting Findings

The final step in the process was to report the findings, highlighting the key themes and their relevance to the use of AI in mental health interventions for children with neurodevelopmental disorders. This stage involved synthesizing the findings into a coherent narrative that described how AI could potentially address the needs of children with ASD and ADHD, as well as the experts' views on the ethical and practical

The coding and decoding system allowed for a thorough and systematic analysis of the interview data, ensuring that the findings accurately reflected the perspectives of the mental health specialists. By categorizing the data into themes of emotion recognition, personalized stress management, and daily observation and intervention, the study was able to provide valuable insights into how AI can be integrated into therapeutic interventions for children with neurodevelopmental disorders. This approach also ensured that all relevant aspects of the data were captured and interpreted in a way that addressed the research questions and supported the conclusions drawn from the study.

DISCUSSION

The findings of this study highlight the transformative potential of artificial intelligence (AI) in supporting mental health interventions for children with neurodevelopmental disorders, particularly autism spectrum disorder (ASD) and Attention Deficit Hyperactivity Disorder (ADHD). The three primary themes that emerged from the analysis of interviews with mental health specialists—emotion recognition systems, personalized stress management applications, and daily observation and intervention suggestions—demonstrate how AI could revolutionize both the detection and treatment of emotional and behavioral challenges in these populations.

Firstly, the theme of emotion recognition systems emerged as one of the most critical areas where AI could make a significant impact. Several specialists noted that AI's ability to detect subtle emotional cues through voice analysis, facial expressions, and behavioral patterns could assist in identifying emotional distress at an early stage. This early detection could lead to timely interventions, which are especially important in neurodevelopmental disorders, where children may struggle to express their emotions verbally or may present with atypical emotional responses (Pepa et al., 2021). The ability of AI to continuously monitor emotional states provides a more nuanced and proactive approach to mental health care, enabling caregivers and clinicians to adjust treatment plans accordingly.

Moreover, the use of personalized stress management applications was seen as an innovative application of AI in the therapeutic context. The specialists in this study emphasized that AI-driven applications could offer tailored interventions that address each child's unique emotional regulation needs. For children with ADHD or ASD, who often have difficulty with self-regulation and coping strategies, personalized AI tools could provide valuable support. These tools can include exercises such as guided relaxation, mindfulness activities, or cognitive-behavioral strategies that are adjusted based on real-time feedback (Lueken & Hahn, 2020). By offering individualized therapy, AI could potentially help children better manage anxiety, stress, and other emotional difficulties, empowering them to take an active role in their emotional well-being.

The third theme, daily observation and intervention suggestions, was also frequently discussed by the specialists. AI systems that monitor children's behaviors and provide real-time recommendations can act as a valuable tool for both parents and therapists. Continuous observation allows AI to detect patterns over time that may not be immediately obvious in clinical settings, offering a comprehensive view of a child's emotional and behavioral state (Barua et al., 2022). Furthermore, real-time suggestions based on AI's analysis could provide immediate intervention strategies, such as prompting caregivers to implement specific coping strategies or adjust the child's environment. This dynamic feedback system could significantly enhance the efficacy of therapeutic interventions, as it allows for constant, individualized support.

While the potential benefits of AI in these three areas are clear, it is important to acknowledge the concerns raised by some participants in the study. One primary concern was the ethical implications of using AI in mental health care, particularly regarding privacy and data security. AI systems often rely on collecting large amounts of data, such as voice recordings or behavioral observations, which could raise concerns about the confidentiality of sensitive information (Fiske et al., 2019). Ensuring that AI tools comply with data protection laws and that families are informed about how their data is used will be essential in mitigating these concerns and promoting trust in AI-based interventions.

Additionally, there were concerns about the potential for over-reliance on AI systems, particularly if they begin to replace human interaction in therapy. Many of the specialists interviewed emphasized that AI should be viewed as a tool to augment, not replace, the expertise of clinicians. As much as AI can provide valuable insights and assistance, it cannot fully replicate the empathy, nuanced understanding, and adaptive decision-making that human therapists bring to their work (Castellani et al., 2023). Furthermore, while AI can offer real-time suggestions, specialists cautioned that these interventions should always be validated and supervised by trained professionals to ensure that they are appropriate for the individual child's needs.

Another limitation discussed was the accessibility of AI-based interventions. Although the potential for AI to improve mental health care for children with neurodevelopmental disorders is great, the cost of implementing such technologies could be a barrier for many families, especially those from low-income backgrounds (Uddin et al, 2019). Additionally, there is the issue of technological literacy; both parents and clinicians need to be adequately trained to use AI tools effectively. Without proper training and support, AI applications may not reach their full potential, and some families may struggle to integrate these technologies into their daily routines.

Despite these challenges, the specialists in this study largely expressed optimism about the future of AI in mental health care. They pointed out that ongoing advancements in AI technology, particularly in machine learning and natural language processing, could improve the accuracy and reliability of emotion recognition and intervention suggestions. As AI systems become more sophisticated, they will likely be better able to understand the complexity of emotional and behavioral challenges in children with ASD and ADHD, offering even more personalized and effective interventions (Vistorte et al., 2024).

Furthermore, AI's ability to continuously monitor children's emotional and behavioral states could contribute to a more holistic approach to mental health care. For example, AI tools could track the effectiveness of interventions over time, providing valuable data that can inform adjustments to treatment plans. This data-driven approach could result in more evidence-based therapies that are tailored to the unique needs of each child (Barua et al., 2022). As such, AI has the potential to support clinicians in developing and refining treatment strategies, ultimately improving outcomes for children with neurodevelopmental disorders.

In terms of practical applications, the integration of AI into existing therapeutic frameworks will require collaboration between mental health professionals, AI developers, and caregivers. AI tools must be designed to be user-friendly and easily adaptable to various clinical settings, while also ensuring that they meet the specific needs of children with neurodevelopmental disorders (Thirupathi et al., 2025). This collaboration will be crucial in ensuring that AI technologies are developed and implemented in a way that maximizes their potential benefits while minimizing any risks.

Finally, the findings from this study suggest that AI holds great promise for improving mental health care for children with neurodevelopmental disorders. The themes of emotion recognition, personalized stress management, and daily observation/intervention suggestions reflect how AI can enhance the detection and treatment of emotional challenges in these children. However, the ethical, accessibility, and implementation challenges highlighted in the study must be addressed to ensure that AI interventions are both effective and equitable. As AI technology continues to advance, it has the potential to play a pivotal role in improving mental health outcomes for children with ASD, ADHD, and other neurodevelopmental disorders, ultimately enhancing their overall quality of life.

CONCLUSION

The integration of artificial intelligence (AI) into mental health interventions for children with neurodevelopmental disorders represents a transformative shift in the way we approach both the detection and management of psychological challenges. Throughout this study, we have explored how AI can significantly enhance the care and support provided to children with ASD and ADHD, offering more personalized, data-driven, and effective treatment strategies. From emotion recognition systems that can detect early signs of distress, to personalized stress management applications that empower children to self-regulate, AI has the potential to revolutionize the landscape of child psychology and therapeutic practices. However, as the study highlights, the promise of AI must be balanced with caution. The ethical concerns surrounding data privacy, the risk of over-reliance on technology, and the accessibility of AI interventions are important considerations that need to be addressed as AI technologies continue to evolve. It is crucial that any AI-driven mental health tools be developed with transparency, ethical guidelines, and a focus on maintaining the human element in therapeutic practice. While AI can provide valuable insights and support, it should always complement, not replace, the expertise and empathy of trained clinicians.

Moreover, the integration of AI into everyday clinical practice will require significant collaboration between mental health professionals, AI developers, and caregivers. This collaborative approach will ensure that the tools developed are not only technologically sound but also practical, user-friendly, and aligned with the specific needs of neurodiverse children. Training for both clinicians and families is essential to ensure the successful implementation of AI tools in therapy, ensuring that these technologies enhance rather than complicate the therapeutic process.

Looking ahead, it is clear that the future of AI in mental health interventions holds tremendous promise. As the technology advances, AI systems will likely become more sophisticated in understanding and responding to the complex emotional and behavioral patterns of children with ASD and ADHD. Continued research and development in this field will unlock new possibilities for creating even more personalized, real-time therapeutic interventions that can lead to improved mental health outcomes and better quality of life for neurodiverse children.

In conclusion, while challenges remain, the potential of AI to improve mental health care for children with neurodevelopmental disorders is undeniable. With careful attention to ethical considerations, accessibility, and the collaborative integration of technology and human expertise, AI has the power to transform the way we understand and support children with ASD, ADHD, and other neurodevelopmental conditions. As we move forward, the promise of AI-driven interventions could

REFERENCES

Argyriadis, A., Drakopoulou, O., Argyriadi, A., Mantsos, E., Katsarou, D., & Patsiaouras, A. (2025). Towards holistic wellness: Strategies for managing mental health and embracing neurodiversity. In Sofologi, M., Katsarou, D., & Efthymiou, E. (Eds.), *Exploring cognitive and psychosocial dynamics across childhood and adolescence* (pp. 1–22). IGI Global.

Barua, P. D., Vicnesh, J., Gururajan, R., Oh, S. L., Palmer, E., Azizan, M. M., Kadri, N. A., & Acharya, U. R. (2022). Artificial intelligence-enabled personalized assistive tools to enhance education of children with neurodevelopmental disorders—A review. *International Journal of Environmental Research and Public Health, 19*(3), 1192. DOI: 10.3390/ijerph19031192 PMID: 35162220

Castellani, A., Benassi, M., & Balboni, G. (2023, June). Ethical artificial intelligence in telerehabilitation of neurodevelopmental disorders: A position paper. In *International Conference on Computational Science and Its Applications* (pp. 87–103). Cham: Springer Nature Switzerland. DOI: 10.1007/978-3-031-37114-1_7

do Rêgo, A. C. M., & Araújo-Filho, I. (2024). Leveraging artificial intelligence to enhance the quality of life for patients with autism spectrum disorder: A comprehensive review. *European Journal of Clinical Medicine, 5*(5), 28–38. DOI: 10.24018/clinicmed.2024.5.5.350

Fiske, A., Henningsen, P., & Buyx, A. (2019). Your robot therapist will see you now: Ethical implications of embodied artificial intelligence in psychiatry, psychology, and psychotherapy. *Journal of Medical Internet Research, 21*(5), e13216. DOI: 10.2196/13216 PMID: 31094356

Gould, K. L., Porter, M., Lyneham, H. J., & Hudson, J. L. (2018). Cognitive-behavioral therapy for children with anxiety and comorbid attention-deficit/hyperactivity disorder. *Journal of the American Academy of Child and Adolescent Psychiatry, 57*(7), 481–490. DOI: 10.1016/j.jaac.2018.03.021 PMID: 29960693

Hansen, B. H., Oerbeck, B., Skirbekk, B., Petrovski, B. É., & Kristensen, H. (2018). Neurodevelopmental disorders: Prevalence and comorbidity in children referred to mental health services. *Nordic Journal of Psychiatry, 72*(4), 285–291. DOI: 10.1080/08039488.2018.1444087 PMID: 29488416

Kasari, C., Sturm, A., & Shih, W. (2018). SMARTer approach to personalizing intervention for children with autism spectrum disorder. *Journal of Speech, Language, and Hearing Research: JSLHR, 61*(11), 2629–2640. DOI: 10.1044/2018_JSLHR-L-RSAUT-18-0029 PMID: 30418492

Liu, F., Ju, Q., Zheng, Q., & Peng, Y. (2024). Artificial intelligence in mental health: Innovations brought by artificial intelligence techniques in stress detection and interventions of building resilience. *Current Opinion in Behavioral Sciences*, *60*, 101452. DOI: 10.1016/j.cobeha.2024.101452

Lueken, U., & Hahn, T. (2020). Personalized mental health: Artificial intelligence technologies for treatment response prediction in anxiety disorders. In *Personalized Psychiatry* (pp. 201–213). Academic Press. DOI: 10.1016/B978-0-12-813176-3.00017-1

Lyu, Y., Liu, D., An, P., Tong, X., Zhang, H., Katsuragawa, K., & Zhao, J. (2024). EMooly: Supporting autistic children in collaborative social-emotional learning with caregiver participation through interactive AI-infused and AR activities. *Proceedings of the ACM on Interactive, Mobile, Wearable and Ubiquitous Technologies*, *8*(4), 1–36. DOI: 10.1145/3699738

Mengi, M., & Malhotra, D. (2022). Artificial intelligence-based techniques for the detection of socio-behavioral disorders: A systematic review. *Archives of Computational Methods in Engineering*, *29*(5), 2811–2855. DOI: 10.1007/s11831-021-09682-8

Panagiotakopoulou, D., Vasileiou, I., & Katsarou, D. (2024). Investigation of sexual education programs for adolescents with autism and the role of parents in providing support. *Materia Socio-Medica*, *36*(2), 155–159. DOI: 10.5455/msm.2024.36.155-159 PMID: 39712329

Pepa, L., Spalazzi, L., Capecci, M., & Ceravolo, M. G. (2021). Automatic emotion recognition in clinical scenarios: A systematic review of methods. *IEEE Transactions on Affective Computing*, *14*(2), 1675–1695. DOI: 10.1109/TAFFC.2021.3128787

Porayska-Pomsta, K., Alcorn, A. M., Avramides, K., Beale, S., Bernardini, S., Foster, M. E., Frauenberger, C., Good, J., Guldberg, K., Keay-Bright, W., Kossyvaki, L., Lemon, O., Mademtzi, M., Menzies, R., Pain, H., Rajendran, G., Waller, A., Wass, S., & Smith, T. J. (2018). Blending human and artificial intelligence to support autistic children's social communication skills. [TOCHI]. *ACM Transactions on Computer-Human Interaction*, *25*(6), 1–35. DOI: 10.1145/3271484

Rosen, T. E., Mazefsky, C. A., Vasa, R. A., & Lerner, M. D. (2018). Co-occurring psychiatric conditions in autism spectrum disorder. *International Review of Psychiatry (Abingdon, England)*, *30*(1), 40–61. DOI: 10.1080/09540261.2018.1450229 PMID: 29683351

Sandipa, B. D., Mitratne, D. M., Isurika, M. D. A., Kandanaarachchi, D. S., Rathnayaka, S. C., & Tissera, W. W. (2023). Artificial intelligence and machine learning-based approach to motivate and assist primary school ADHD children. *International Research Journal of Innovations in Engineering and Technology*, *7*(9), 89–96. DOI: 10.47001/IRJIET/2023.709010

Song, C., Jiang, Z. Q., Liu, D., & Wu, L. L. (2022). Application and research progress of machine learning in the diagnosis and treatment of neurodevelopmental disorders in children. *Frontiers in Psychiatry*, *13*, 960672. DOI: 10.3389/fpsyt.2022.960672 PMID: 36090350

Talaat, F. M., Ali, Z. H., Mostafa, R. R., & El-Rashidy, N. (2024). Real-time facial emotion recognition model based on kernel autoencoder and convolutional neural network for autism children. *Soft Computing*, *28*(9-10), 1–14. DOI: 10.1007/s00500-023-09477-y

Thirupathi, L., Kaashipaka, V., Dhanaraju, M., & Katakam, V. (2025). AI and IoT in mental health care: From digital diagnostics to personalized, continuous support. In *Intelligent Systems and IoT Applications in Clinical Health* (pp. 271–294). IGI Global.

Uddin, M., Wang, Y., & Woodbury-Smith, M. (2019). Artificial intelligence for precision medicine in neurodevelopmental disorders. *NPJ Digital Medicine*, *2*(1), 112. DOI: 10.1038/s41746-019-0191-0 PMID: 31799421

Vistorte, A. O. R., Deroncele-Acosta, A., Ayala, J. L. M., Barrasa, A., López-Granero, C., & Martí-González, M. (2024). Integrating artificial intelligence to assess emotions in learning environments: A systematic literature review. *Frontiers in Psychology*, *15*, 1387089. DOI: 10.3389/fpsyg.2024.1387089 PMID: 38966729

Wankhede, N. L., Kale, M. B., Shukla, M., Nathiya, D., Roopashree, R., Kaur, P., & Koppula, S. (2024). Leveraging AI for the diagnosis and treatment of autism spectrum disorder: Current trends and future prospects. *Asian Journal of Psychiatry*, *101*, 104241. DOI: 10.1016/j.ajp.2024.104241 PMID: 39276483

Weiss, J. A., Riosa, P. B., Mazefsky, C. A., & Beaumont, R. (2017). Emotion regulation in autism spectrum disorder. In *Emotion Regulation and Psychopathology in Children and Adolescents* (pp. 235–258).

Chapter 7
Balancing AI and Human Interaction:
Impact of AI Interaction on Well-Being

Sanam Soomro
https://orcid.org/0000-0003-2955-4798
Jiangsu University, China

Mingyue Fan
https://orcid.org/0000-0001-9678-0205
Jiangsu University, China

Safia Soomro
https://orcid.org/0009-0002-3190-4187
Sukkur IBA University, Pakistan

Erum Naseer
Sukkur IBA University, Pakistan

Sonia Najam Shaikh
https://orcid.org/0000-0001-7365-1064
Jiangsu University, China

Suman Najam Shaikh
https://orcid.org/0000-0002-1874-3836
University of Putra Malaysia, Malaysia

ABSTRACT

As artificial intelligence (AI) becomes increasingly integrated into workplaces and daily life, its impact on human well-being has emerged as a critical area of research. This chapter explores the dual role of AI in enhancing productivity and efficiency while addressing the psychological, emotional, and social implications it brings to individuals and organizations. This chapter discusses how AI can improve well-being by automating repetitive tasks, providing personalized healthcare solutions, and supporting employee engagement. However, the chapter also highlights key challenges, including AI anxiety, job displacement, privacy concerns, and the ethical risks of bias in decision-making. Drawing on theories such as the Technology Acceptance Model and Human-Technology Interaction and socio technical theory, this chapter discusses how the optimal balance between AI and human interaction

DOI: 10.4018/979-8-3373-5072-1.ch007

can be achieved.

INTRODUCTION

Over the last few years, Artificial intelligence has emerged as a potential tool that can drastically change organizational processes and reshape workforce dynamics. This widespread adoption shows the central role of AI in contemporary organizations. However, achieving successful AI adoption presents a distinct challenge. While the use of AI and more specifically machine learning has increased dramatically, and while at current, 80% of large organizations have adopted AI at least in some capacity, many organizations across the globe struggle to move beyond isolated solutions and achieve holistic integration across their business functions (Ghosh et al., 2019). However, AI, being the enabler of productivity and efficiency, also brings unique challenges, particularly in balancing technological capabilities with essential human qualities like creativity, empathy, and ethical judgment. The adoption of AI enhances efficiency, and decision-making, and allows human workers to focus on creative and strategic tasks. However, AI's rapid Adoption poses challenges, such as job security concerns and the need for lifelong learning (Arslan et al., 2021; Rampersad, 2020). Due to global disruptions, organizations are reacting quickly to survive, by introducing technological innovation that offers growth and development opportunities to employees. The idea of AI has great potential but its successful application requires the human factor (Chen, 2024). The evolving technological landscape, despite offering immense opportunities, can induce anxiety among employees(Chakraborty, 2024; Pektaş, 2024). AI anxiety may cause stress, mental fatigue, doubt, and feelings of ineffectiveness.

Artificial intelligence is being developed at a very fast pace and has caused significant changes in work organizations, and societal culture transforming how we live, work, and interact(Gohil, 2023; Rajagopal et al., 2022). The potential benefits of AI applications are higher productivity and growth but there are important questions about the impact of AI on people's lives in particular(George, 2024; Khogali & Mekid, 2023). Research shows the connection between improved well-being and AI utilization, by assuming routine work and thus reducing the workload of employees. However, along with these advantages, researchers also observed such challenges as job displacement, "AI anxiety", and growing surveillance at work, all of which can negatively impact employees' mental and emotional health. According to the World Economic Forum (*The Future of Jobs Report 2023*, 2023)14 million jobs, or roughly 2% of current employment could be interrupted due to AI automation, which is causing employees high rates of anxiety about the future of work. The study conducted by the MIT Sloan Management Review found that nearly 61% of surveyed workers felt nervous or uncertain about AI's impact on their roles (MIT Review, 2020). The concept of "AI anxiety" has emerged as a recognized response, describing the fear or discomfort many employees feel toward automation and AI-driven changes. As the integration of artificial intelligence increases, such concerns go beyond worry about job security, skill relevance, applicability of skills, and the general concern over decisions being made by machines. As, it is expected that, with AI interventions increasing, this is especially critical as AI is projected to take on more cognitive tasks, potentially reshaping the nature of human work itself.

This chapter explores the delicate balance between AI and human interaction, emphasizing how this balance impacts well-being. We will delve into the socio-technical systems theory to understand how organizations can design AI-human collaborations that enhance productivity without compromising employee satisfaction. Through a close look at both benefits and challenges, practical strategies, and ethical considerations, this chapter aims to provide a nuanced perspective on how organizations can harness AI responsibly to support and uplift the human workforce.

AI and its Impact on Well-Being

The impact of AI on human well-being extends far beyond its technical capabilities. The socio-technological applications of AI technologies such as virtual assistants, healthcare diagnostics, and even automation of the workplaces, which are vast and are gradually becoming part of people's daily lives, have a great impact on the psychological, emotional, and social well-being of human(Schrape, 2025; Vasiliu & Yavetz, 2024). Even though AI provides innovative solutions for improving the quality of lives of people and their communities, its effect on individual and communal experiences, and connections, represents a number of critical questions(George & George, 2024; Hsu et al., 2022). Getting real insight into how AI can enhance or diminish well-being is helpful for guiding how it will be incorporated into society in the future. AI must be integrated in ways that prioritize mental health, promote a balanced workload, and ensure that the transition into an AI-driven workforce does not leave behind those who struggle to adapt(Ojo et al., 2025; Olawade et al., 2024). Organizations need to create an environment in which AI compliments human capabilities rather than replacing them. Organizations need to ensure that the impact of AI on well-being remains positive. AI is likely to reduce work stress, by adopting AI to perform tasks that involve routine tasks such as data entry, scheduling, and customer queries, it allows employees to focus on more challenging and creative tasks at the workplace. This reduces cognitive load, increases job satisfaction, and improves the quality of work and personal life and well-being(Kelly et al., 2020; Ripp, 2021). AI-powered tools that help manage workload distribution or identify the early symptoms of burnout in employees can contribute to changes in behavior, this enables organizations to take proactive measures. This shift not only improves individual well-being but also fosters healthier workplace cultures.(Dey, 2024; Kaaria, 2024). AI promotes social well-being due to its contribution to communication and connection. Social applications, virtual assistants, and chatbots make the connection between people easier, regardless of where the people are located or what time it is. In this regard, AI enhances social connections and may also help decrease loneliness, especially for vulnerable populations like the elderly or those with disabilities.

The fast pace at which AI has become part of people's daily lives may lead to psychological strain and pressure. As, AI can automate many simple tasks which may create anxiety about job replacement as a result of automation in fields like manufacturing(Estlund, 2021; Tschang & Almirall, 2021), retail, and customer service may leave workers feeling uncertain about their job security and prospects. Artificial intelligence is a monumental phenomenon, its impact on well-being is complex and multifaceted. On one hand, AI has known benefits including an increase in the quality of life, an increase in productivity, and better social attainments, but on the other hand, it has some associated drawbacks such as its negative impact on mental health, risk-related to privacy, and effects on the societal well-being.

Key Definitions

Artificial Intelligence

Artificial Intelligence is defined as the designing of machines that can do activities that require intelligence.

Well-Being

Well-being involves the physical psychological emotional and social dimensions of life. It also includes so much more than being healthy like having a good job, relationships, and having a high level of happiness and overall life satisfaction.

Anxiety

It is defined as an emotional experience that is associated with feelings of apprehension, concern, or fear for a future event or for what might happen.

Efficiency

Efficiency is the intrinsic capability that makes it possible for a particular individual, a group of individuals, or an organization to realize a given aim using the least number of resources in terms of time and finances.

Job Replacement

That is the act of substituting a human being's job or task with a new approach such as machine algorithms, automation, or artificial intelligence (AI).

Technostress

Technostress is the stress that comes with the inability to integrate into new technologies.

THEORETICAL CONCEPTS

There are several widely accepted models in the domain of Human Technology Interaction and they can be applied and put to use in order to help when designing and assessing the human technology interaction specifically as it relates to AI systems. Performance impact models theories, or paradigms employed in the attempt to moderate the evaluation and analysis of the effects of some variables including technology, change within organizational designs and structures, and employee behaviors. While addressing the relationship between interactions with intelligent technologies and overall performance, the models of combining AI competencies with human talent provide an understanding of how improved results in terms of productivity, efficiency, innovation, morale, and organizational performance can be achieved. Some of the models and related theories are discussed below.

Human-Technology Interaction (HTI) Model

Human-Technology Interaction is an approach to technology development and enhancement that is important to the economic performance of technologies(Soch et al., 2022). HTI research targets improving the actualization of information technologies in contexts that are more functional, usable, and meaningful to people(Enstroem et al., 2024). It informs about and enables methods people employ the technology in business, in the home as well as in many other contexts. As AI and advanced technologies pervade work and daily life, technology-based performance prediction models of HTI provide means for identifying how technology can impact performance, proactivity, workload, and affective well-being(Colaiacovo,

2024). It prescribes pointers and approaches for the application of technology into the operations of an organization to build and enrich human capabilities. Applying HTI models in the case of AI adoption means making sure that AI amplifies human roles instead of negating them.

Core Components of HTI Models

- ***Usability***: How much extent the experience with the technology products can be easily controlled. Usability concentrates on the concept that the system enables effective, accurate, and pleasant interactions. Usability in the context of AI systems means creating interfaces that are easy to use and allow to interpret easily without profound IT knowledge.
- ***User Experience (UX)***: It covers everything a user feels, thinks, does, and prefers while using technology, including emotional responses, satisfaction, and perceived utility. The role of UX is significant in artificial intelligence to embrace since the users should feel comfortable with the technology for effective adoption.
- ***Task Fit***: This aspect examines the effectiveness of the technology in enabling the users to carry out their work. HTI models determine whether a technology is a boon or bane to productivity, especially beneficial in artificial intelligence, a process where some tasks might be automated or augmented
- ***Intellectual Load***: The mental effort required to use a technology. Information overload reduces comprehension, leads to frustration, and errors, and reduces efficiency. As for the HTI models, the primary objective is to design technology that minimizes unnecessary complexity and thus is easy to master.
- ***Adaptability***: HTI models also take into consideration if a technology is user-centric and if it considers the user's capabilities. This is because adaptive AI systems can learn from user behaviors and subsequently enhance the interfaces' recommendations to lead to better interrelation experiences.

Applications of HTI Model in AI Adoption

- ***User-Centric AI Design***: HTI models place a particular focus on consumer need satisfaction through friendly and timely responses. AI chatbots should use natural language processing to understand customer queries so that customer service agents can be freed of extra burden.
- ***Enhancing Decision-Making***: HTI models, especially cognitive engineering approaches, guide the design of AI tools that provide clear insights and visualizations, enabling users to make informed decisions without feeling overwhelmed by data.

- ***Minimizing Technostress***: By ensuring AI interfaces are spontaneous frequent and task-relevant. HTI models take measures to minimize technostress, which negatively impacts the adoption and performance rates.
- ***Adaptive Learning Systems***: AI systems leveraging HTI principles can be intelligent, meaning they can learn a user's experience level or even their suggested changes. This flexibility can be illustrated with artificial intelligence-enabled educational platforms that customize content based on a learner's progress.

Benefits of Human-Technology Interaction Models

Incorporating the concept of HTI models with AI, the general user experience improves making using the technology more convenient, efficient, and enjoyable to use(Pyae et al., 2023). For the same activity if an AI tool is easy to adopt and aligns well with the contextual task, it enhances productivity rather than creating additional challenges or cognitive demands(Al Naqbi et al., 2024). It promotes acceptance of AI by incorporating the needs and capacities of its users and application in the design and functioning of AI minimizes errors and increases safety by making it easier for users to interpret AI outputs accurately.

Challenges in Human-Technology Interaction with AI

- ***The complexity of AI***: Traditional AI systems are highly technical, using algorithms and database processing not readily understandable to the average consumer. The current HTI models have the ambition to do so, but they might struggle when AI roles are too complicated.
- ***Balancing Automation and Control***: It's challenging to balance automation with user control, particularly in high-stakes environments like finance or healthcare, where users must understand and potentially override AI decisions.
- ***Cultural and Individual Differences:*** The use of AI for recommendation varies with user backgrounds, experiences, and technology use, implying that there could be no best approach. HTI models call for flexibility in system design, however, achieving this remains complex.

Socio-Technical Systems Theory

Socio-technical systems (STS) theory is an organizational model that focuses on the interdependence between the social (human factors) environment and the technical (technological) environment of working systems to achieve the overall efficiency as well as the well-being of people in the work subsystem(Sony & Naik, 2020). STS theory boasts of the fact that it focuses on both social and technical developments at the same time rather than at different times. It also assumes that the design and performance of an organizational system can be enhanced only through integrating the social and technical elements(Thomas, 2024). The theory states that social and technical systems in an organization are more effective when both systems are aligned and designed(Hess & Sovacool, 2020).

Here's an in-depth look at the key aspects of STS theory, its applications, and relevance especially in contexts like AI adoption:

Core Concepts of Socio-Technical Systems Theory

- ***Social System***: The social work system includes work team, communication, work satisfaction, the organizational culture of a work team, relation to trust, worker involvement, and health. The social system emphasizes teamwork, communication, job satisfaction, and the organizational culture that fosters trust, engagement, and employee well-being.
- ***Technical System***: This involves the instruments and technology, techniques and activities, approaches and methods, equipment and system, and facilities and systems employed in achieving organizational objectives. This will include elements such as AI models like machine learning, automation systems, Data processing tools, and other digital resources.
- ***Joint Optimization***: According to STS theory, the social as well as the technical systems should be optimized. The theory is further expounded to mean that the idea of optimizing performance within a system is not a product of either the technology aspect of the system or the human component, but instead a result of forming the system in such a way that individuals and technology are integrated with each other.

Applications of STS Theory in AI Adoption

When applying STS theory to the adoption of AI in organizations, several key factors can help balance AI capabilities with human skills to improve performance and employee satisfaction(Chowdhury et al., 2022; Yu et al., 2022):

- ***Redesigning Roles:*** AI can automate repetitive tasks, freeing human employees from routine work and empowering them to do creative and interpersonal work. Such redesigned roles would supplement and enhance human strength and job satisfaction rather than replace human roles entirely.

- ***Enhancing Job Satisfaction:*** Therefore, when applied selectively, AI can contribute greatly to increasing the level of perceptions of the meaningfulness of work and decrease the level of feelings of replacement anxiety. In this approach is the feeling of working together with the technology, which is in harmony, aligning with STS's emphasis on well-being.
- ***Building Trust and Transparency:*** STS for the adoption of AI in organizations requires a clear declaration of what AI will do, why it will do it, and what it cannot do. The use of AI should make people feel it can help them do the job better and should not make them feel threatened, which corresponds to STS's human-centered focus.
- ***Feedback Loops:*** Encouraging employee feedback in AI systems makes the technical system consistent with the social system. If the AI systems disrupt organizational processes or create stressful conditions, such information is useful for necessary adjustments.

Benefits of Socio-Technical Systems Theory in AI Implementation

There is improved performance on the socio-technical system by leaving data-intensive work to the AI tools, while people work on tasks that require their judgment, creativity, or ethical reasoning. It focuses on happiness, self-esteem, and turnover by minimizing the chance of stress or burnout due to AI integration by organizing an employee's work assignment(Loureiro et al., 2023). Therefore, the culture that should be promoted by organizations is the culture of acceptance of human insight as well as technology; this makes it easy for organizations to adapt to change as influenced by technology.

Challenges and Considerations

Implementing STS in AI adoption requires careful consideration of challenges like:

- ***Resistance to Change:*** Organizations could potentially experience some level of employee rejection of AI if they fear it will replace their jobs. STS theory addresses this by engaging the employees in the design and implementation process.
- ***Complexity of Integration***: It is challenging even for experienced practitioners to appropriately balance social and technical factors given the dynamic nature of AI. Organizations may need ongoing assessment to maintain an optimal balance.
- ***Ethical Concerns:*** Ethical factors to be captured for any AI system include; Ensuring that the AI systems incorporate ethical values that meet the organi-

zational ethics. An STS approach guarantees that applications of technology are relevant to human interest as well as ethical.

Technology Acceptance Model (TAM)

The Technology Acceptance Model (TAM) was developed by Fred Davis in the year 1986(Santi & Erdani, 2021). TAM is a theoretical model that provides a theoretical perspective on how and why individuals adopt and use a specific technology, due to its effectiveness in predicting the usage intention of new technological inventions(Martín-García et al., 2022). It is one of the most popular models to measure the user acceptance of technology in various fields such as business, healthcare, education, information system, and many more(Yadegari et al., 2024). TAM on the other hand is useful to explain how adoption can be achieved in not only professional usage but consumer usage as well.

Core Components of TAM

TAM consists of two primary factors that drive an individual's intention to use a technology.

- ***Perceived Usefulness (PU):*** The degree to which an individual believes that using a specific technology utility of the specific technology in enhancing performance or ease of tasks.
- ***Perceived Ease of Use (PEOU):*** The degree to which the individual feels that the use of the technology will not involve any effort. If a technology is easy to use it means that the users will always have positive attitudes towards that particular technology and use it regularly.

Applications of TAM

TAM and its extended versions are applied across a wide range of domains:

- ***Workplace Technology***: Applied to forecast the probability of the employee acceptance of new systems that include enterprise software, customer relationship management (CRM) systems, and communication tools.
- ***Healthcare***: Helps to assess the adoption of telemedicine, electronic health records, and health-monitoring applications.
- ***Education***: May be used to evaluate the extent of adoption of telemedicine, e-health records, and health-monitoring applications.

- ***Consumer Technology***: Measures acceptance attitudes towards smart devices, social media, and mobile apps.

Benefits of TAM and Extended TAM

TAM's simple structure makes it useful for analyzing user adoption behavior, especially in organizational contexts where ease of use and perceived usefulness are of paramount concern to organizational users(Isiaku & Adalier, 2024; Mohd Amir et al., 2020). TAM can be used by developers and organizations to identify key areas such as simplifying interfaces or emphasizing benefits that can improve user adoption rates(Ishengoma, 2024). More parameters can be added to the proposed model to consider the given influence, for example, social pressure, experience, or enjoyment; therefore, it can be applicable in any field.

Challenges and Limitations of TAM

- ***Simplicity***: While the simplicity of TAM is a strength. In simplified, the model may not capture the real situation in environments where the users are many and characterized by dynamic behaviors by providing an overly simple and elegant description of problems.
- ***Lack of Focus on Emotional Factors***: Basic TAM does not take into account the affective states such as anxiety/ excitement resulting from the applications of AI/automation in technology adoption.
- ***Limitations with Mandatory Use***: TAM assumes that users assume that the use of a particular technology is voluntary. It will be useful when demands to use technology are compulsory, and the role of subjective norms and resistance should be examined more thoroughly.
- ***Evolving Contexts***: As technologies and user expectations evolve, TAM has to be updated frequently to accommodate new changes, which can add complexity to its application.

UNDERSTANDING CAPABILITIES AND LIMITATIONS OF AI

Capabilities of AI

AI has shifted traditional roles and introduced new opportunities for productivity and efficiency. However, the real excitement is in pursuing how AI recreates not only what work is accomplished but how and by whom is it accomplished. In the dynamic setting of today's workplace, AI is a competent partner for human workers.

The fact is that programs that independently make tentative and alert about possible future changes, can transform such sectors as marketing, finance, and logistics. Employers now make better decisions, detect new trends in the market, and interact with customers more individually, thus making the corporation more flexible(Sima et al., 2020). However, as AI integrates deeper into work environment objectives, it raises some questions about the future of work roles and human relevance. It's crucial to acknowledge that AI automation typically targets specific tasks within roles rather than entire jobs, coexisting with other tasks that remain untouched by automation. (Brynjolfsson et al., 2018) Found that while many tasks across various industries could potentially be automated, there are no occupations where all tasks could be replaced by AI. It is argued that the current passive view often fails to see how the technology can, and perhaps should be adjusted to the competency, needs, and value of humans. Research indicates that the theoretical framework could play a role in explaining how a combination of technology and human skill could support the overall well-being and productivity of human beings (Dubey et al., 2019). A positive view of technology can make people acquire the skills that are required in the use of technology appropriately. In contrast, where training initiatives do not already exist in organizations, resentment of AI among employees is created (Bhattacharyya & Nair, 2019). This shift not only challenges traditional job structures but also opens the door for new career paths focused on overseeing, guiding, and enhancing AI systems. In some places, this shift has redesigned education for skill acquisition where training focuses on how to interact with AI tools and use them as an extension of their capabilities.

The rise of AI in workplaces also fuels discussions on work-life balance and the well-being of employees. When it comes to advantages and disadvantages, AI can alleviate repetitive workload and reduce stress, however, issues like job insecurity, having too much surveillance, and constant examination or monitoring of their work, these issues may have a detrimental effect on the morale of employees. Therefore, organizations must navigate this shift carefully, and the best ways to meet new increases in productivity are through the use of artificial intelligence while maintaining an employee-focused, positive work culture. AI is now a reality in many organizations and people's daily lives, the change from simple administrative work to the most complicated work has been brought by AI (Singh et al., 2024). AI can efficiently organize and interpret large amounts of data quickly and accurately identifying patterns, and performing repetitive tasks with speed and accuracy that far exceed human capabilities. Unlike humans, AI systems can operate continuously without fatigue, ensuring consistent performance and availability around the clock(Baruwal Chhetri et al., 2024; Shneiderman, 2020). In consumer relations, AI chatbots can simultaneously answer thousands of questions, all at once, and this is invaluable. Almost every company has tasks that are repetitive, from simple typing of data to complex tasks in a manufacturing assembly line, and can be effectively handled by AI(Boysen et al., 2022; Sotskov, 2023). AI can automate a wide range of repetitive tasks, from simple data entry to more complex functions like inventory management or predictive maintenance in manufacturing. It can analyze user preferences and behaviors which makes it possible for it to develop highly personalized experiences. However, AI also has its limitations that have to be carefully considered as it gets deployed in various aspects of work and daily life. The limitation of AI is analyzed below.

Limitations of AI

- **Lack of Emotional Intelligence and Contextual Understanding**: While AI can work with data and patterns, it cannot recognize emotions, cultural factors, and social signals. This can lead to issues in job areas that demand one to have interpersonal skills in areas of social, counseling, conflict solving and counseling, conflict resolution, or caregiving, where human connection and emotional understanding are critical.
- **Bias and Ethical Concerns**: AI systems are trained on past data, and so if the data itself is biased, is the model. This is particularly concerning in areas such as hiring, law enforcement, and lending, where biased AI decisions could disadvantage certain groups based on gender, race, or socioeconomic status. For instance, studies have demonstrated that facial recognition algorithms produce worse results when identifying people especially, people of color, recruitment algorithms can also perpetuate bias due to skewed training data. Addressing these biases requires a multifaceted approach from expanding the sources of data to creating reliable approaches to the AI-models auditing for their bias. Ensuring fairness, transparency, and ethical use of AI requires constant oversight, and addressing these challenges remains a critical limitation.
- **Dependence on Quality Data**: The outcome of AI extremely depends on the quality and quantity of data sets it has been trained on. When data is of low quality or datasets are missing some data, they produce wrong predictions or may lead to wrong results. Thus, this reliance on data can limit AI's usefulness in situations where comprehensive or clean data is unavailable.
- **Limited Creativity and Adaptability**: AI works according to the constructed algorithms and trained data configuration and is consequently incapable of coping with new scenarios that are out of its jurisdiction. AI can make the best out of the existing data or the map where it exists. It struggles with generating truly original ideas, improvising in unexpected scenarios, or adapting to rapidly changing environments tasks where human creativity and flexibility are key.

- **Security and Privacy Risks**: AI owns and incorporates large stocks of personal and sensitive data hence it poses a threat to privacy and data security. Because AI has the potential to monitor, track, and even predict an individual's behaviors, the line between personalization and surveillance becomes increasingly blurry. AI applied to consumers' services, like Advertising or smart homes technologies might impair private life. However, personal information leakage or malicious use of personal information through the use of artificial intelligence could have serious consequences that undermine public trust. The most pressing concerns that make the case for well-designed security frameworks are hacking, insider threats, abuse of artificial intelligence systems, and unauthorized access to someone's data highlighting the need for robust security frameworks. Ensuring that data is used responsibly, with consent and transparency, is crucial in mitigating these risks. As, AI systems gather and process users' data, new ethical challenges connected with the data users' consent and privacy emerge.

It is important to understand these limitations as a way of attaining the best way of interacting with artificial intelligence. Knowing when and where AI increases the value and when human input is inevitable allows an organization to develop a synergy of AI and human-centered work models. This approach not only boosts output but also focuses on interests and well-being, AI compliments the human workforce instead of replacing them.

ACHIEVING THE OPTIMAL BALANCE

As artificial intelligence becomes an integral part of modern workplaces, the key to optimizing employee-machine relationships has become an art as much as a science. The real issue is not whether or not AI should be implemented but instead how AI should be implemented in such a way that can support the work being done by people, and build upon the strengths of people without overshadowing the unique qualities that humans bring like empathy, creativity, and complex problem-solving. A balanced approach to AI-human collaboration involves more than simply dividing tasks between machines and people(Jiang et al., 2022). It's about creating workflows that leverage AI to handle repetitive, data-heavy tasks while empowering employees to engage in strategic thinking, building relationships with customers, and creativity(Joo et al., 2022). The cooperation is not only efficient; it also increases the interest of the workers and makes it possible for them to focus on some valuable aspects of their employment which may be diminished if they perform routine tasks without the participation of their co-workers. Imagine the increasing popularity of the hybrid work models where AI provides day-to-day operations and allows employees to focus on tasks that require human judgment and insight. As a result, AI becomes a useful tool for maximizing productivity, not a replacement.

AI and Human Hybrid Work Models

The hybrid work models show various versatile approaches with augmented collaboration of AI skills and human cognitive abilities in many different fields. By thoughtfully blending AI efficiency with human insight, creativity, and judgment, these models offer a harmonized form of work for the future. Here are a few hybrid work models that integrate both human expertise and AI capabilities, aiming to balance productivity, innovation, and human engagement effectively.

- **AI-Augmented Decision-Making Teams:** In this model, AI systems analyze large data sets and provide insights or predictions, enabling teams to make more informed, data-driven decisions. For example, in finance or healthcare, AI assists in risk assessment or diagnostics, while human experts apply judgment and ethical considerations, tailoring recommendations to unique situations.
- **Human-in-the-Loop (HITL) Systems:** This model automates information processing and the completion of routine tasks through AI control, though people must be ready to address matters as and when they occur. For example, in customer service, AI is used to deal with frequent queries, but refer complex or sensitive queries to the care team. This ensures efficiency while retaining a high level of personalized, empathetic service.
- **Collaborative AI for Creative Projects:** AI tools can create concepts, predictions, or recommendations for designs that can inspire human creative workers or provide them with new points of view. For instance, in marketing and design, AI can determine consumer preferences and suggest content themes that consumers would likely be interested in but human creatives think of unique messaging, and emotional appeal that connect with the customers.
- **Predictive Maintenance Teams:** This model is frequently utilized in manufacturing industries; this model employs the use of AI for usage patterns and environmental analysis to assess the maintenance requirements for the equipment. Informed by these insights, human technicians undertake required corrective measures so that there is minimum disruption and safe effective functioning.
- **AI-Driven Training and Development**: The AI system can analyze certain aspects of performance and come up with certain conclusions such as the areas in which the employees lack certain skills, and therefore require training

in those areas. Human managers, in turn, apply them proactively in tailoring developmental interventions whereby employees receive a combination of coaching and skills exposure and feedback, enabling human capital to grow along the strategic directions of the organization.

- **Customer Relationship Management (CRM) with AI Insights**: In sales and marketing, AI analyzes customer data to predict buying patterns or identify potential leads whereas, on the human side, you obtain genuine interactions, negotiate deals with clients, unique appeals that make every customer feel special. This balance improves customer satisfaction and paves the way for the improvement of loyalty.
- **AI-Enhanced Hiring Processes**: AI automates initial recruitment steps by scanning resumes, determining key skills, and proposing possible candidates for some positions while HRs interview candidates, evaluate organizational fit, and make the final decision. With this model, recruitment is accelerated but without sacrificing the human judgment necessary to select the best candidates.
- **Intelligent Robotic Process Automation (RPA)**: This model deals with automating high-volume, repetitive tasks, such as data entry or compliance checks, by means of RPA. The employees gain more time for high-level decision-making and manage the roles and responsibilities of such RPA systems to maintain high-end accuracy and smooth workflow.
- **AI-Integrated Project Management**: AI tools help project managers by; estimating timelines and schedules as well as analyzing potential risks based on data from previous projects. Human project managers then rely on such information to organize resources smartly organize the workforce and adjust plans as new project dynamics unfold.
- **Healthcare Diagnostics with Human Oversight**: In the medical field AI helps to diagnose illnesses by scanning images or patients' histories for abnormalities. However, these results are confirmed by the physicians, who consider the patient's history and other context factors to make the final diagnostic and treatment decisions, ensuring holistic patient care.

However, achieving this balance isn’t without its challenges. Over-reliance on AI can risk separating employees or devaluing roles that AI can’t fully replace, especially those involving empathy and nuanced understanding. High-performing organizations are those that embrace the operational constraints of AI, while at the same time promoting a workplace culture of embracing the operational AI and supporting employees as they increase their ability to integrate the technology into their work. It might be understood as the striving for the best balance of people and artificial intelligence in the environment that must be profitable for both parties(Bilen

& Hervé, 2024). It is an evolutionary one, that is a process that calls for vision, acknowledging the dignity of people at work, and a good understanding of how AI futures the world of work. This balance will decide how artificial intelligence champions the new and reshapes the future of work, not as an eradication of human input but by enhancing it in ways we are just beginning to explore. An augmentation of it in ways we have not fully appreciated.

CHALLENGES AND ETHICAL CONSIDERATIONS

Every time a new role is created by AI to innovate and transform industries, new concerns, and ethical dilemmas are brought along(Aldoseri et al., 2024). On the one hand, AI is set to deliver unmatched efficiency and productivity and, on the other hand, it provokes precise societal and ethical questions about fairness, accountability, and the long-term impacts on individuals and society. It is crucial to understand how these challenges can be managed effectively as the technology and applications of intelligent systems grow more on a day-by-day basis. The prospects of AI about its ability to perform most of the work possible have created a situation where the future of work and the displacement of workers are regarded as a major concern(Kolade & Owoseni, 2022). While AI can improve productivity and reduce costs for businesses, it also has the potential to make certain roles obsolete. AI can bring efficiency, and effectiveness and often leads to making certain roles obsolete. The manufacturing industry, transport, and industries that involve numerous workers directly interacting with consumers will experience reduced workforce due to capital-intensive and efficient machine control systems that will be made possible by artificial intelligence. Moreover, the skills gap between those who can adapt to AI-driven work environments and those who cannot could exacerbate social inequalities(Kyriakidou et al., 2025). On one hand, AI creates new opportunities for employees within tech, data, and AI management industries; on the other hand, it is important to train the workers for such shifts and provide them with proper support(Kaasinen et al., 2020). As AI systems become more complex and embedded, the ability to understand why the AI has made a particular decision also known as "explainability" is also much more complicated. This lack of transparency can pose significant challenges when AI is used to make high-stakes decisions, such as in healthcare diagnoses or criminal sentencing(Bagaric et al., 2021). If a system makes the wrong decision, to determine who was at fault be it the developers who designed the system, the organization that employed the technology, or the AI itself is relatively complex. General guidelines and checks and balances on who is developing these systems are crucial to maintaining that these systems are responsible, explainable, and equitable. This also means ensuring that any AI systems used can be explained to the users who depend on them so that the rationale behind decisions can be easily understood and challenged when necessary.

AI is being used in the planning process and as it becomes more self-directing, many human beings are wondering how much decision-making ability they should turn over to machines(Farrow, 2022; Knox et al., 2020). In the meanwhile, the delegation of critical decision-making processes to AI poses risks of undersigning human agency and offering conclusive reliance on AI that is always swift and based only on relevant information. The problem with delegating decisions to AI is that the more we rely on it the more vulnerable we are to making mistakes or being manipulated by those systems(Candrian & Scherer, 2022). Businesses must take into account the ethical implications of how to have human control of the autonomous process, the ability to guarantee that the process has substantial human participation, and the risk associated with the reliance on autonomous AI systems. AI also has practical concerns in applications like self-driving cars, drones, and robotics, raising complex ethical dilemmas. For example, how should an autonomous vehicle react in a life-threatening situation where a decision must be made about whom to harm? Should AI systems prioritize human life over property? These ethical questions delve into deep philosophical territory about human values, moral decision-making, and the role of machines in critical life-and-death situations. Ensuring that AI will act in a way that will be compliant with norms and ethical standards will be a crucial step in making people accept the idea of having an autonomous system. While AI can propose high efficiency in terms of productivity and critically lower certain environmental impacts in some industries, a significant amount of energy is needed to train and run large-scale AI models (Waltersmann et al., 2021). Although the field is quite new, a recent issue that has been brought up and has implications regarding AI and the ethics of the future is the environmental impact of AI, particularly the carbon footprint associated with data centers and the hardware needed to support AI models. As, AI advances, it will be critical with advancing AI to strike a balance between advancing technology as well as offering environmental sustainability objectives. Organizations and researchers need to flow resources into efficient artificial intelligence solutions and related hardware, ensuring that any efficiency has the least possible negative impact on the environment.

AI's rise presents both remarkable opportunities and significant ethical challenges. Navigating these challenges requires collaboration involving technologists, policymakers, businesses, and ethicists to establish frameworks that prioritize fairness, transparency, accountability, and human dignity. Addressing these concerns in advance it will become certain that AI will be used further in a benevolent manner and will help to create a future in which technology and people thrive together.

CONCLUSION

The higher the level of decision-making implemented in the AI, the more vulnerable we are to mistakes or control by those systems. For this purpose, the threat of over-reliance on AI, the need for making human supervision and intervention meaningful, and the need to justify the extent of AI autonomy require ethical considerations. There is a need for the development of AI systems with an emphasis on the well-being of human beings so that the technologies will be in a position to benefit society. This includes the creation of AI systems with ethical considerations as the main goal of their work, and the main goal of the design of algorithms is the transparency of algorithms, the choice is non-biased, and aligned with human values. AI developers and adopting companies or organizations should focus on AI solutions that are aimed at improving profound human emotions and well-being, offering solutions for equality, and enabling access to the needed resources. Therefore, integrating well-being at the core of both AI engineering and use, the direction beneficial to people's well-being, in general, would be attainable and promote individual and social well-being in society. Integrating the role of AI and human resources is not just for the enhancement of organizational productivity but also for maintaining the worth of human capital in the workforce. This balance is important bearing in mind that AI is being integrated into the workplace as a tool to enhance productivity, innovation as well as better health and well-being of workers.

For future research, careful attention needs to be paid to the consequences AI will have on the overall workforce and employee psychological well-being, in addition to gaining a better understanding of the strategies for addressing ethical risks associated with AI adoption. In the future, the research should aim at properly managing human AI partnerships as a way of enhancing work arrangements in the face of emerging technologies around the globe. Also, it is high time to shift focus to the psychological effects that AI might have, and how to contain such effects as AI anxiety, job replacement, and emotional loneliness and on the other part, while also exploring how AI can be used to promote well-being. Workforce reskilling will be essential as AI transforms industries, with a focus on preparing employees for the new roles and skill sets required for successful AI-human collaboration. Lastly, as AI reshapes societal structures, future research should anticipate and address long-term social and cultural changes, ensuring that AI enhances the human experience without exacerbating existing challenges. By focusing on these areas, we can ensure that AI contributes positively to both individual well-being and societal progress.

REFERENCES

Al Naqbi, H., Bahroun, Z., & Ahmed, V. (2024). Enhancing Work Productivity through Generative Artificial Intelligence: A Comprehensive Literature Review. *Sustainability (Basel)*, *16*(3), 3. Advance online publication. DOI: 10.3390/su16031166

Aldoseri, A., Al-Khalifa, K. N., & Hamouda, A. M. (2024). AI-Powered Innovation in Digital Transformation: Key Pillars and Industry Impact. *Sustainability (Basel)*, *16*(5), 5. Advance online publication. DOI: 10.3390/su16051790

Arslan, A., Cooper, C., Khan, Z., Golgeci, I., & Ali, I. (2021). Artificial intelligence and human workers interaction at team level: A conceptual assessment of the challenges and potential HRM strategies. *International Journal of Manpower*, *43*(1), 75–88. DOI: 10.1108/IJM-01-2021-0052

Bagaric, M., Svilar, J., Bull, M., Hunter, D., & Stobbs, N. (2021). *The Solution to the Pervasive Bias and Discrimination in the Criminal Justice: Transparent Artificial Intelligence* (SSRN Scholarly Paper No. 3795911). Social Science Research Network. https://papers.ssrn.com/abstract=3795911

Baruwal Chhetri, M., Tariq, S., Singh, R., Jalalvand, F., Paris, C., & Nepal, S. (2024). Towards Human-AI Teaming to Mitigate Alert Fatigue in Security Operations Centres. *ACM Trans. Internet Technol.*, *24*(3), 12:1-12:22. DOI: 10.1145/3670009

Bhattacharyya, S. S. S., & Nair, S. (2019). Explicating the future of work: Perspectives from India. *Journal of Management Development*, *38*(3), 175–194. DOI: 10.1108/JMD-01-2019-0032

Bilen, E., & Hervé, J. (2024). *When AI Gives Bad Advice: Critical thinking in human-AI collaborations* (SSRN Scholarly Paper No. 5040466). Social Science Research Network. DOI: 10.2139/ssrn.5040466

Boysen, N., Schulze, P., & Scholl, A. (2022). Assembly line balancing: What happened in the last fifteen years? *European Journal of Operational Research*, *301*(3), 797–814. DOI: 10.1016/j.ejor.2021.11.043

Brynjolfsson, E., Mitchell, T., & Rock, D. (2018). What Can Machines Learn, and What Does It Mean for Occupations and the Economy? *AEA Papers and Proceedings. American Economic Association*, *108*, 43–47. DOI: 10.1257/pandp.20181019

Candrian, C., & Scherer, A. (2022). Rise of the machines: Delegating decisions to autonomous AI. *Computers in Human Behavior*, *134*, 107308. DOI: 10.1016/j.chb.2022.107308

Chakraborty, A. (2024). Navigating Career Anxiety in the Modern Age: Understanding Its Roots and Remedies. *International Journal of Interdisciplinary Approaches in Psychology, 2*(1), 13:24-13:24.

Chen, C. (2024). Influence of Employees' Intention to Adopt AI Applications and Big Data Analytical Capability on Operational Performance in the High-Tech Firms. *Journal of the Knowledge Economy, 15*(1), 3946–3974. DOI: 10.1007/s13132-023-01293-x PMID: 40478985

Chowdhury, S., Budhwar, P., Dey, P. K., Joel-Edgar, S., & Abadie, A. (2022). AI-employee collaboration and business performance: Integrating knowledge-based view, socio-technical systems, and organizational socialization framework. *Journal of Business Research, 144*, 31–49. DOI: 10.1016/j.jbusres.2022.01.069

Colaiacovo, B. (2024). *TECHNOLOGY-DRIVEN WORK ENVIRONMENTS: AN ATTRIBUTIONAL PERSPECTIVE ON EMPLOYEES¿ WELL-BEING*. https://tesidottorato.depositolegale.it/handle/20.500.14242/112816

Dey, D. N. C. (2024). *Harmonizing The Threads of Well-Being: AI (Artificial Intelligence), Spirituality, Healthcare, And Management* (SSRN Scholarly Paper No. 5002655). Social Science Research Network. DOI: 10.2139/ssrn.5002655

Dubey, R., Gunasekaran, A., Childe, S. J., Blome, C., & Papadopoulos, T. (2019). Big Data and Predictive Analytics and Manufacturing Performance: Integrating Institutional Theory, Resource-Based View and Big Data Culture. *British Journal of Management, 30*(2), 341–361. DOI: 10.1111/1467-8551.12355

Enstroem, R., Kang, P. S., & Bhawna, B. (2024). The harmonized information-technology and organizational performance model (HI-TOP). *International Journal of Organizational Analysis, ahead-of-print*(ahead-of-print). DOI: 10.1108/IJOA-03-2024-4403

Estlund, C. (2021). *Automation Anxiety: Why and How to Save Work*. Oxford University Press. DOI: 10.1093/oso/9780197566107.001.0001

Farrow, E. (2022). Determining the human-to-workforce ratio – Exploring future organizational scenarios and the implications for anticipatory workforce planning. *Technology in Society, 68*, 101879. DOI: 10.1016/j.techsoc.2022.101879

George, D. A. S. (2024). Automated Futures: Examining the Promise and Peril of AI on Jobs, Productivity, and Work-Life Balance. *Partners Universal Innovative Research Publication, 2*(6), 6. Advance online publication. DOI: 10.5281/zenodo.14544519

George, D. A. S., & George, A. S. H. (2024). Towards a Super Smart Society 5.0: Opportunities and Challenges of Integrating Emerging Technologies for Social Innovation. *Partners Universal International Research Journal*, *3*(2), 2. Advance online publication. DOI: 10.5281/zenodo.11522048

Ghosh, B., Daugherty, P. R., Wilson, H. J., & Burden, A. (2019). *Taking a Systems Approach to Adopting AI.*

Gohil, M. G. (2023). A study on the impact of Artificial Intelligence (AI), automation, and digital transformation on society. *Revista Review Index Journal of Multidisciplinary*, *3*(4), 4. Advance online publication. DOI: 10.31305/rrijm2023.v03.n04.004

Hess, D. J., & Sovacool, B. K. (2020). Sociotechnical matters: Reviewing and integrating science and technology studies with energy social science. *Energy Research & Social Science*, *65*, 101462. DOI: 10.1016/j.erss.2020.101462

Hsu, Y.-C., Huang, T.-H., Verma, H., Mauri, A., Nourbakhsh, I., & Bozzon, A. (2022). Empowering local communities using artificial intelligence. *Patterns (New York, N.Y.)*, *3*(3), 100449. Advance online publication. DOI: 10.1016/j.patter.2022.100449 PMID: 35510187

Ishengoma, F. (2024). Revisiting the TAM: Adapting the model to advanced technologies and evolving user behaviors. *The Electronic Library*, *42*(6), 1055–1073. DOI: 10.1108/EL-06-2024-0166

Isiaku, L., & Adalier, A. (2024). Determinants of business intelligence systems adoption in Nigerian banks: The role of perceived usefulness and ease of use. *Information Development*, *02666669241307024*, 02666669241307024. Advance online publication. DOI: 10.1177/02666669241307024

Jiang, N., Liu, X., Liu, H., Lim, E. T. K., Tan, C.-W., & Gu, J. (2022). Beyond AI-powered context-aware services: The role of human–AI collaboration. *Industrial Management &amp. Industrial Management & Data Systems*, *123*(11), 2771–2802. DOI: 10.1108/IMDS-03-2022-0152

Joo, B.-K., Yim, J.-H., Jin, Y. S., & Han, S. J. (2022). Empowering leadership and employee creativity: The mediating roles of work engagement and knowledge sharing. *European Journal of Training and Development*, *47*(9), 881–899. DOI: 10.1108/EJTD-02-2022-0016

Kaaria, A. G. (2024). Artificial Intelligence and Employee Well-Being: Balancing Technological Progressions with Human-Centric Workplace Strategies, a Research Agenda. *East African Journal of Information Technology*, *7*(1), 1. Advance online publication. DOI: 10.37284/eajit.7.1.2281

Kaasinen, E., Schmalfuß, F., Özturk, C., Aromaa, S., Boubekeur, M., Heilala, J., Heikkilä, P., Kuula, T., Liinasuo, M., Mach, S., Mehta, R., Petäjä, E., & Walter, T. (2020). Empowering and engaging industrial workers with Operator 4.0 solutions. *Computers & Industrial Engineering*, *139*, 105678. DOI: 10.1016/j.cie.2019.01.052

Kelly, M., Soles, R., Garcia, E., & Kundu, I. (2020). Job Stress, Burnout, Work-Life Balance, Well-Being, and Job Satisfaction Among Pathology Residents and Fellows. *American Journal of Clinical Pathology*, *153*(4), 449–469. DOI: 10.1093/ajcp/aqaa013 PMID: 32080717

Khogali, H. O., & Mekid, S. (2023). The blended future of automation and AI: Examining some long-term societal and ethical impact features. *Technology in Society*, *73*, 102232. DOI: 10.1016/j.techsoc.2023.102232

Knox, J., Williamson, B., & Bayne, S. (2020). Machine behaviourism: Future visions of 'learnification' and 'datafication' across humans and digital technologies. *Learning, Media and Technology*, *45*(1), 31–45. DOI: 10.1080/17439884.2019.1623251

Kolade, O., & Owoseni, A. (2022). Employment 5.0: The work of the future and the future of work. *Technology in Society*, *71*, 102086. DOI: 10.1016/j.techsoc.2022.102086

Kyriakidou, O., Goumas, B., Manteli, M., & Tasoula, E. (2025). AI and the Future of Work: Bridging Divides for Marginalised Workers. In *AI and Diversity in a Datafied World of Work: Will the Future of Work be Inclusive?* (world; Vol. 12, pp. 205–224). Emerald Publishing Limited. DOI: 10.1108/S2051-233320250000012023

Loureiro, S. M. C., Bilro, R. G., & Neto, D. (2023). Working with AI: Can stress bring happiness? *Service Business*, *17*(1), 233–255. DOI: 10.1007/s11628-022-00514-8

Martín-García, A. V., Redolat, R., & Pinazo-Hernandis, S. (2022). Factors Influencing Intention to Technological Use in Older Adults. The TAM Model Aplication. *Research on Aging*, *44*(7–8), 573–588. DOI: 10.1177/01640275211063797 PMID: 34962846

Mohd Amir, R. I., Mohd, I. H., Saad, S., Abu Seman, S. A., & Tuan Besar, T. B. H. (2020). Perceived Ease of Use, Perceived Usefulness, and Behavioral Intention: The Acceptance of Crowdsourcing Platform by Using Technology Acceptance Model (TAM). In Kaur, N., & Ahmad, M. (Eds.), *Charting a Sustainable Future of ASEAN in Business and Social Sciences* (pp. 403–410). Springer., DOI: 10.1007/978-981-15-3859-9_34

Ojo, Y., Makinde, O. A., Babatunde, O. V., Babatunde, G., & Okeowo, S. (2025). Evaluating AI-Driven Mental Health Solutions: A Hybrid Fuzzy Multi-Criteria Decision-Making Approach. *AI*, *6*(1), 1. Advance online publication. DOI: 10.3390/ai6010014

Olawade, D. B., Wada, O. Z., Odetayo, A., David-Olawade, A. C., Asaolu, F., & Eberhardt, J. (2024). Enhancing mental health with Artificial Intelligence: Current trends and future prospects. *Journal of Medicine, Surgery, and Public Health*, *3*, 100099. DOI: 10.1016/j.glmedi.2024.100099

Pektaş, T. (2024). THE IMPACT OF ARTIFICIAL INTELLIGENCE ANXIETY ON EMPLOYEES: A COMPREHENSIVE REVI. *International Journal of Education Technology and Scientific Researches*, *26*, 26. Advance online publication. DOI: 10.35826/ijetsar.733

Pyae, A., Ravyse, W., Luimula, M., Pizarro-Lucas, E., Sanchez, P. L., Dorado-Diaz, I. P., & Thaw, A. K. (2023). Exploring User Experience and Usability in a Metaverse Learning Environment for Students: A Usability Study of the Artificial Intelligence, Innovation, and Society (AIIS). *Electronics (Basel)*, *12*(20), 20. Advance online publication. DOI: 10.3390/electronics12204283

Rajagopal, N. K., Qureshi, N. I., Durga, S., Ramirez Asis, E. H., Huerta Soto, R. M., Gupta, S. K., & Deepak, S. (2022). Future of Business Culture: An Artificial Intelligence-Driven Digital Framework for Organization Decision-Making Process. *Complexity*, *2022*(1), 7796507. DOI: 10.1155/2022/7796507

Rampersad, G. (2020). Robot will take your job: Innovation for an era of artificial intelligence. *Journal of Business Research*, *116*, 68–74. DOI: 10.1016/j.jbusres.2020.05.019

Review, M. S. M. (2020). *How AI Is Transforming the Organization*. MIT Press. DOI: 10.7551/mitpress/12588.001.0001

Ripp, J. (2021). Cognitive Load as a Mediator of the Relationship Between Workplace Efficiency and Well-Being. *Joint Commission Journal on Quality and Patient Safety*, *47*(2), 74–75. DOI: 10.1016/j.jcjq.2020.12.002 PMID: 33358324

Santi, I. H., & Erdani, B. (2021). *TECHNOLOGY ACCEPTANCE MODEL (TAM)*. Penerbit NEM.

Schrape, J.-F. (2025). *Artificial Intelligence and Social Action: A techno-sociological contextualization* (Vols. 2025–03). Universität Stuttgart, Fak. 10 Wirtschafts- und Sozialwissenschaften, Institut für Sozialwissenschaften Abt. VI Organisations- und Innovationssoziologie.

50. Shneiderman, B. (2020). Human-Centered Artificial Intelligence: Reliable, Safe & Trustworthy. *International Journal of Human-Computer Interaction, 36*(6), 495–504. DOI: 10.1080/10447318.2020.1741118

Sima, V., Gheorghe, I. G., Subić, J., & Nancu, D. (2020). Influences of the Industry 4.0 Revolution on the Human Capital Development and Consumer Behavior: A Systematic Review. *Sustainability (Basel), 12*(10), 10. Advance online publication. DOI: 10.3390/su12104035

Singh, M., Naval, P., Patil, N., Tiwari, M., Ashok, V., & Katikar, S. M. (2024). Understanding the Strengths and Limitations of AI for Data Access Optimization. *2024 15th International Conference on Computing Communication and Networking Technologies (ICCCNT)*, 1–6. DOI: 10.1109/ICCCNT61001.2024.10724814

Soch, N. N., Hogan, M., Harney, O., Hanlon, M., Brady, C., & McGrattan, L. (2022). *Developing a Utopian Model of Human-Technology Interaction: Collective Intelligence Applications in Support of Future Well-Being*. DOI: 10.5325/utopianstudies.33.1.0054

Sony, M., & Naik, S. (2020). Industry 4.0 integration with socio-technical systems theory: A systematic review and proposed theoretical model. *Technology in Society, 61*, 101248. DOI: 10.1016/j.techsoc.2020.101248

Sotskov, Y. N. (2023). Assembly and Production Line Designing, Balancing and Scheduling with Inaccurate Data: A Survey and Perspectives. *Algorithms, 16*(2), 2. Advance online publication. DOI: 10.3390/a16020100

The Future of Jobs Report 2023. (2023). World Economic Forum. https://www.weforum.org/publications/the-future-of-jobs-report-2023/

Thomas, A. (2024). Digitally transforming the organization through knowledge management: A socio-technical system (STS) perspective. *European Journal of Innovation Management, 27*(9), 437–460. DOI: 10.1108/EJIM-02-2024-0114

Tschang, F. T., & Almirall, E. (2021). Artificial Intelligence as Augmenting Automation: Implications for Employment. *The Academy of Management Perspectives, 35*(4), 642–659. DOI: 10.5465/amp.2019.0062

Vasiliu, V., & Yavetz, G. (2024). Who's afraid of AI? Socio-technological perspectives on artificial intelligence in the workforce: an Israeli case study. *Aslib Journal of Information Management, ahead-of-print*(ahead-of-print). DOI: 10.1108/AJIM-12-2023-0562

Waltersmann, L., Kiemel, S., Stuhlsatz, J., Sauer, A., & Miehe, R. (2021). Artificial Intelligence Applications for Increasing Resource Efficiency in Manufacturing Companies—A Comprehensive Review. *Sustainability (Basel)*, *13*(12), 12. Advance online publication. DOI: 10.3390/su13126689

Yadegari, M., Mohammadi, S., & Masoumi, A. H. (2024). Technology adoption: An analysis of the major models and theories. *Technology Analysis and Strategic Management*, *36*(6), 1096–1110. DOI: 10.1080/09537325.2022.2071255

Yu, X., Xu, S., & Ashton, M. (2022). Antecedents and outcomes of artificial intelligence adoption and application in the workplace: The socio-technical system theory perspective. *Information Technology &amp. Information Technology & People*, *36*(1), 454–474. DOI: 10.1108/ITP-04-2021-0254

ADDITIONAL READING

Alter, S. (2022). Understanding artificial intelligence in the context of usage: Contributions and smartness of algorithmic capabilities in work systems. *International Journal of Information Management*, *67*, 102392. DOI: 10.1016/j.ijinfomgt.2021.102392

Appelbaum, S. H. (1997). Socio-technical systems theory: An intervention strategy for organizational development. *Management Decision*, *35*(6), 452–463. DOI: 10.1108/00251749710173823

Gupta, D., Singhal, A., Sharma, S., Hasan, A., & Raghuwanshi, S. (2023). Humans' Emotional and Mental Well-Being under the Influence of Artificial Intelligence. *Journal for ReAttach Therapy and Developmental Diversities*, *6*(6s), 184–197.

Nazareno, L., & Schiff, D. S. (2021). The impact of automation and artificial intelligence on worker well-being. *Technology in Society*, *67*, 101679. DOI: 10.1016/j.techsoc.2021.101679

Safdar, N. M., Banja, J. D., & Meltzer, C. C. (2020). Ethical considerations in artificial intelligence. *European Journal of Radiology*, *122*, 108768. DOI: 10.1016/j.ejrad.2019.108768 PMID: 31786504

Chapter 8
Applications of Artificial Intelligence Use in Therapeutic Interventions: A Multidisciplinary Approach

Lara Carneiro
https://orcid.org/0000-0002-4385-5290
United Arab Emirates University, UAE

Ana Gomes
https://orcid.org/0009-0005-6230-1399
New York University, Abu Dhabi, UAE

ABSTRACT

Mental health care faces challenges such as limited access, stigma, and resource shortages. Artificial Intelligence (AI) offers solutions such as early diagnosis, personalized therapies, through virtual platforms, and machine-learning database. AI allows improvement of therapeutic outcomes and shows potential for reducing disparities worldwide. Applications like chatbots and health apps can enhance support through real-time engagement and data-driven insights. In hybrid care models, AI can assist therapists and patients by providing valuable data insights, support decision making, and provide personalized care and accurate real-time feedback. However, concerns about the lack of human interaction, trust, and empathy persist. Ethical concerns around privacy, consent, and bias must be addressed. Regulatory frameworks, such as the EU's AI Act, aim to ensure safe and ethical AI use. For successful integration, ongoing research, funding, professional training,

DOI: 10.4018/979-8-3373-5072-1.ch008

and interdisciplinary collaboration are essential.

INTRODUCTION

Artificial Intelligence: A Brief Introduction

The growth of artificial intelligence (AI) has undeniably been instrumental in shaping the development of the internet (Liu et al., 2017). Over the past decade, AI has become increasingly integrated into society, playing a more prominent role in people's everyday lives (Dwivedi et al., 2023). This introduction explores the concept of AI. Before defining "AI," it is important to clarify the concept of "intelligence."

There are different ways of conceiving intelligence (Sternberg, 2021). It can be viewed as a psychometric trait like general intelligence (g), an information-processing construct such as working memory, a biological attribute rooted in the brain, or even as a developmental process that evolves over time (Sternberg, 1990). Howard Gardner's "Theory of Multiple Intelligence," took a distinct approach to intelligence (Julita, 2024). According to Gardner's theory, there are eight distinct types of intelligence: linguistic, logical-mathematical, spatial, musical, bodily-kinesthetic, naturalistic, interpersonal, and intrapersonal intelligence (Davis et al., 2011; Gardner, 2011). Defining human intelligence in a way that gains broad consensus has proven difficult, a challenge similarly reflected in the varied interpretations of AI within computer science (Gignac & Szodorai, 2024).

AI represents a modern branch of technological science dedicated to exploring and advancing theories, methodologies, technologies, and application systems designed to replicate, enhance, and elevate human intelligence (Huawei Technologies, 2023).

The modern origins of AI can be traced to the Turing Test introduced by Alan M. Turing, often regarded as "the Father of Artificial Intelligence," in 1950 (Guo, 2015; Huawei Technologies, 2023; Turing, 1950). It has been more than 75 years since he published his groundbreaking paper, 'Computing Machinery and Intelligence,' in Mind (Turing, 1950). In Turing´s paper, several questions were raised, one of which was whether computers could ever be considered capable of "thinking". He also introduced various criteria, including his Imitation Game, to help determine if a computer could be regarded as "intelligent" (Luger & Chakrabarti, 2017).

Based on his premise, if a computer can converse with humans without being recognized as a machine, it is considered to possess intelligence (Huawei Technologies, 2023).

While AI as a concept has only existed for a few decades, its theoretical foundations and supporting technologies have evolved over a much longer period (Russell & Norvig, 2011). The current success of AI is the result of progress in related fields and the combined efforts of scientists across generations (Huawei Technologies, 2023).

Therefore, AI has been hailed as the "fourth industrial revolution", bringing transformative global impacts across various fields, including public health (Murphy et al., 2021).

Indeed, AI has become a groundbreaking force, including its impactful application in mental healthcare (Olawade et al., 2024), and the convergence of AI and mental healthcare fields marks a significant transformation in medical care (E. Lee et al., 2021).

AI can be broadly defined as a field of study that integrates computer science, engineering, and related disciplines to create machines capable of performing behaviors that would be considered intelligent if observed in humans (House of Lords, 2018).

AI draws from a variety of disciplines, including mathematics (to develop algorithms), biology, philosophy, psychology, neuroscience (to explore the human mind and behavior), statistics (to manage and analyze large datasets), and, most importantly, computer science (to execute algorithms and apply concepts in practice; Ghosh & Arunachalam, 2021).

AI generally refers to a computerized system: hardware (such as an Amazon Echo running the Alexa digital assistant software) or software (such as Google Assistant running on Android devices or Siri running on Apple devices) that can perform tasks or reasoning processes that we usually associate with intelligence in a human being (Cho et al., 2015; Vaidyam et al., 2019).

This chapter explores the expanding role of AI in mental health, emphasizing its contributions, applications, and multidisciplinary approach.

Section 1 begins by exploring the interplay between AI and mental health (1). It then analyzes how AI-driven applications are transforming mental health care, highlighting various AI tools currently utilized in this field (2). Finally, the section addresses ethical considerations surrounding the use of AI in mental health (3).

Section 2 explores the application of AI as a multidisciplinary approach in therapy, highlighting its role in psychological practice (1). The section further investigates how AI supports mental health professionals by enhancing diagnostics and treatment processes (2). It distinguishes AI from cognitive computing, discussing the benefits and risks associated with these technologies (3). It also examines the effectiveness of AI in delivering evidence-based computerized cognitive behavioral therapy (CBT; 4).

THE INTERPLAY OF AI AND MENTAL HEALTH

Background

According to the World Health Organization (WHO, 2022a), action toward prevention and early intervention in mental health is urgently needed and indisputable.

Mental health care faces numerous challenges, including limited access to services, stigma, shortages of trained professionals, inadequate financial resources, the digital divide, and delays in early diagnosis (McGinty, 2023; Wainberg et al., 2017).

The global rise in mental health challenges has reached pandemic proportions, accounting for around 16% of the total disease burden worldwide (Arias et al., 2022). Major conditions like depression and anxiety lead to an estimated annual economic loss of 1 trillion USD due to reduced productivity, underscoring the critical need for effective interventions (The Lancet Global Health, 2020).

For instance, the WHO has set the "triple billion" target, aiming to ensure that 1 billion more people benefit from universal health coverage, are better protected from health emergencies, and experience improved health and wellbeing. The WHO (2025a) believes that AI can play a key role in achieving these goals.

The number of publications on mental health and AI has grown significantly in recent years (S. Zhou et al., 2022). In mental healthcare, where understanding complex human behaviors and emotions is crucial, AI has the potential to revolutionize the field by offering insights and solutions that were previously unattainable through conventional methods (Nilsen et al., 2022).

Various tools are currently under development. These include digital tracking of depression and mood via keyboard interaction, speech, voice, facial recognition, sensors, and interactive chatbots (Eltahawy et al., 2024; Firth et al., 2017; Fitzpatrick et al., 2017; Karkosz et al., 2024).

AI systems can also detect micro-expressions and subtle facial feature changes that could reveal underlying psychological conditions (Zhao & X. Li, 2019). Micro-expressions are a form of non-verbal communication that unintentionally reveal a person's true emotions (Navukkarasu et al., 2023).

Chatbots can be especially beneficial for individuals who feel uneasy sharing their emotions with another person (Vaidyam et al., 2019). For instance, veterans, who frequently hesitate to share their experiences after a tour of duty, were much more likely to engage with a chatbot when informed it was a virtual therapist rather than being operated by a human (Lucas et al., 2014). This approach shows promise in improving access to necessary care (Tanielian & Jaycox, 2008).

Additionally, machine learning has been explored by clinical psychology and psychiatry (Dwyer et al., 2018) to predict the efficacy of antidepressant medication (Chekroud et al., 2016), characterising depression (Wager & Woo, 2017), and predicting depression (Yoo et al., 2024) and suicide (Walsh et al., 2017). AI can also help to differentiate overlapping clinical presentations (Dwyer et al., 2018). Examples include the identification of unipolar versus bipolar depression (Redlich et al., 2014) or the differentiation between different types of Alzheimer´s (Xue et al., 2024).

AI is a transformative tool, enabling advanced detection methods, personalized therapies, and virtual therapeutic platforms. It can potentially expand healthcare access, reduce stigma, and enhance treatment outcomes (Johnson et al., 2021). A significant application of AI in mental health awareness is the analysis and regulation of social media data. Platforms such as Twitter and Instagram offer a rich source of user-generated content that can be leveraged to assess public sentiment on mental health topics. AI-driven sentiment analysis algorithms can identify emotions conveyed in posts, allowing researchers and mental health organizations to track changes in public discourse and identify critical topics requiring focused awareness (Mowery et al., 2017).

AI has also become a powerful tool for the early detection and diagnosis of mental health disorders (Abd-alrazaq et al., 2022). The primary diagnostic tools used by mental health professionals to identify and classify mental disorders based on symptom type, intensity, and duration are the Diagnostic and Statistical Manual of Mental Disorders (DSM; Regier et al., 2013) and the International Classification of Diseases (ICD; WHO, 2025b). The DSM system is more commonly used by researchers, whereas the ICD serves as a legally required health data standard (Stein et al., 2022). Although these tools are widely used, they have certain limitations (Tutun et al., 2022).

Despite the availability of numerous diagnostic guidelines and tools, many mental health professionals continue to face challenges in diagnosing patients accurately and efficiently.

As a result, recent literature has emphasized the need for further research into advanced technologies, such as AI, to develop decision support systems (DSSs; Balcombe & De Leo, 2021). These systems aim to assist mental health professionals in making evidence-based treatment decisions and to support policymakers in implementing digital mental health solutions.

AI Applications in Mental Health Care

The integration of AI into mental health care has led to the development of innovative tools designed to improve emotional well-being and enhance therapeutic outcomes.

This section highlights some examples of AI-powered solutions currently used in mental health care, categorized into chatbot-based therapy, emotional health apps, and smart mental health tools.

Chatbot-based therapy

- **Woebot**. (n.d). *Woebot*. https://woebothealth.com

Operates on a rules-based system. Its dialogues are crafted by conversational writers who incorporate principles from CBT, Interpersonal Psychotherapy (IPT), and Dialectical Behavioral Therapy (DBT), with input from clinical experts;

- **Betterhelp**. (n.d). BetterHelp. https://www.betterhelp.com

It's a multimodal digital psychotherapy platform that links individuals to licensed therapists. It utilizes AI for therapist-patient matching and provides access to a wide variety of therapeutic methods, such as CBT and psychodynamic therapy;

- **Youper. (n.d). Youper.**https://www.youper.ai/

It's a mental health chatbot app that uses CBT and Positive Psychology techniques to help users manage their mental health. YOUPER combines psychology and AI to understand users' emotional needs and engage in natural conversations.

Emotional Health Apps

- **Superbetter**. (n.d.) *SuperBetter.*https://superbetter.com

This app is designed to boost resilience and help users reach their goals through a gamified approach. It features a range of challenges and rewards to keep users motivated and track their progress. SUPERBETTER presents a promising model for disseminating evidence-based practices (Chou et al., 2017);

- **Calm.** (n.d). *Calm*. https://www.calm.com

It's an app that provides guided meditation and mindfulness exercises. It also includes relaxation and sleep support features, such as sleep stories and soothing ambient sounds.

Smart Mental Health Tools

- **Kintsugi**. (n.d). *Kintsugi Health.*https://www.kintsugihealth.com

Employs facial and voice analysis to deliver real-time emotional insights to therapists, supporting the early identification of emotional distress (Olawade et al., 2024);

- **Mindstrong Health**. (n.d). *Mindstrong Health.* https://mindstrong.health/

Uses AI to analyze smartphone keyboard interactions during teletherapy sessions, offering therapists valuable insights into a patient's emotional state (Tom Gruber, 2025).

To sum up, chatbots (Marcelle et al., 2019; Mehta et al., 2021), emotional health apps (Huberty et al., 2019), and smart mental health tools (Melnyk et al., 2022) represent a promising innovation for mental health care apps, offering the potential to deliver effective and accessible evidence-based therapies. However, as this technology is still in its early stages, limited information is available about newly developed apps, their features, and their effectiveness (Casu et al., 2024; Huberty et al., 2019; Koh et al., 2022).

Ethical Considerations in AI for Mental Health

AI in mental healthcare offers several benefits such as improved diagnostics, personalized treatment and increased access to mental health support (Thakkar et al., 2024).

While AI holds promise for advancing health equity, it is crucial to address its ethical implications to minimize potential harms, especially for the most vulnerable populations (Murphy et al., 2021).

Ensuring the responsible and effective use of AI in mental healthcare requires careful attention to ethical considerations (Olawade et al., 2024). Striking a balance between the benefits of AI and ethical issues is essential to ensure these technological advancements are used responsibly and prioritize the well-being of patients (Khawaja & Bélisle-Pipon, 2023).

The application of AI in healthcare, especially in sensitive domains like mental health, presents complex ethical challenges, including concerns about privacy, consent, transparency, accountability, bias, and the risk of unintended harm (Thakkar et al., 2024).

Another key challenge in the field is the lack of clear and comprehensive regulatory frameworks to govern the use of AI in mental health (Rodrigues, 2020). Regulatory frameworks for AI are essential to mitigate risks and promote AI's ethical, secure, and effective application in healthcare and population health (Schmidt et al., 2024).

A recent review explored the regulatory shortcomings and potential health risks associated with AI-powered wellness apps, particularly their management of mental health crises in the absence of adequate oversight (De Freitas & Cohen, 2024). According to the authors, most wellness apps powered by generative AI are unlikely to undergo evaluation by the Food and Drug Administration (FDA) or other health authorities.

In February 2024, the Council and the European Parliament (EP, 2024) agreed on the Artificial Intelligence Regulation (AI Act, AIA). This regulation evaluates AI applications to ensure they are used ethically and responsibly, promoting the development of safe and lawful AI across the EU's single market (Cancela-Outeda, 2024). This is especially crucial for the healthcare sector, as other current harmonization laws, like the Medical Device Regulation, do not specifically address medical AI applications (F. Busch et al., 2024).

Below, we will explore some key issues, including privacy and confidentiality, informed consent, bias and fairness, transparency, explainability, accountability, autonomy and human agency.

Privacy and Confidentiality

AI systems frequently process vast amounts of sensitive personal data, making it essential to handle this information securely and uphold individuals' privacy rights (Khalid et al., 2023; Villegas-Ch & García-Ortiz, 2023). Managing personal data in AI requires implementing policies and practices that safeguard individual privacy (Villegas-Ch & García-Ortiz, 2023).

Various techniques and approaches are used to protect privacy in AI. Some of them include:

1. Data anonymization techniques can be employed to remove or mask personally identifiable information from datasets used in AI, ensuring that the data cannot be directly linked to specific individuals (S. Li et al., 2021);

2. Minimizing the collection of personal information involves reducing the gathering of unnecessary data in AI systems. This can be achieved by limiting the amount of personal data collected and utilizing techniques such as aggregation and tokenization to minimize the exposure of personally identifiable information (Younis et al., 2024);
3. Use of differential privacy techniques: Differential privacy is a technique that adds controlled noise to the data so that the AI results do not reveal sensitive information about specific individuals. This protects an individual's data privacy without compromising the model's utility (Villegas-Ch & García-Ortiz, 2023).

In the process of developing AI systems, it is essential to adopt an approach that emphasizes privacy. This means considering privacy issues in all phases of the AI lifecycle, from data collection to model deployment, to address privacy challenges adequately.

Informed Consent

Informed consent is the quintessential document maintained by professionals in the provision of mental health services (Bradshaw et al., 2014). It is vital to ensure individuals are fully informed about how their data will be used, along with the potential risks and benefits of AI-based interventions. Securing informed consent before implementation is crucial (Solaiman et al., 2024; Ursin et al., 2021). Patients should be informed about how their data will be used and the possible implications of AI-driven mental health interventions. Informed consent is particularly important considering the sensitive nature of mental health data (Rigby, 2019).

Obtaining consent for applications used outside medical systems could present significant challenges (Fiske et al., 2019). For example, an elderly person or someone with intellectual disabilities may struggle to understand the nature or function of a robot installed at home to monitor their activities, potentially leading to privacy violations (Vandemeulebroucke et al., 2018).

Bias and Fairness

Some researchers have highlighted the potential of AI to reduce existing biases within healthcare systems (Murphy et al., 2021). Examples of this potential include minimizing human error (Markowetzs et al., 2014) and addressing cognitive biases in healthcare providers' treatment decisions—such as recency, anchoring, or availability biases (Paul et al., n.d.).

The recency effect is a cognitive bias in which those items, ideas, or arguments that came last are remembered more clearly than those that came first (Turvey & Freeman, 2012).

- Example: A mental health professional who recently diagnosed a patient with borderline personality disorder (BPD) might overidentify the same condition in another patient exhibiting some overlapping symptoms, even if the broader clinical picture suggests generalized anxiety disorder (GAD) instead.

To reduce recency bias, AI systems could analyze large datasets to provide evidence-based probabilities, ensuring clinicians focus on the most statistically likely conditions rather than overemphasizing recent cases (G. Smith & Rustagi, 2020).

Another cognitive bias is anchoring bias, wherein physicians focus on a single—often initial—piece of information when formulating a diagnosis without sufficiently adjusting to later information (Croskerry, 2020).

- Example: A psychiatrist may anchor their diagnosis on a patient's initial report of “feeling sad all the time” and diagnose depression without adequately exploring other symptoms, potentially missing a bipolar disorder diagnosis that includes hypomanic episodes.

To address anchoring bias, AI tools that track symptom progression could prompt clinicians to reconsider initial diagnoses and explore alternative explanations as new data emerges (Zheng et al., 2024).

Availability Bias leads to diagnostic errors and arises when clinicians are overly influenced by cases they remember most vividly, even if those cases are rare or atypical (P. Li et al., 2020).

- Example: A therapist who recently treated a high-profile case of post-traumatic stress disorder (PTSD) might overestimate its prevalence and prematurely diagnose PTSD in a patient reporting sleep disturbances, ignoring other possibilities such as insomnia or generalized anxiety disorder.

To counteract availability bias, AI could highlight less memorable but more common conditions, helping clinicians avoid overdiagnosis of rare disorders based on vivid past experiences (Ly et al., 2023).

Transparency, Explainability, and Accountability

All algorithms utilized in mental health must be transparent and explainable. Patients and healthcare providers need to comprehend how AI systems make decisions to promote accountability and foster trust (Thakkar et al., 2024).

The involvement of AI systems in mental healthcare treatment raises important questions about accountability and liability. A common question being raised is who should be held responsible for errors in the use of AI technology in clinical and at-home care delivery. The question has frequently emerged due to the complexity of AI processes, which are often difficult for many individuals to understand and explain, limiting the ability of the output of AI systems (House of Lords, 2018) to be critically assessed.

Autonomy and Human Agency

The integration of AI into mental health care has raised critical questions about autonomy and human agency (Alowais et al., 2023). Autonomy, defined as the ability to make independent decisions guided by one's own values and beliefs, is a cornerstone of ethical practice in mental health (Prunkl, 2024).

Human agency, closely linked to autonomy, refers to an individual's capacity to act intentionally and make meaningful choices. In the context of AI-driven mental health solutions, these concepts become both vital and complex. Although AI technologies can enhance decision-making processes, human oversight remains crucial to ensure that interventions are consistent with users' preferences and values (Fanni et al., 2023; Love, 2023).

To summarize, AI in mental healthcare provides improved diagnostics, personalized treatments, and enhanced access to support, but ethical concerns must be addressed to protect vulnerable populations. Key ethical challenges include privacy, informed consent, transparency, bias, accountability, and unintended harm, necessitating frameworks like the EU's AI Act. Privacy can be safeguarded with data anonymization, differential privacy, and limited data collection. Informed consent is critical in mental health to ensure individuals understand data use and risks. Transparency and accountability are vital for trust and oversight, ensuring AI interventions align with patient autonomy and values.

THE APPLICATION OF AI AS A MULTIDISCIPLINARY APPROACH IN THERAPY

Background

Several studies have been shown an increase in the prevalence of mental disorders in the global population, highly amplified by the Covid-19 pandemic (Busetta et al., 2021; Kola et al., 2021; Kopelovich et al., 2021; Lim et al., 2022; Nochaiwong et al., 2021; Santomauro et al., 2021; Wang et al., 2020; Williams & Cooper, 2020), and pointing to a particular concern during adolescence and early adulthood (Dick & Ferguson, 2015; Divin et al., 2018; Goodwin et al., 2020; Gustavson et al., 2018; Kieling et al., 2011; Melcher & Tourous, 2020; Niermann et al., 2021; Patel et al., 2018). Worldwide mental health services have been lacking in efficient responses to the increase in mental health disease mainly due to: (1) the severe shortage of mental health practitioners (Barrón-Velázquez et al., 2024; Looi et al., 2024; Satiani et al., 2018; WHO, 2022b; Yellowlees, 2022); (2) the direct consequences of economic breakdown (Cuellar et al., 2020; Islam et al., 2022; Martinez et al., 2020; Silva et al., 2020); (3) the geographic location and accessibility (WHO, 2022b); and (4) the individual's subjective stigma around mental health and willingness to request formal support (Aktan et al., 2022; Corrigan 2020). These factors have brought a negative impact on the available mental health support to the general population and, consequently, an increased need for the development of new ways of delivering appropriate mental health support worldwide. The development of innovative responses to the growing crisis has become crucial, tailoring mental health intervention alternatives to the traditional psychotherapeutic setting.

The widespread adoption of smartphones (Business Wire, 2012; Krebs & Duncan, 2015; N. Shah, 2014; A. Smith, 2013) has been the first response to reduce the negative impacts of the above-mentioned factors. Mobile Mental Health (mHealth) has been an emergent alternative response, integrating telemedicine or telehealth (A. Busch et al., 2021; Dong & Bouey, 2020; Hohman et al., 2022), texting applications, mental health smartphone applications, social media (Figueroa & Aguilera, 2020), interactive audio and/or video interfaces, patient remote monitoring, online mental health surveys, telephone-based hotlines, and online mental health educational materials (Ojha & Syed, 2020). However, to date, the effectiveness of these resources has been inconsistent in research (Lecomte et al., 2020). The inconsistent findings have origins in the quality and veracity of evidence-based information delivered, drop-out rates, and usability factors (Alqahtani & Orji, 2019; Huckvale et al., 2020; Lecomte et al., 2020; Roepke et al., 2015; Vaidyam et al., 2019). A systematic review exposes a dissonance between the use and adherence to mental health apps in research (44% to 99%) and real-world settings (1% to 29%; Fleming et al., 2018).

Although there are more than 20,000 mental health and wellness apps worldwide (Clay, 2021; Torous & Roberts, 2017) created to support mental wellbeing, they are mostly focused on delivering information and exercises in a self-help manner, limiting any potential connection, one of the key predictors of treatment response (Torous et al., 2019).

Application of AI in Psychological Practice

The use of AI chatbots has expanded applications for psychological support and therapy that include talk-based therapies for mild to moderate mental health problems, social interaction, assistance with coping with mental and physical conditions, facilitating communication with humans, and eliminating time and space constraints (Kuhail et al., 2024). AI chatbots, such as chat GPT, show the potential to reduce the stigma of face-to-face therapy, and consequently improve help seeking behavior for psychological support, especially in the age range of young adulthood (Hoffman et al., 2024) and adolescence (Alfano et al., 2023). YOUPER is another example of AI chatbot that aims to understand users´ emotional needs and engage in natural conversations. This chatbot shows a decrease in symptoms of anxiety in the first two weeks of app use, results that were maintained in the subsequent two weeks (Mehta et al., 2021). The same study suggested similar results to symptoms of depression, with a slight increase in symptoms after two weeks of app use. According to the recent work of I. Lee and Hahn (2024), chatbot messages are perceived as more effective if considered human-like minds by their users, including when chatbots provide either informational or emotional support. AI has been explored with the goal of identifying and predicting the risk of relapse, symptoms improvement, remission after treatment, and disease progression, as well as supporting therapists with the development of accurate assessments, and decision-making about diagnosis, prognosis and treatment plans, through data collection (Richards, 2024). It promotes remote access and increases the rate of participation in therapy (Aktan et al., 2022). Since machine learning uses multi-site databases, including sophisticated biological, genetic, and linguistic characteristics, it has the potential for diagnostic and prognostic prediction in the mental health field. Studies using hybrid AI have found significant predictive rates of depression (accuracy of 80% to 90% (Li et al., 2019; Yan et al., 2023), suicide risk (accuracy of 65% to 85%), clinical remission for drug abuse (rate of 65%), responsiveness to CBT for anxiety-related disorders (precision of 59% to 75%), use of antidepressants treatment response for depression (accuracy of 25%), decision of tree for treatment selection (accuracy of 85%; Tahan & Saleem, 2023), accurate predictions of attention deficit hyperactivity disorder (ADHD) diagnosis in research setting (accuracy of 70% to 80%; Tachmazidis et al., 2021), accurate referrals of complex ADHD cases to clinical experts (accuracy of 81.37% to 93.61%; T. Chen et al., 2023), identification of subgroups of Autism Spectrum Disorders (ASD) based on kinetic characteristics of walking patterns (accuracy of 82.5%; Hasan et al., 2017), and the list continues. It is therefore important to consider how the integration of AI in the psychotherapeutic context may bring benefits.

Standard language-the-board, or Natural Language Processing (NLP) procedures used in AI chatbots have shown promising results in identifying linguistic alterations indicative of reflective moments. It provides early warning indicators, treatment and monitoring of post-partum depression, in countries which present constricted access to mental health services, such as India (P. Shah & Yadav, 2024). In a pilot study using a chatbot (WOEBOT) to provide CBT-based intervention for mild depression symptoms in athletes, there was a reduction of depression symptoms due to the chatbot (Qi, 2024). Although these results require further analysis due to the sample small size, other studies have presented similar conclusions regarding the improvement of symptoms of depression, anxiety, psychosis, autism, and schizophrenia with the use of AI chatbots that deliver CBT and other forms of treatment (Eid et al., 2023; Holohan & Fiske, 2021; Omarov et al., 2023; Zafar, 2024). Community-based clinics that complement mental health services with an AI platform specializing in behavioral treatment, such as Eleos Health, show more effectiveness in reducing anxiety and depression symptoms than standard therapy (Sadeh-Sharvit et al., 2023). AI chatbots seem to be effective in reducing symptoms when delivering CBT and Mindfulness Based Stress-Reduction (MBSR) treatment to individuals with depression and high levels of stress, respectively (Y. Li et al., 2024; Molli, 2022). Early symptom detection of PTSD diagnosis, as well as personalized treatment plans and patient monitoring, including intervention in crisis, have also been facilitated by AI, such as PTSD Coach app (Wan et al., 2025).

Additionally, AI use can enhance the accuracy in the detection of depression and anxiety, with a cost-effective advantage, which enables the faster identification of suicidal ideation, although ethical concerns should be considered (Barua et al., 2024). Chatbots that deliver real-time 24/7 support and personalized interventions for moderate anxiety (mindfulness exercises, breathing techniques and cognitive restructuring), show an average symptom reduction of 21.15%, which tends to decrease with chatbot use over time (Manole et al., 2024). AI high-performance learning, through Deep Neural Networks (DNNs), has shown great potential in extracting raw multimodal data, such as speech, behavior/motion, fMRI, and EEG data, to develop accurate predictions of psychosis and early diagnosis in schizophrenia (Cortes-Briones et al., 2022). AI-driven tools have also been shown to be promising in supporting precise and objective clinical assessment for schizophrenia diagnosis, traditionally dependent on patient self-report, to establish personalized therapeutic and adequate drug treatment, and to manage schizophrenia symptoms by close monitoring (Melo et al., 2024). The accuracy of ADHD diagnosis in children is usually considered poor and time-consuming by professionals. Adding non-traditional methods to the traditional assessment, such as EEG (electroencephalography) and brain functional information, can significantly increase the accuracy and precision of the ADHD diagnosis (Moghaddari et al., 2020; Tang et al., 2022). AI is capable of assessing and processing data from several sources, such as eye focus, facial expression, 3D body posture, and other functional information, to facilitate test results, abnormal behavior analysis, diagnostic aid conclusions, and treatment recommendations for ADHD (Mengi & Malhotra, 2022; Zhang et al., 2021). AI mobile applications allow behavioral monitoring and data collection, cognitive training programs with combined use of biofeedback and neurofeedback, personalized treatment plans, behavioral therapy support, physiological monitoring, and feedback on ADHD symptoms management/coping (Frolli et al., 2023). There is a potential for time and cost reduction in the evaluation and diagnosis of ASD, as well as early detection, rapid support in the diagnostic process based on each child's characteristics, and monitoring of mood and behaviors to improve therapeutic intervention, with the use of AI (Anagnostopoulou et al., 2020; Banna et al., 2020; Shahamiri & Thabtah., 2020). Equally, there have been several studies highlighting the use of AI for the diagnosis of Alzheimer's disease and other neurodegenerative diseases, through multi-data processing (Bi et al., 2021; Filippini et al., 2020). Overall, applied AI in the mental health sector presents an important role in diagnostics, treatment and patient management, as well as multimodal data analysis, and clinical research for medicinal and intervention enhancement (Zeb et al., 2024).

Advancements of AI in Supporting Mental Health Professionals

The use of mental health AI applications as hybrid care, supplementing in-person therapeutic interventions, has been found to: improve self-management (Chandrashekar, 2018); increase rate participation and accessibility (Aktan et al., 2022); promote psychoeducation, evidence-based coping skills and emotional support (Alanezi, 2024); and provide monitoring of treatment progress and interaction between formal therapy sessions (Husnain et al., 2024). Considering the use of AI as part of hybrid care seems to be a more appealing approach (Prescott & Hanley, 2023). Automated data collection allows the acquirement and processing of information and, consequently, the generation of fully automated prediction models of patients for mental health conditions, reported alliance and symptom ratings, based on behavioral markers, such as body and facial movements, and linguistic features (Aafjes-van Doorn, 2024). Advances in the field of AI, particularly of NLP and audio analysis provide indications about psychological states and are consistently highly rated as having higher quality than human transcripts, supporting the integration of AI chatbots for individuals experiencing mild to moderate psychological challenges (D'Alfonso, 2020). Several studies between 2014 and 2023 have shown positive results of the use of AI for suicide prediction and prevention. With NLP (natural language processing), ML (machine learning), DL (deep learning), and social suicidal prediction tools, that include browsing habits from social media to determine suicide risk, it has been possible to identify patients at risk (Lejeune et al., 2022; Atmakuru et al., 2025; D'Hotman & Loh, 2020).

It has been demonstrated that routinely collecting patients' feedback to therapists and client's self-report, can reduce dropouts and improve symptomatic outcomes since treatment can be readjusted whenever progress fails to occur (de Jong et al., 2021). This method, known as routine outcome monitoring (ROM), is considered demanding and completion rates are inconsistent when done without AI support (Aafjes-van Doorn, 2024). Overall, applied AI in the mental health sector presents an important role in diagnostics, treatment and patient management, as well as multimodal data analysis, and clinical research for medicinal and intervention enhancement (Zeb et al., 2024).

However, some important components of AI chatbots for therapeutic purposes are missing, such as therapeutic alliance. Research has been consensual that the success of psychotherapeutic interventions varies according to the therapeutic alliance (Baier et al., 2020; Falkenström et al., 2013). Moreover, successful therapeutic outcomes require specific factors such as trust, boundaries and expectations, confidential and ethical setting conditions, and attunement-rupture-repair processes, that can only be performed by trained psychotherapists (Molden, 2024). Additionally, therapy aims to work on the person's unified belief system by integrating new information based on social, dialectic and normative discursive practice, which AI can only simulate by offering different definitions or descriptions, without truly understanding the relevant nuances of a particular individual, undermining the delivery of successful support (Sedlakova & Trachsel, 2023). Another limitation of AI in therapy is the inability to use or understand empathy or emotions, limiting the understanding of human language. Even though recent studies showed that a human-AI collaboration outperformed humans with empathetic conversations and has shown an advanced understanding of the theory of mind, simply mimicking empathy responses may not be enough (Ojha & Syed, 2020). Another concern of the use of AI alone is the risk of exacerbation of symptoms. Overly engaging with (and attributing real emotions to AI) may exacerbate delusional thinking in patients with schizophrenia and increase social isolation in the elderly and individuals with substance use disorders (Joseph & Babu, 2024). Even though Conversational AI (CAI) is based on data processing and evaluation that mimic agent-like features, it can impact how individuals acquire an understanding of themselves and the world, potentially causing shifts in values and concepts, more than only providing evidence-based information to the user (Sedlakova & Trachsel, 2023). Therefore, it is important to underline that the process of transference in hybrid care can pose potential risk to patients, since AI virtual therapists are not moral agents nor have consciousness or responsibility (Molden, 2024). Additionally, basing information on algorithms may lead to an over focus in diagnostic models, such as DSM-V, not considering personal expectations and cultural differences (Molden, 2024). Consisten with this information, mental health chatbots also present limitations to mental health emergency requests, such as immediate harm or suicidal ideation (Koutsouleris et al., 2022). Another branch of concern is related to ethical practice. Using AI in the therapeutic setting for mental health, based on the multi-data processing aspect, raises ethical challenges related to dignity protection and data privacy, therefore presenting risks to the clients (Alfano et al., 2023). The potential risks of user privacy create a boundary where users with higher privacy concerns are less likely to disclose information, creating a significant impact on how therapeutic AI should be designed and regulated (A. Chen et al., 2024).

AI, Computerized Cognitive Behavioral Therapy (CCBT) and Cognitive Computing in Mental Health

When turning attention to patients, it is important to consider that traditional therapy may pose restrictions in access, costs and stigma, so other forms of CBT delivery to patients have been investigated for many years. AI has developed to integrate several stages of CBT treatment providing different support in the pre-treatment, therapeutic process and post-treatment. In the pre-treatment stage AI can support with the Mental Health Assessment, Personalized Treatment Selection and Client Psychoeducation (Jiang et al., 2024). During the treatment stage, therapists can benefit from AI augmentation of therapeutic strategies and tools, real-time monitoring and feedback to the patient and the therapist, early prediction of CBT outcomes and evaluation of therapists and clients. Finally, for the pot-treatment AI can provide information about treatment response and relapse prediction. Another example is the benefits of self-help CBT bibliotherapy reported in research that brought increased interest in the development of other approaches with the use of digital technology (McKendree-Smith et al., 2003). The potential of AI integration in mental health services as a hybrid care is known as Computerized Cognitive Behavioral Therapy (CCBT). CCBT is an evidence-based computer interface for self-management support that uses specific software, such as 'Stressbusters', 'Master your mood online', 'CATCH-IT', 'BRAVE online', 'Cool Teens' and 'MoodGYM', and 'Beating the Blues', among others. It offers the benefits of CBT through computer led response with limited involvement of the therapist (Kaltenthaler et al., 2004). It is mainly delivered through software packages designed for specific patient groups, which means that access to a computer, smartphone or the internet is a mandatory requirement (Kaltenthaler et al., 2006). The patients have access to a specific number of multimedia sessions with assigned homework to be completed in between the sessions, with weekly progress being automatically reported to a mental health professional (T. Richardson et al., 2010). CCBT is designed as short-term CBT therapy, that uses text, audio files and video clips to deliver content such as psychoeducation, cognitive restructuring, and behavior activation anywhere and anytime (T. Zhou et al., 2016). Due to its nature, CCBT shows the potential to be delivered to a greater number of people worldwide, including in remote areas. In fact, according to research, CCBT may be more acceptable to populations living in remote or rural areas compared with populations that live in urban areas (Vallury et al., 2015). Different forms of CCBT delivery have been proposed, including the use of games and gamification with CBT techniques for depression, anxiety and stress disorders, with positive results for patient engagement, motivation and treatment adherence (Amer et al., 2024). These programs deliver adequate quality, security and efficacy, access to coping strategies, and are especially reliable when selected by clinicians and used as a complement to traditional therapy (Wright et al., 2019).

More research is necessary to find conclusive results about the effectiveness of CCBT compared with CBT delivered by a therapist. The use of CCBT may lead to a reduction of the therapist's time, in comparison to traditional one-on-one therapy (Kaltenthaler et al., 2008). However, CCBT shows more promising results when the program delivered is supported by a clinical or other helping professional (Andersson & Cuijpers, 2009; Rajeshkumar et al., 2024). It shows potential effectiveness in the treatment of depression, anxiety, phobias and panic disorders, at different levels (Kaltenthaler et al., 2006; Wright et al., 2022). It shows mild to moderate efficacy for insomnia as a short-term low-intensity treatment (Cheng & Dizon, 2012), and improvements in social anxiety (Helgadóttir et al., 2014), as well as a reduction in alcohol use and adherence to treatment for alcohol use disorders (Kiluk et al., 2016). CCBT has also been found to deliver substantial evidence of therapeutic alliance features in programs designed for the treatment of depression (Barazzone et al., 2012). However, CCBT presents concerns about acceptability, efficiency and accessibility that should be taken into account (Waller & Gilbody, 2009) and other forms of therapy delivery using AI should be considered. Other challenges include a lack of medical diagnostic capability, insufficient levels of personalization and poor interactivity (Jiang et al., 2024). It is also important to consider that older populations may be less adherent to CCBT, although more studies in this population need to be developed for consistent results (Crabb et al., 2012).

AI was initially developed based on suppositions about human performance, lacking correlative studies, application and testing, and ignoring the exploration of psychological effects (Tahan & Saleem, 2023). Only in recent years has there been an increase in the use of AI applied to the mental health sector, and it remain limited. Therefore, it is important to highlight that AI is programmed to perform specific tasks independently, using algorithms, creating final decisions that mimic human intelligence, but are unable to learn or adapt to actual human needs. Studying how the brain works has enhanced a better understanding of human behavior. This includes how people respond to things around them, the origin of emotionally balanced behaviors, and processes such as motivation and feelings (Rodríguez et al., 2011). In that line of investigation, cognitive computing uses more developed algorithm models based on the calculation of mathematical principles of brain functioning (neurobiological facts), with the ability to mimic processes of perception, memory, language, intelligence and consciousness (Chen & Jiang, 2019). It provides pertinent information that allows humans to make the final decision for themselves (M. Richardson, 2021). As explained by Haleem and Javaid (2024), "*Cognitive computing enhances human decision-making by integrating reasoning, machine learning, speech, natural language processing (NLP), and human-computer interaction (...) facilitates the analysis of clinical and genetic data to forecast diseases, tailor therapies, and elevate drug development*". Platforms like IBM Watson and Microsoft Cognitive Services exemplify this approach, offering accessible cloud-based cognitive tools that integrate AI techniques to assist clinicians and researchers (Sheth et al., 2019).

CONCLUSION

By analyzing large health data sets and identifying patterns, AI allows early detection and preventive intervention to at-risk populations, reduction of healthcare costs, increased access to healthcare providers and services, and the creation of personalized effective treatment options for clients (Abdullah & Yusuf, 2023). However, it is important to highlight how the lack of human interaction leads to the lack of trust and dropout of hybrid care (Miner et al., 2019), and how only mental health professionals can perform critical tasks, such as risk management and intervention, with empathy and compassion (Roa et al., 2021).

Considering the potential and obstacles of the use of AI in the mental health field, an important debate needs to be raised on how clinicians can consider to use AI as an integrative part of mental health services, specifically, as hybrid care. To date, AI has been proposed as a consulting tool for workflow and decision-making, while the therapist maintains control over the treatment and management aspects of the client (Tahan, 2023). With the focus on quality control and patient monitoring, AI insights from data can provide in-session support to the therapist and increase engagement in therapy for patients who usually struggle with traditional one-to-one therapy (Molden, 2024). The same author brings to life different levels of hybrid care to consider, including: AI app-based exercises which are introduced by the therapist as a key part of the treatment and the therapist is responsible for the intervention and risk assessment; AI is part of the therapy providing feedback insight to the therapist for quality control; and the use of AI which has virtual therapist while the human therapist maintains overall responsibility and proceeds with regular pre-agreed check-ins. Lin and colleagues (2023) propose a virtual psychotherapy AI companion that not only supports the client but also the therapists, by providing real-time feedback and treatment strategy recommendations in the therapeutic setting.

The therapeutic alliance is a predictor of a patient's disclosure in the psychotherapeutic setting and is also the main vehicle for diagnosis and treatment inference (Farber, 2003). However, patients with different symptoms/concerns or diagnoses may vary in their availability for self-disclosure, such as patients with binge drinking behavior (Miner et al., 2019). According to Torous et al. (2019) a digital therapeutic alliance can be developed if the specific elements of therapeutic alliance in the traditional setting are present, such as the definition of achievable therapeutic goals, specific tasks, and emotional bonds.

The use of AI-assisted therapy as a complement to traditional psychotherapy offers many advantages and allows effective and personalized care if ethical concerns are addressed and ongoing research on ethical guidelines is developed (Husnain et al., 2024). Different fronts and needs must be involved in the process of developing and implementing usable hybrid mental health care with AI-based technology, therefore the involvement and participation of patients, therapists and administrators, among others, is crucial (Yule et al., 2024). In the study of Aktan and colleagues (2022), it was found that 55% of the participants perceived AI-based psychotherapy positively, mental health professionals were more likely to reject this option, and the belief of the effectiveness of AI-based psychotherapy was the most important factor in developing positive attitudes towards AI in the psychotherapy setting. Similar conclusions have been reached in the literature where patients report the use of AI practices as important for the treatment, while therapists show overall concern about the clinical relevance of AI in mental health care (Westbye et al., 2024). Literature has also shown that the younger population has a growing interest in a more digitally accessible and less judgmental type of psychotherapy, which raises new questions on how AI-based therapies should be included as a complement to traditional psychotherapy, especially for this age group, given its characteristics (Alfano et al., 2023). Therefore, mandatory training for professionals may increase the potential of patient care in real-time in a collaborative hybrid setting, and is likely to support clinicians in administrative tasks, monitoring and risk assessment and to support clients in receiving highly personalized and trustworthy treatment (Ojha & Syed, 2020). The effective use of AI in the mental health field requires health professionals to have access to specific training, therefore funds should be considered for outreach and education programs of AI-based interventions, especially among disproportionate communities (Abdullah & Yusuf, 2023). Future developments in AI applied to mental health care, should consider enhancements in NLP algorithms, personalized drug and therapy design, and advanced genomic brain functional analysis, while ensuring ethical and data protection, algorithmic transparency and interdisciplinary collaboration (Zeb et al., 2024). The use of AI designed for emergencies in war zones has also rise attention for the need of functional AI in offline mode, AI co-pilot that support humanitarian volunteers providing personalized counseling, and even personalized therapy with Chat GPT-2 through LLM (large language model) for war areas that lack mental health support (*Anonymous*, 2024).

Overall, applied AI in the mental health sector presents an important role in diagnostics, treatment and patient management, as well as multimodal data analysis, and clinical research for medicinal and intervention enhancement (Zeb et al., 2024).

REFERENCES

Aafjes-van Doorn, K. (2024). Feasibility of artificial intelligence-based measurement in psychotherapy practice: Patients' and clinicians' perspectives. *Counseling Psychology Review, 25. Article, 1280*, 1–11. DOI: 10.1002/capr.12800

Abd-alrazaq, A., Alhuwail, D., Schneider, J., Toro, C. T., Ahmed, A., Alzubaidi, M., Alajlani, M., & Househ, M. (2022). The performance of artificial intelligence-driven technologies in diagnosing mental disorders: An umbrella review. *npj. Digital Medicine*, *5*(87), 1–12. DOI: 10.1038/s41746-022-00631-8 PMID: 35798934

Abdula, A., & Yusuf, M. (2023). The effectiveness of AI-Based Interventions in Reducing Healthcare Inequalities: A comprehensive Review. *Journal of Contemporary Healthcare Analytics*, *7*(1), 1–30. https://publications.dlpress.org/index.php/jcha/article/view/4

Aktan, M. E., Turhan, Z., & Dolu, I. (2022). Attitudes and perspectives towards the preferences for artificial intelligence in psychotherapy. *Computers in Human Behavior, 133. Computers in Human Behavior, 107273*, 107273. Advance online publication. DOI: 10.1016/j.chb.2022.107273

Alanezi, F. (2024). Assessing the effectiveness of ChatGPT in delivering mental health support: A qualitative study. *Journal of Multidisciplinary Healthcare*, *31*(17), 461–471. DOI: 10.2147/JMDH.S447368 PMID: 38314011

Alfano, L., Malcotti, I., & Ciliberti, R. (2023). Psychotherapy, artificial intelligence and adolescents: Ethical aspects. *Journal of Preventive Medicine and Hygiene*, *64*, E438–E442. DOI: 10.15167/2421-4248/jpmh2023.64.4.3135 PMID: 38379752

Alowais, S. A., Alghamdi, S. S., Alsuhebany, N., Alqahtani, T., Alshaya, A. I., Almohareb, S. N., Aldairem, A., Alrashed, M., Bin Saleh, K., Badreldin, H. A., Al Yami, M. S., Al Harbi, S., & Albekairy, A. M. (2023). Revolutionizing healthcare: The role of artificial intelligence in clinical practice. *BMC Medical Education*, *23*(1), 689. DOI: 10.1186/s12909-023-04698-z PMID: 37740191

Alqahtani, F., & Orji, R. (2019, June 9-12). *Usability issues in mental health applications* [Conference session]. Proceedings of the UMAP'19 adjunct publication of the 27th conference on user modeling, adaptation and personalization, Larnaca, Cyprus. https://www.researchgate.net/publication/333740636_Usability_Issues_in_Mental_Health_Applications

Amer, N., Abdelrazek, S., Eladrosy, W., El-Bakry, H., & Shohieb, S. (2024). Computer-based cognitive behavioral therapy intervention for depression, anxiety, and stress disorders: A systematic review. *International Journal of Cognitive Therapy*, *17*(4), 885–918. DOI: 10.1007/s41811-024-00225-0

Anagnostopoulou, P., Alexandropoulou, V., Lorentzou, G., Lykothanasi, A., Ntaountaki, P., & Drigas, A. (2020). Artificial intelligence in autism assessment. *International Journal of Emerging Technologies in Learning*, *15*(6), 95–107. DOI: 10.3991/ijet.v15i06.11231

Andersson, G., & Cuijpers, P. (2009). Internet-based and other computerized psychological treatments for adult depression: A meta-analysis. [A]. *Cognitive Behaviour Therapy*, *38*(4), 196–205. DOI: 10.1080/16506070903318960 PMID: 20183695

Anonymous. (2024). *Innovating AI for humanitarian action in emergencies.* In *Proceedings of the AAAI Conference on Artificial Intelligence.* https://openreview.net/pdf?id=CLJxxqSKNJ

Arias, D., Saxena, S., & Verguet, S. (2022). Quantifying the global burden of mental disorders and their economic value. *eClinicalMedicine, 54. EClinicalMedicine, 101675*, 101675. Advance online publication. DOI: 10.1016/j.eclinm.2022.101675 PMID: 36193171

Atmakuru, A., Shahini, A., Chakraborty, S., Seoni, S., Salvi, M., Hafeez-Baig, A., Rashid, S., Tan, R., Barua, P., Molinari, F., & Acharya, U. (2025). Artificial intelligence-based suicide prevention and prediction: A systematic review (2019–2023). Information Fusion, Volume 114,102673, ISSN 1566-2535, DOI: 10.1016/j.inffus.2024.102673

Baier, A. L., Kline, A. C., & Feeny, N. C. (2020). Therapeutic alliance as a mediator of change: A systematic review and evaluation of research. *Clinical Psychology Review, 82. Clinical Psychology Review, 101921*, 101921. Advance online publication. DOI: 10.1016/j.cpr.2020.101921 PMID: 33069096

Balcombe, L., & De Leo, D. (2021). Digital mental health challenges and the horizon ahead for solutions. *JMIR Mental Health*, *8*(3), e26811. Advance online publication. DOI: 10.2196/26811 PMID: 33779570

Banna, M. H., Ghosh, T., Taher, K. A., Kaiser, M. S., & Mahmud, M. (2020). A monitoring system for patients of autism spectrum disorder using artificial intelligence. In Mahmud, M., Vassanelli, S., Kaiser, M. S., & Zhong, N. (Eds.), Lecture notes in computer science: Vol. 12241. *Brain informatics* (pp. 251–262). Springer., DOI: 10.1007/978-3-030-59277-6_23

Barazzone, N., Cavanagh, K., & Richards, D. (2012). Computerized cognitive behavioural therapy and the therapeutic alliance: A qualitative enquiry. *British Journal of Clinical Psychology, 51*(4), 396–417. DOI: 10.1111/j.2044-8260.2012.02035.x PMID: 23078210

Barrón-Velázquez, E., Mendoza-Velásquez, J., Mercado-Lara, A., Quijada-Gaytán, J., & Flores-Vázquez, J. (2024). The mental health provider shortage in the Mexican. Public sector: 2023 estimates of psychiatrists and psychologists. *Salud Mental, 47*(4), 179–187. DOI: 10.17711/SM.0185-3325.2024.023

Barua, P., Vicnesh, J., Lih, O., Palmer, E., Yamakawa, T., Kobayashi, M., & Acharya, U. (2024). Artificial intelligence assisted tools for the detection of anxiety and depression leading to suicidal ideation in adolescents: A review. *Cognitive Neurodynamics, 18*(1), 1–22. DOI: 10.1007/s11571-022-09904-0 PMID: 36467993

Bi, X., Liu, W., Liu, H., & Shang, Q. (2021). Artificial intelligence-based MRI images for brain in prediction of Alzheimer's disease. *Journal of Healthcare Engineering. Journal of Healthcare Engineering, 8198552*, 1–7. DOI: 10.1155/2021/8198552 PMID: 34712461

Bradshaw, K. M., Donohue, B., & Wilks, C. (2014). A review of quality assurance methods to assist professional record keeping: Implications for providers of interpersonal violence treatment. *Aggression and Violent Behavior, 19*(3), 242–250. DOI: 10.1016/j.avb.2014.04.010 PMID: 24976786

Busch, A., Sugarman, D., Horvitz, E., & Greenfield, S. (2021). Telemedicine for treating mental health and substance use disorders: Reflections since the pandemic. *Neuropsychopharmacology : Official Publication of the American College of Neuropsychopharmacology, 46*(6), 1068–1070. DOI: 10.1038/s41386-021-00960-4 PMID: 33479513

Busch, F., Kather, J. N., Johner, C., Moser, M., Truhn, D., Adams, L. C., & Bressem, K. K. (2024). Navigating the European Union artificial intelligence act for healthcare. *npj. Digital Medicine, 7*(210), 1–6. DOI: 10.1038/s41746-024-01213-6 PMID: 39134637

Busetta, G., Campolo, M., Fiorillo, F., Pagani, L., Panarello, D., & Augello, V. (2021). Effects of COVID-19 lockdown on university students' anxiety disorder in Italy. *Genus, 77*(25), 1–16. DOI: 10.1186/s41118-021-00135-5 PMID: 34658399

Business Wire. (2012). *Strategy analytics: Worldwide smartphone population tops 1 billion in Q3 2012*. Business Wire. https://www.businesswire.com/news/home/20121017005479/en/Strategy-Analytics-Worldwide-Smartphone-Population-Tops-1-Billion-in-Q3-2012

Cancela-Outeda, C. (2024). The EU's AI act: A framework for collaborative governance. *Internet of Things, 27. Internet of Things : Engineering Cyber Physical Human Systems, 101291*, 101291. Advance online publication. DOI: 10.1016/j.iot.2024.101291

Casu, M., Triscari, S., Battiato, S., Guarnera, L., & Caponnetto, P. (2024). AI chatbots for mental health: A scoping review of effectiveness, feasibility, and applications. *Applied Sciences, 14*(13). *Applied Sciences (Basel, Switzerland), 5889*(13), 5889. Advance online publication. DOI: 10.3390/app14135889

Chandrashekar, P. (2018). Do mental health mobile apps work: Evidence and recommendations for designing high-efficacy mental health mobile apps. *mHealth, 4*, 6. DOI: 10.21037/mhealth.2018.03.02 PMID: 29682510

Chekroud, A. M., Zotti, R. J., Shehzad, Z., Gueorguieva, R., Johnson, M. K., Trivedi, M. H., Cannon, T. D., Krystal, J. H., & Corlett, P. R. (2016). Cross-trial prediction of treatment outcome in depression: A machine learning approach. *The Lancet. Psychiatry, 3*(3), 243–250. DOI: 10.1016/S2215-0366(15)00471-X PMID: 26803397

Chen, A., Evans, R., & Zeng, R. (2024). Editorial: Coping with an AI-saturated world: Psychological dynamics and outcomes of AI-mediated communication. *Frontiers in Psychology, 15. Frontiers in Psychology, 1479981*, 1479981. Advance online publication. DOI: 10.3389/fpsyg.2024.1479981 PMID: 39351112

Chen, M., & Jiang, S. (2019). Analysis and research on mental health college students based on cognitive computing. *Cognitive Systems Research, 56*, 151–158. DOI: 10.1016/j.cogsys.2019.03.003

Chen, T., Tachmazidis, I., Batsakis, S., Adamou, M., Papadakis, E., & Antoniou, G. (2023). Diagnosing attention deficit hyperactivity disorder (ADHD) using artificial intelligence: A clinical study in the UK. *Frontiers in Psychiatry, 14. Frontiers in Psychiatry, 1164433*, 1164433. Advance online publication. DOI: 10.3389/fpsyt.2023.1164433 PMID: 37363182

Cheng, S., & Dizon, J. (2012). Computerised cognitive behavioural therapy for insomnia: A systematic review and meta-analysis. *Psychotherapy and Psychosomatics, 81*(4), 206–216. DOI: 10.1159/000335379 PMID: 22585048

Cho, J., Lee, K., Shin, E., Choy, G., & Do, S. (2015). How much data is needed to train a medical image deep learning system to achieve necessary high accuracy? *ArXiv*, 1-10. https://doi.org//arXiv.1511.06348DOI: 10.48550

Chou, T., Bry, L. J., & Comer, J. S. (2017). Multimedia field test: Evaluating the creative ambitions of SuperBetter and its quest to gamify mental health. *Cognitive and Behavioral Practice*, *24*(1), 115–120. DOI: 10.1016/j.cbpra.2016.10.002

Clay, R. A. (2021, January 1). *Mental health apps are gaining traction*. American Psychological Association. https://www.apa.org/monitor/2021/01/trends-mental-health-apps

Corrigan, P. (2020). Effect of contact-based interventions on stigma and discrimination. *Psychiatric Services (Washington, D.C.)*, *71*(12), 1324–1325. DOI: 10.1176/appi.ps.711203 PMID: 33256526

Cortes-Briones, J., Tapia-Rivas, N., D'Souza, D., & Estevez, P. (2022). Going deep into schizophrenia with artificial intelligence. *Schizophrenia Research*, *245*, 122–140. DOI: 10.1016/j.schres.2021.05.018 PMID: 34103242

Crabb, R., Cavanagh, K., Proudfoot, J., Learmonth, D., Rafie, S., & Weingardt, K. (2012). Is computerized cognitive-behavioural therapy a treatment option for depression in late-life? A systematic review. *British Journal of Clinical Psychology*, *51*(4), 459–464. DOI: 10.1111/j.2044-8260.2012.02038.x PMID: 23078214

Croskerry, P. (2020). *The cognitive autopsy: A root cause analysis of medical decision making*. Oxford University Press., DOI: 10.1093/med/9780190088743.001.0001

Cuellar, A., Mark, T., Sharfstein, S., & Huskamp, H. (2020). How to mitigate the mental health care consequences of the COVID-19 financial crisis. *Psychiatric Services (Washington, D.C.)*, *71*(12), 1317–1319. DOI: 10.1176/appi.ps.202000329 PMID: 32988321

D'Alfonso, S. (2020). AI in mental health. *Current Opinion in Psychology*, *36*, 112–117. DOI: 10.1016/j.copsyc.2020.04.005 PMID: 32604065

D'Hotman, D., & Loh, E. (2020). AI enabled suicide prediction tools: A qualitative narrative review. *BMJ Health & Care Informatics*, *27*(3), e100175. DOI: 10.1136/bmjhci-2020-100175 PMID: 33037037

Davis, K., Christodoulou, J., Seider, S., & Gardner, H. (2011). The theory of multiple intelligences. In Sternberg, R. J., & Kaufman, S. B. (Eds.), *The Cambridge handbook of intelligence* (pp. 485–503). Cambridge University Press., DOI: 10.1017/CBO9780511977244.025

De Freitas, J., & Cohen, I. G. (2024). The health risks of generative AI-based wellness apps. *Nature Medicine*, *30*(5), 1–7. DOI: 10.1038/s41591-024-02943-6 PMID: 38684859

De Jong, K., Conijn, J. M., Gallagher, R. A. V., Reshetnikova, A. S., Heij, M., & Lutz, M. C. (2021). Using progress feedback to improve outcomes and reduce drop-out, treatment duration, and deterioration: A multilevel meta-analysis. *Clinical Psychology Review, 85. Clinical Psychology Review, 102002*, 102002. Advance online publication. DOI: 10.1016/j.cpr.2021.102002 PMID: 33721605

Dick, B., & Ferguson, B. (2015). Health for the world's adolescents: A second chance in the second decade. *The Journal of Adolescent Health, 56*(1), 3–6. DOI: 10.1016/j.jadohealth.2014.10.260 PMID: 25530601

Dong, L., & Bouey, J. (2020). Public mental health crisis during COVID-19 pandemic, China. *Emerging Infectious Diseases, 26*(7), 1616–1618. DOI: 10.3201/eid2607.200407 PMID: 32202993

Dwivedi, Y. K., Sharma, A., Rana, N. P., Giannakis, M., Goel, P., & Dutot, V. (2023). Evolution of artificial intelligence research in *Technological Forecasting and Social Change*: Research topics, trends, and future directions. *Technological Forecasting and Social Change, 192. Technological Forecasting and Social Change, 122579*, 122579. Advance online publication. DOI: 10.1016/j.techfore.2023.122579

Dwyer, D. B., Falkai, P., & Koutsouleris, N. (2018). Machine learning approaches for clinical psychology and psychiatry. *Annual Review of Clinical Psychology, 7*(14), 91–118. DOI: 10.1146/annurev-clinpsy-032816-045037 PMID: 29401044

Eid, M., Yundong, W., Mensah, G., & Pudasaini, P. (2023). Treating psychological depression utilising artificial intelligence: AI for precision medicine- focus on procedures. *Mesopotamian Journal of Artificial Intelligence in Healthcare,* 76–81. https://doi.org/DOI: 10.58496/MJAIH/2023/015

Eltahawy, L., Essig, T., Myszkowski, N., & Trub, L. (2024). Can robots do therapy?: Examining the efficacy of a CBT bot in comparison with other behavioral intervention technologies in alleviating mental health symptoms. *Computers in Human Behavior: Artificial Humans, 2*(1). *Article, 100035*(1), 100035. Advance online publication. DOI: 10.1016/j.chbah.2023.100035

European Parliament. (2024). *Artificial intelligence act*. https://www.europarl.europa.eu/doceo/document/TA-9-2024-0138_EN.pdf

Falkenström, F., Granström, F., & Holmqvist, R. (2013). Therapeutic alliance predicts symptomatic improvement session by session. *Journal of Counseling Psychology, 60*(3), 317–328. DOI: 10.1037/a0032258 PMID: 23506511

Fanni, R., Steinkogler, V. E., Zampedri, G., & Pierson, J. (2023). Enhancing human agency through redress in artificial intelligence systems. *AI & Society*, *38*(2), 537–547. DOI: 10.1007/s00146-022-01454-7 PMID: 35692234

Farber, B. (2003). Patient self-disclosure: A review of the research. *Journal of Clinical Psychology*, *59*(5), 589–600. DOI: 10.1002/jclp.10161 PMID: 12696134

Figueroa, C., & Aguilera, A. (2020). The need for a mental health technology revolution in the COVID-19 pandemic. *Frontiers in Psychiatry*, *11*(523), 523. Advance online publication. DOI: 10.3389/fpsyt.2020.00523 PMID: 32581891

Filippini, C., Perpetuini, D., Cardone, D., Chiarelli, A. M., & Merla, A. (2020). Thermal infrared imaging and artificial intelligence techniques can support mild Alzheimer disease diagnosis. *Proceedings of the Digital Innovations for Learning and Neurodevelopmental Disorders*, *2804*, 1–9. https://ceur-ws.org/Vol-2804/short2.pdf

Firth, J., Torous, J., Nicholas, J., Carney, R., Pratap, A., Rosenbaum, S., & Sarris, J. (2017). The efficacy of smartphone-based mental health interventions for depressive symptoms: A meta-analysis of randomized controlled trials. *World Psychiatry; Official Journal of the World Psychiatric Association (WPA)*, *16*(3), 287–298. DOI: 10.1002/wps.20472 PMID: 28941113

Fiske, A., Henningsen, P., & Buyx, A. (2019). Your robot therapist will see you now: Ethical implications of embodied artificial intelligence in psychiatry, psychology, and psychotherapy. *Journal of Medical Internet Research, 21*(5). *Journal of Medical Internet Research, 13216*(5), e13216. Advance online publication. DOI: 10.2196/13216 PMID: 31094356

Fitzpatrick, K. K., Darcy, A., & Vierhile, M. (2017). Delivering cognitive behavior therapy to young adults with symptoms of depression and anxiety using a fully automated conversational agent (Woebot): A randomized controlled trial. *JMIR Ment Health, 4*(2). *JMIR Mental Health, 19*(2), e19. Advance online publication. DOI: 10.2196/mental.7785 PMID: 28588005

Fleming, T., Bavin, L., Lucassen, M., Stasiak, K., Hopkins, S., & Merry, S. (2018). Beyond the trial: Systematic review of real-world uptake and engagement with digital self-help interventions for depression, low mood, or anxiety. *Journal of Medical Internet Research, 20*(6). *Article, 199*. Advance online publication. DOI: 10.26686/wgtn.12331259

Frolli, A., Saviano, E., Ricci, M., Sica, S., & Romano, M. (2023). Artificial intelligence in ADHD treatment: A brief narrative review. *Proceedings of the Digital Innovations for Learning and Neurodevelopmental Disorders*, *3751*, 1–9. https://ceur-ws.org/Vol-3751/paper1.pdf

Gardner, H. E. (2011). *Frames of mind: The theory of multiple intelligences*. Basic Books.

Ghosh, M., & Arunachalam, T. (2021). Introduction to artificial intelligence. In Srinivasa, K. G., Siddesh, G. M., & Sekkar, S. R. M. (Eds.), *Artificial intelligence for information management: A healthcare perspective* (pp. 23–44). Springer., DOI: 10.1007/978-981-16-0415-7_2

Gignac, G. E., & Szodorai, E. T. (2024). Defining intelligence: Bridging the gap between human and artificial perspectives. *Intelligence, 104*. *Intelligence*, *101832*, 101832. Advance online publication. DOI: 10.1016/j.intell.2024.101832

Goodwin, R. D., Weinberger, A. H., Kim, J. H., Wu, M., & Galea, S. (2020). Trends in anxiety among adults in the United States, 2008–2018: Rapid increases among young adults. *Journal of Psychiatric Research*, *130*, 441–449. DOI: 10.1016/j.jpsychires.2020.08.014 PMID: 32905958

Guo, T. (2015). Alan Turing: Artificial intelligence as human self-knowledge. *Anthropology Today*, *31*(6), 3–7. DOI: 10.1111/1467-8322.12209

Gustavson, K., Knudsen, A. K., Nesvåg, R., Knudsen, G. P., Vollset, S. E., & Reichborn-Kjennerud, T. (2018). Prevalence and stability of mental disorders among young adults: Findings from a longitudinal study. *BMC Psychiatry, 18*. *BMC Psychiatry*, *65*(1), 65. Advance online publication. DOI: 10.1186/s12888-018-1647-5 PMID: 29530018

Haleem, A., & Javaid, M. (2024). Role of Cognitive Computing in enhancing innovative healthcare solutions. *Advances in Biomarker Sciences and Technology*, *6*, 152–165. DOI: 10.1016/j.abst.2024.08.002

Hasan, C., Jailani, R., Tahir, N., Yassin, I., & Rizman, Z. (2017). Automated classification of autism spectrum disorders gait patterns using discriminant analysis based on kinematic and kinetic gait features. *Journal of Applied Environmental and Biological Sciences*, *7*(1), 50–156. https://www.researchgate.net/publication/312505554_Automated_Classification_of_Autism_Spectrum_Disorders_Gait_Patterns_Using_Discriminant_Analysis_Based_on_Kinematic_and_Kinetic_Gait_Features

Helgadóttir, F., Menzies, R., Onslow, M., Packman, A., & O'Brian, S. (2014). A standalone internet cognitive behavior therapy treatment for social anxiety in adults who stutter: CBTpsych. *Journal of Fluency Disorders*, *41*, 47–54. DOI: 10.1016/j.jfludis.2014.04.001 PMID: 25173456

Hoffman, B., Oppert, M., & Owen, M. (2024). Understanding young adults' attitudes towards using AI chatbots for psychotherapy: The role of self-stigma. *Computers in Human Behavior: Artificial Humans*, *2*(2), 100086. DOI: 10.1016/j.chbah.2024.100086

Hohman, J., Martinez, K., Anand, A., Rood, M., Martyn, T., Rose, S., & Rothberg, M. (2022). Use of direct-to-consumer telemedicine to access mental health services. *Journal of General Internal Medicine*, *37*(11), 2759–2767. DOI: 10.1007/s11606-021-07326-y PMID: 35091925

Holohan, M., & Fiske, A. (2021). "Like I'm talking to a real person": Exploring the meaning of transference for the use and design of ai-based applications in psychotherapy. *Frontiers in Psychology*, *12*(720476), 1–9. DOI: 10.3389/fpsyg.2021.720476 PMID: 34646209

House of Lords. (2018). *AI in the UK: Ready, willing and able?* House of Lords Select Committee on Artificial Intelligence Report of Session 2017-2019. https://publications.parliament.uk/pa/ld201719/ldselect/ldai/100/100.pdf

Huawei Technologies Co. Ltd. (2023). A general introduction to artificial intelligence. In Huawei Technologies Co., Ltd (Ed.), *Artificial intelligence technology* (pp. 1-41). Springer, Posts & Telecom Press. https://doi.org/DOI: 10.1007/978-981-19-2879-6_1

Huberty, J., Green, J., Glissmann, C., Larkey, L., Puzia, M., & Lee, C. (2019). Efficacy of the mindfulness meditation mobile app "calm" to reduce stress among college students: Randomized controlled trial. *JMIR mHealth and uHealth, 7*(6). *JMIR mHealth and uHealth*, *14273*(6), e14273. Advance online publication. DOI: 10.2196/14273 PMID: 31237569

Huckvale, K., Nicholas, J., Torous, J., & Larsen, M. (2020). Smartphone apps for the treatment of mental health conditions: Status and considerations. *Current Opinion in Psychology*, *36*, 65–70. DOI: 10.1016/j.copsyc.2020.04.008 PMID: 32553848

Husnain, A., Ahmad, A., Saeed, A., & Din, S. (2024). Harnessing AI in depression therapy: Integrating technology with traditional approaches. *International Journal of Science and Research Archive*, *12*(02), 2585–2590. DOI: 10.30574/ijsra.2024.12.2.1512

Islam, Z., Gangat, S., Mohanan, P., Rahmat, Z., El Chbib, D., Marfani, W., & Essar, M. (2022). Mental health impacts of Lebanon's economic crisis on healthcare workers amidst COVID-19. *The International Journal of Health Planning and Management*, *37*(2), 1160–1165. DOI: 10.1002/hpm.3324 PMID: 34476840

Jiang, M., Yu, Y., Zhao, Q., Li, J., Song, C., Qi, H., Zhai, W., Luo, D., Wang, X., Fu, G., & Yang, B. (2024). AI-enhanced cognitive behavioral therapy: Deep learning and large language models for extracting cognitive pathways from social media texts. *ArXiv*, 1-10. https://arxiv.org/pdf/2404.11449

Jiang, M., Zhao, Q., Li, J., Wang, F., He, T., Cheng, X., Yang, B., Ho, G., & Fu, G. (2024). *A Generic Review of Integrating Artificial Intelligence in Cognitive Behavioral Therapy*. arXiv (retrieved from https://arxiv.org/abs/2407.19422). https://doi.org//arXiv.2407.19422DOI: 10.48550

Johnson, K. B., Wei, W. Q., Weeraratne, D., Frisse, M. E., Misulis, K., Rhee, K., Zhao, J., & Snowdon, J. L. (2021). Precision medicine, AI, and the future of personalized health care. *Clinical and Translational Science*, *14*(1), 86–93. DOI: 10.1111/cts.12884 PMID: 32961010

Joseph, A., & Babu, A. (2024). Transference and the psychological interplay in AI-enhanced mental healthcare. *Frontiers in Psychiatry, 15. Frontiers in Psychiatry, 1460469*, 1460469. Advance online publication. DOI: 10.3389/fpsyt.2024.1460469 PMID: 39224481

Julita, J. M. (2024). Gardner's theory of multiple intelligences: The basis for creating a new learning approach appropriate for teaching home economics at Hondagua National High School. *Psychology and Education: A Multidisciplinary Journal, 19*(2), 120-131. https://ssrn.com/abstract=4802063

Kaltenthaler, E., Brazier, J., Nigris, E., Tumur, I., Ferriter, M., Beverley, C., Parry, G., Rooney, G., & Sutcliffe, P. (2006). Computerised cognitive behaviour therapy for depression and anxiety update: A systematic review and economic evaluation. *Health Technology Assessment*, *10*(33), 168. DOI: 10.3310/hta10330 PMID: 16959169

Kaltenthaler, E., Parry, G., & Beverley, C. (2004). Computerized cognitive behavior therapy: A systematic review. *Behavioural and Cognitive Psychotherapy*, *32*(1), 31–55. DOI: 10.1017/S135246580400102X

Kaltenthaler, E., Parry, G., Beverley, C., & Ferriter, M. (2008). Computerised cognitive–behavioural therapy for depression: A systematic review. *The British Journal of Psychiatry*, *193*(3), 181–184. DOI: 10.1192/bjp.bp.106.025981 PMID: 18757972

Karkosz, S., Szymański, R., Sanna, K., & Michalowski, J. (2024). Effectiveness of a web-based and mobile therapy chatbot on anxiety and depressive symptoms in subclinical young adults: Randomized controlled trial. *JMIR Formative Research, 8. JMIR Formative Research, 47960*, e47960. Advance online publication. DOI: 10.2196/47960 PMID: 38506892

Khalid, N., Qayyum, A., Bilal, M., Al-Fuqaha, A., & Qadir, J. (2023). Privacy-preserving artificial intelligence in healthcare: Techniques and applications. *Computers in Biology and Medicine, 158. Computers in Biology and Medicine, 106848*, 106848. Advance online publication. DOI: 10.1016/j.compbiomed.2023.106848 PMID: 37044052

Khawaja, Z., & Bélisle-Pipon, J. C. (2023). Your robot therapist is not your therapist: Understanding the role of AI-powered mental health chatbots. *Frontiers in Digital Health*, *5*, 1–13. DOI: 10.3389/fdgth.2023.1278186 PMID: 38026836

Kieling, C., Baker-Henningham, H., Belfer, M., Conti, G., Ertem, I., Omigbodun, O., Rohde, L., Srinath, S., Ulkuer, N., & Rahman, A. (2011). Child and adolescent mental health worldwide: Evidence for action. *Lancet*, *378*(9801), 1515–1525. DOI: 10.1016/S0140-6736(11)60827-1 PMID: 22008427

Kiluk, B., Devore, K., Buck, M., Nich, C., Frankforter, T., LaPaglia, D., Yates, B., Gordon, M., & Carroll, K. (2016). Randomized trial of Computerized cognitive behavioral therapy for alcohol use disorders: Efficacy as a virtual stand-alone and treatment add-on compared with standard outpatient treatment. *Alcohol, Clinical and Experimental Research*, *40*(9), 1991–2000. DOI: 10.1111/acer.13162 PMID: 27488212

Koh, J., Tng, G. Y. Q., & Hartanto, A. (2022). Potential and pitfalls of mobile mental health apps in traditional treatment: An umbrella review. *Journal of Personalized Medicine, 12*(9). *Journal of Personalized Medicine*, *1376*(9), 1376. Advance online publication. DOI: 10.3390/jpm12091376 PMID: 36143161

Kola, L., Kohrt, B. A., Hanlon, C., Naslund, J. A., Sikander, S., Balaji, M., Benjet, C., Cheung, E. Y. L., Eaton, J., Gonsalves, P., Hailemariam, M., Luitel, N. P., Machado, D. B., Misganaw, E., Omigbodun, O., Roberts, T., Salisbury, T. T., Shidhaye, R., Sunkel, C., & Patel, V. (2021). COVID-19 mental health impact and responses in low-income and middle-income countries: Reimagining global mental health. *The Lancet. Psychiatry*, *8*(6), 535–550. DOI: 10.1016/S2215-0366(21)00025-0 PMID: 33639109

Kopelovich, S. L., Monroe-DeVita, M., Buck, B. E., Brenner, C., Moser, L., Jarskog, L. F., Harker, S., & Chwastiak, L. A. (2021). Community mental health care delivery during the COVID-19 pandemic: Practical strategies for improving care for people with serious mental illness. *Community Mental Health Journal*, *57*(3), 405–415. DOI: 10.1007/s10597-020-00662-z PMID: 32562033

Koutsouleris, N., Hauser, T. U., Skvortsova, V., & De Choudhury, M. (2022). From promise to practice: Towards the realisation of AI-informed mental health care. *The Lancet. Digital Health, 4*(11), 829–840. DOI: 10.1016/S2589-7500(22)00153-4 PMID: 36229346

Krebs, P., & Duncan, D. T. (2015). Health app use among US mobile phone owners: A national survey. *JMIR mHealth and uHealth, 3*(4). *JMIR mHealth and uHealth, 101*(4), e101. Advance online publication. DOI: 10.2196/mhealth.4924 PMID: 26537656

Kuhail, M., Alturki, N., Thomas, J., Alkhalifa, A., & Alshardan, A. (2024). Human-human vs human-AI therapy: An empirical study. *International Journal of Human-Computer Intercation*, 1-12. https://doi.org/DOI: 10.1080/10447318.2024.2385001

Lecomte, T., Potvin, S., Corbière, M., Guay, S., Samson, C., Cloutier, B., Francoeur, A., Pennou, A., & Khazaal, Y. (2020). Mobile apps for mental health issues: Meta-review of meta-analyses. *JMIR mHealth and uHealth, 8*(5), 17458. Advance online publication. DOI: 10.2196/17458 PMID: 32348289

Lee, E. E., Torous, J., De Choudhury, M., Depp, C. A., Graham, S. A., Kim, H., Paulus, M. P., Krystal, J. H., & Jeste, D. V. (2021). Artificial intelligence for mental health care: Clinical applications, barriers, facilitators, and artificial wisdom. *Biological Psychiatry: Cognitive Neuroscience and Neuroimaging, 6*(9), 856–864. DOI: 10.1016/j.bpsc.2021.02.001 PMID: 33571718

Lee, I., & Hahn, S. (2024). On the relationship between mind perception and social support of chatbots. *Frontiers in Psychology, 15. Frontiers in Psychology, 1282036*, 1282036. Advance online publication. DOI: 10.3389/fpsyg.2024.1282036 PMID: 38510306

Lejeune, A., Le Glaz, A., Perron, P-A., Sebti, J., Baca-Garcia, E., Walter, M., Lemey, C., & Berrouiguet, S. (2022). Artificial intelligence and suicide prevention: A systematic review. European Psychiatry, 65(1), e19, 1–8 DOI: 10.1192/j.eurpsy.2022.8

Li, P., Cheng, Z. Y., & Liu, G. L. (2020). Availability bias causes misdiagnoses by physicians: Direct evidence from a randomized controlled trial. *Internal Medicine (Tokyo, Japan), 59*(24), 3141–3146. DOI: 10.2169/internalmedicine.4664-20 PMID: 32788532

Li, S., Iqbal, M., Bashir, A. K., & Wang, X. (2021). Privacy preservation in artificial intelligence-enabled healthcare analytics. *Human-centric Computing and Information Sciences*, 1-13. https://orca.cardiff.ac.uk/id/eprint/167919/1/HCIS_T2023_Final_pr.pdf

Li, X., Zhang, X., Zhu, J., Mao, W., Sun, S., Wang, Z., Xia, C., & Hu, B. (2019). Depression recognition using machine learning methods with different feature generation strategies. *Artificial Intelligence in Medicine, 99. Artificial Intelligence in Medicine, 101696*, 101696. Advance online publication. DOI: 10.1016/j.artmed.2019.07.004 PMID: 31606115

Li, Y., Chung, T., Lu, W., He, M., & Mei, X. (2024). Chatbot-based mindfulness-based stress reduction program for university students with depressive symptoms: Intervention development and pilot evaluation. *Journal of the American Psychiatric Nurses Association*, •••, 1–14. DOI: 10.1177/10783903241302092 PMID: 39704086

Lim, H. C., Kolangde, S., Mohan, D., Hezam, A., Amatur, M., & Yusof, S. M. (2022). Artificial intelligence concepts for mental health application development: Therapy for mental health care. *American Journal of Multidisciplinary Research and Innovation*, *1*(6), 127–135. DOI: 10.54536/ajmri.v1i6.1038

Liu, F., Shi, Y., & Li, P. (2017). Analysis of the relation between artificial intelligence and the internet from the perspective of brain science. *Procedia Computer Science*, *122*, 377–383. DOI: 10.1016/j.procs.2017.11.383

Looi, J., Allison, S., Bastiampillai, T., Hensher, M., Kisely, S., & Robson, S. (2024). Australian specialised mental healthcare labour shortages: Potential interventions for consideration and further research. *Australasian Psychiatry*, *32*(5), 446–449. DOI: 10.1177/10398562241267138 PMID: 39110758

Love, C. S. (2023). "Just the Facts Ma'am": Moral and ethical considerations for artificial intelligence in medicine and its potential to impact patient autonomy and hope. *The Linacre Quarterly*, *90*(4), 375–394. DOI: 10.1177/00243639231162431 PMID: 37974568

Lucas, G. M., Gratch, J., King, A., & Morency, L. P. (2014). It's only a computer: Virtual humans increase willingness to disclose. *Computers in Human Behavior*, *37*, 94–100. DOI: 10.1016/j.chb.2014.04.043

Luger, G. F., & Chakrabarti, C. (2017). From Alan Turing to modern AI: Practical solutions and an implicit epistemic stance. *AI & Society*, *32*(3), 321–338. DOI: 10.1007/s00146-016-0646-7

Ly, D. P., Shekelle, P. G., & Song, Z. (2023). Evidence for anchoring bias during physician decision-making. *JAMA Internal Medicine*, *183*(8), 818–823. DOI: 10.1001/jamainternmed.2023.2366 PMID: 37358843

Manole, A., Cârciumaru, R., Brinzas, R., & Manole, F. (2024). Harnessing AI in anxiety management: A chatbot-based intervention for personalized mental health support. *Information (Basel), 15*(12), 768. DOI: 10.3390/info15120768

Marcelle, E. T., Nolting, L., Hinshaw, S. P., & Aguilera, A. (2019). Effectiveness of a multimodal digital psychotherapy platform for adult depression: A naturalistic feasibility study. *JMIR mHealth and uHealth, 7*(1). *JMIR mHealth and uHealth, 10948*(1), e10948. Advance online publication. DOI: 10.2196/10948 PMID: 30674448

Markowetz, A., Blaszkiewicz, K., Montag, C., Switala, C., & Schlaepfer, T. E. (2014). Psycho-informatics: Big data shaping modern psychometrics. *Medical Hypotheses, 82*(4), 405–411. DOI: 10.1016/j.mehy.2013.11.030 PMID: 24529915

Martinez, A., Co, M., Lau, J., & Brown, J. (2020). Filipino help-seeking for mental health problems and associated barriers and facilitators: A systematic review. *Social Psychiatry and Psychiatric Epidemiology, 55*(11), 1397–1413. DOI: 10.1007/s00127-020-01937-2 PMID: 32816062

McGinty, B. (2023). The future of public mental health: Challenges and opportunities. *The Milbank Quarterly, 101*(S1), 532–551. DOI: 10.1111/1468-0009.12622 PMID: 37096616

McKendree-Smith, N., Floyd, M., & Scogin, F. (2003). Self-administered treatments for depression: A review. *Journal of Clinical Psychology, 59*(3), 275–288. DOI: 10.1002/jclp.10129 PMID: 12579545

Mehta, A., Niles, A. N., Vargas, J. H., Marafon, T., Couto, D. D., & Gross, J. J. (2021). Acceptability and effectiveness of artificial intelligence therapy for anxiety and depression (Youper): Longitudinal observational study. *Journal of Medical Internet Research, 23*(6). *Journal of Medical Internet Research, 26771*(6), e26771. Advance online publication. DOI: 10.2196/26771 PMID: 34155984

Melcher, J., & Torous, J. (2020). Smart phone apps for college mental health: A concern for privacy and quality of current offerings. *Psychiatric Services (Washington, D.C.), 71*(11), 1114–1119. DOI: 10.1176/appi.ps.202000098 PMID: 32664822

Melnyk, B. M., Hoying, J., & Tan, A. (2022). Effects of the MINDSTRONG© CBT-based program on depression, anxiety and healthy lifestyle behaviors in graduate health sciences students. *Journal of American College Health, 70*(4), 1001–1009. DOI: 10.1080/07448481.2020.1782922 PMID: 32672515

Melo, A., Romão, J., & Duarte, T. (2024). Artificial intelligence and schizophrenia: Crossing the limits of the human brain. In Hocaoglu, C. (Ed.), *New Approaches to the Management and Diagnosis of Schizophrenia* (pp. 1–18). IntechOpen., DOI: 10.5772/intechopen.1004805

Mengi, M., & Malhotra, D. (2022). Artificial intelligence-based techniques for the detection of socio-behavioral disorders: A systematic review. *Archives of Computational Methods in Engineering*, *29*(5), 2811–2855. DOI: 10.1007/s11831-021-09682-8

Miner, A., Shah, N., Bullock, K., Arnow, B., Bailenson, J., & Hancock, J. (2019). Key considerations for incorporating conversational AI in psychotherapy. *Frontiers in Psychiatry, 10. Frontiers in Psychiatry*, *746*, 746. Advance online publication. DOI: 10.3389/fpsyt.2019.00746 PMID: 31681047

Moghaddari, M., Lighvan, M., & Danishvar, S. (2020). Diagnose ADHD disorder in children using convolutional neural network based on continuous mental task EEG. *Computer Methods and Programs in Biomedicine, 197. Computer Methods and Programs in Biomedicine*, *105738*, 105738. Advance online publication. DOI: 10.1016/j.cmpb.2020.105738 PMID: 32927404

Molden, H. (2024). AI, automation and psychotherapy – A proposed model for losses and gains in the automated therapeutic encounter. *European Journal of Psychotherapy & Counselling*, *26*(1-2), 48–66. DOI: 10.1080/13642537.2024.2318628

Molli, V. (2022). Effectiveness of AI-based chatbots in mental health support: A systematic review. *Journal of Healthcare AI and ML*, *9*(9), 1–11. https://journalpublication.wrcouncil.org/index.php/JHAM/article/view/10

Mowery, D., Smith, H., Cheney, T., Stoddard, G., Coppersmith, G., Bryan, C., & Conway, M. (2017). Understanding depressive symptoms and psychosocial stressors on twitter: A corpus-based study. *Journal of Medical Internet Research, 19*(2). *Journal of Medical Internet Research*, *48*(2), e48. Advance online publication. DOI: 10.2196/jmir.6895 PMID: 28246066

Murphy, K., Di Ruggiero, E., Upshur, R., Willison, D. J., Malhotra, N., Cai, J. C., Malhotra, N., Lui, V., & Gibson, J. (2021). Artificial intelligence for good health: A scoping review of the ethics literature. *BMC Medical Ethics*, *22*(14), 1–17. DOI: 10.1186/s12910-021-00577-8 PMID: 33588803

Navukkarasu, A., Varnam, M. P., & Jayasankar, T. (2023). Facial micro emotion detection and classification using swarm intelligence based modified convolutional network. *Expert Systems with Applications, 233. Expert Systems with Applications*, *120947*, 120947. Advance online publication. DOI: 10.1016/j.eswa.2023.120947

Niermann, H., Voss, C., Pieper, L., Venz, J., Ollmann, T., & Beesdo-Baum, K. (2021). Anxiety disorders among adolescents and young adults: Prevalence and mental health care service utilization in a regional epidemiological study in Germany. *Journal of Anxiety Disorders, 83. Journal of Anxiety Disorders, 102453*, 102453. Advance online publication. DOI: 10.1016/j.janxdis.2021.102453 PMID: 34303082

Nilsen, P., Svedberg, P., Nygren, J., Frideros, M., Johansson, J., & Schueller, S. (2022). Accelerating the impact of artificial intelligence in mental healthcare through implementation science. *Implementation Research and Practice, 3. Implementation Research and Practice, 26334895221112033*, 26334895221112033. Advance online publication. DOI: 10.1177/26334895221112033 PMID: 37091110

Nochaiwong, S., Ruengorn, C., Thavorn, K., Hutton, B., Awiphan, R., Phosuya, C., Ruanta, Y., Wongpakaran, N., & Wongpakaran, T. (2021). Global prevalence of mental health issues among the general population during the coronavirus disease-2019 pandemic: A systematic review and meta-analysis. *Scientific Reports, 11. Scientific Reports, 10173*(1), 10173. Advance online publication. DOI: 10.1038/s41598-021-89700-8 PMID: 33986414

Ojha, R., & Syed, S. (2020). Challenges faced by mental health providers and patients during the coronavirus 2019 pandemic due to technological barriers. *Internet Interventions, 21. Internet Interventions : the Application of Information Technology in Mental and Behavioural Health, 100330*, 100330. Advance online publication. DOI: 10.1016/j.invent.2020.100330 PMID: 32542180

Olawade, D. B., Wada, O. Z., Odetayo, A., David-Olawade, A. C., Asaolu, F., & Eberhardt, J. (2024). Enhancing mental health with artificial intelligence: Current trends and future prospects. *Journal of Medicine, Surgery, and Public Health, 3. Journal of Medicine, Surgery, and Public Health, 100099*, 100099. Advance online publication. DOI: 10.1016/j.glmedi.2024.100099

Omarov, B., Zhumanov, Z., Gumar, A., & Kuntunova, L. (2023). Artificial intelligence enabled mobile chatbot psychologist using AI and cognitive behavioral therapy. *(IJACSA). International Journal of Advanced Computer Science and Applications, 14*(6), 137–146. DOI: 10.14569/IJACSA.2023.0140616

Patel, V., Saxena, S., Lund, C., Thornicroft, G., Baingana, F., Bolton, P., Chisholm, D., Collins, P., Cooper, J., Eaton, J., Herrman, H., Herzallah, M., Huang, Y., Jordans, M., Kleinman, A., Medina-Mora, M., Morgan, E., Niaz, U., Omigbodun, O., & UnÜtzer, J. Ü. (2018). The Lancet Commission on global mental health and sustainable development. *Lancet, 392*(10157), 1553–1598. DOI: 10.1016/S0140-6736(18)31612-X PMID: 30314863

Paul, Y., Hickok, E., Sinha, A., & Tiwari, U. (n.d.). Artificial intelligence in the healthcare industry in India. *The Centre for Internet and Society*, 1-45. https://cis-india.org/internet-governance/files/ai-and-healtchare-report

Prescott, J., & Hanley, T. (2023). Therapists' attitudes towards the use of AI in therapeutic practice: Considering the therapeutic alliance. *Mental Health and Social Inclusion*, *27*(2), 177–185. DOI: 10.1108/MHSI-02-2023-0020

Prunkl, C. (2024). Human autonomy at risk? An analysis of the challenges from AI. *Minds and Machines*, *34*(26), 1–21. DOI: 10.1007/s11023-024-09665-1

Qi, Y. (2024). Pilot quasi-experimental research on the effectiveness of the Woebot AI chatbot for reducing mild depression symptoms among athletes. *International Journal of Human-Computer Interaction*. Advance online publication. DOI: 10.1080/10447318.2023.2301256

Rajeshkumar, L., Mishkind, M., Coleman, J., Pahwa, M., LaPreze, D., Solenske, S., & Wright, J. (2024). Computer-assisted Cognitive Behavior Therapy and mobile apps for depression and anxiety: Evidence-based digital tools for clinical practice. *Journal of Psychiatric Practice*, *30*(6), 389–399. DOI: 10.1097/PRA.0000000000000815 PMID: 39655965

Redlich, R., Almeida, J. J., Grotegerd, D., Opel, N., Kugel, H., Heindel, W., Arolt, V., Phillips, M. L., & Dannlowski, U. (2014). Brain morphometric biomarkers distinguishing unipolar and bipolar depression. A voxel-based morphometry-pattern classification approach. *JAMA Psychiatry*, *71*(11), 1222–1230. DOI: 10.1001/jamapsychiatry.2014.1100 PMID: 25188810

Regier, D. A., Kuhl, E. A., & Kupfer, D. J. (2013). The DSM-5: Classification and criteria changes. *World Psychiatry; Official Journal of the World Psychiatric Association (WPA)*, *12*(2), 92–98. DOI: 10.1002/wps.20050 PMID: 23737408

Richardson, M. (2021, December 13). *Cognitive computing vs. AI: What's the difference?* Spiceworks. https://www.spiceworks.com/tech/artificial-intelligence/articles/cognitive-computing-vs-ai/

Richardson, T., Stallard, P., & Velleman, S. (2010). Computerised cognitive behavioural therapy for the prevention and treatment of depression and anxiety in children and adolescents: A systematic review. *Clinical Child and Family Psychology Review*, *13*(3), 275–290. DOI: 10.1007/s10567-010-0069-9 PMID: 20532980

Rigby, M. J. (2019). Ethical dimensions of using artificial intelligence in health care. *AMA Journal of Ethics*, *21*(2), 121–124. DOI: 10.1001/amajethics.2019.121

Roa, T., Biller-Andorno, N., & Trachsel, M. (2021). The ethics of artificial intelligence in psychotherapy. In Trachsel, M., Gaab, J., Biller-Andorno, N., Tekin, Ş., & Sadler, J. Z. (Eds.), *The Oxford handbook of psychotherapy ethics/Online 2020* (pp. 744–758). Oxford University Press., DOI: 10.1093/oxfordhb/9780198817338.013.91

Rodrigues, R. (2020). Legal and human rights issues of AI: Gaps, challenges and vulnerabilities. *Journal of Responsible Technology*, *4*, 100005. DOI: 10.1016/j.jrt.2020.100005

Rodríguez, L., Ramos, F., & Wang, Y. (2011). Cognitive computational models of emotions. *International Journal of Software Science and Computational Intelligence*, *4*(2), 75–84. DOI: 10.1109/COGINF.2011.6016124

Roepke, A. M., Jaffee, S. R., Riffle, O. M., McGonigal, J., Broome, R., & Maxwell, B. (2015). Randomized controlled trial of SuperBetter, a smartphone-based/internet-based self-help tool to reduce depressive symptoms. *Games for Health Journal*, *4*(3), 235–246. DOI: 10.1089/g4h.2014.0046 PMID: 26182069

Russell, S., & Norvig, P. (2011). *Artificial intelligence: A modern approach* (3rd ed.). Pearson.

Sadeh-Sharvit, S., Camp, T., Horton, S., Hefner, J., Berry, J., Grossman, E., & Hollon, S. (2023). Effects of an artificial intelligence platform for behavioral interventions on depression and anxiety symptoms: Randomized clinical trial. *Journal of Medical Internet Research, 25, Article* e46781. https://doi.org/DOI: 10.31234/osf.io/97pdj

Santomauro, D., Herrera, A., Shadid, J., Zheng, P., Ashbaugh, C., Pigott, D. M., Abbafati, C., Adolph, C., Amlag, J. O., Aravkin, A. Y., Bang-Jensen, B. L., Bertolacci, G. J., Bloom, S. S., Castellano, R., Castro, E., Chakrabarti, S., Chattopadhyay, J., Cogen, R. M., Collins, J. K., & Ferrari, A. J. (2021). Global prevalence and burden of depressive and anxiety disorders in 204 countries and territories in 2020 due to the COVID-19 pandemic. *Lancet*, *398*(10312), 1700–1712. DOI: 10.1016/S0140-6736(21)02143-7 PMID: 34634250

Satiani, A., Niedermier, J., Satiani, B., & Svendsen, D. (2018). Projected workforce of psychiatrists in the United States: A population analysis. *Psychiatric Services (Washington, D.C.)*, *69*(6), 710–713. DOI: 10.1176/appi.ps.201700344 PMID: 29540118

Schmidt, J., Schutte, N. M., Buttigieg, S., Novillo-Ortiz, D., Sutherland, E., Anderson, M., de Witte, B., Peolsson, M., Unim, B., Pavlova, M., Stern, A. D., Mossialos, E., & van Kessel, R. (2024). Mapping the regulatory landscape for artificial intelligence in health within the European Union. *NPJ Digital Medicine, 7*(1). *NPJ Digital Medicine*, *229*(1), 229. Advance online publication. DOI: 10.1038/s41746-024-01221-6 PMID: 39191937

Sedlakova, J., & Trachsel, M. (2023). Conversational artificial intelligence in psychotherapy: A new therapeutic tool or agent? *The American Journal of Bioethics*, *23*(5), 4–13. DOI: 10.1080/15265161.2022.2048739 PMID: 35362368

Shah, N. (2014). *Market monitor: Q1 2014: Smartphones now 95% of total handset revenues*. Counterpoint Technology Market Research. https://www.counterpointresearch.com/insight/market-monitor-q1-2014-smartphones-now-95-of-total-handset-revenues

Shah, P., & Yadav, K. (2024). From detection to recovery: The promise of AI in managing postpartum depression in India. *E3S Web of Conferences, 556. Article, 01047*, 01047. Advance online publication. DOI: 10.1051/e3sconf/202455601047

Shahamiri, S., & Thabtah, F. (2020). Autism AI: A new autism screening system based on artificial intelligence. *Cognitive Computation*, *12*(4), 766–777. DOI: 10.1007/s12559-020-09743-3

Sheth, A., Yip, H. Y., Iyengar, A., & Tepper, P. (2019). Cognitive services and intelligent chatbots: Current perspectives and special issue introduction. *IEEE Internet Computing*, *23*(2), 6–12. DOI: 10.1109/MIC.2018.2889231 PMID: 33746506

Silva, M., Resurrección, D. M., Antunes, A., Frasquilho, D., & Cardoso, G. (2020). Impact of economic crises on mental health care: A systematic review. *Epidemiology and Psychiatric Sciences*, *29*(e7), 1–13. DOI: 10.1017/S2045796018000641 PMID: 30419997

Smith, A. (2013, June 5). *Smartphone ownership 2013*. Pew Research Center. https://www.pewresearch.org/internet/2013/06/05/smartphone-ownership-2013/

Smith, G., & Rustagi, I. (2020). Mitigating bias in artificial intelligence: An equity fluent leadership playbook. *Berkeley Haas Center for Equity, Gender and Leadership*, 1-67. https://haas.berkeley.edu/wp-content/uploads/UCB_Playbook_R10_V2_spreads2.pdf

Solaiman, B., Malik, A., & Ghuloum, S. (2024). Monitoring mental health: Legal and ethical considerations of using artificial intelligence in psychiatric wards. *American Journal of Law & Medicine*, *49*(2-3), 250–266. DOI: 10.1017/amj.2023.30 PMID: 38344795

Stein, D. J., Shoptaw, S. J., Vigo, D. V., Lund, C., Cuijpers, P., Bantjes, J., Sartorius, N., & Maj, M. (2022). Psychiatric diagnosis and treatment in the 21st century: Paradigm shifts versus incremental integration. *World Psychiatry; Official Journal of the World Psychiatric Association (WPA)*, *8*(21), 393–414. DOI: 10.1002/wps.20998 PMID: 36073709

Sternberg, R. J. (1990). *Metaphors of mind: Conceptions of the nature of intelligence*. Cambridge University Press.

Sternberg, R. J. (2021). Adaptive intelligence: Intelligence is not a personal trait but rather a person × task × situation interaction. *Journal of Intelligence*, *9*(4), 1–9. DOI: 10.3390/jintelligence9040058 PMID: 34940380

Tachmazidis, I., Chen, T., Adamou, M., & Antoniou, G. (2021). A hybrid AI approach for supporting clinical diagnosis of attention deficit hyperactivity disorder (ADHD) in adults. *Health Information Science and Systems*, *9*(1), 1–8. DOI: 10.1007/s13755-020-00123-7 PMID: 33235709

Tahan, M. (2023). Robot-based psychological intervention program for the prevention of child sexual abuse: An overview. *Neuropsychopharmacologia Hungarica*, *25*(1), 18–25. DOI: 10.17504/protocols.io.36wgq3dnxlk5/v1 PMID: 37262332

Tahan, M., & Saleem, T. (2023). Application of artificial intelligence for diagnosis, prognosis and treatment in psychology: A review. *Neuropsychiatria i Neuropsychologia.*, *18*(1–2), 36–45. DOI: 10.5114/nan.2023.129070

Tang, Y., Sun, J., Wang, C., Zhong, Y., Jiang, A., Liu, G., & Liu, X. (2022). ADHD classification using auto-encoding neural network and binary hypothesis testing. *Artificial Intelligence in Medicine, 123. Artificial Intelligence in Medicine, 102209*, 102209. Advance online publication. DOI: 10.1016/j.artmed.2021.102209 PMID: 34998510

Tanielian, T., & Jaycox, L. H. (2008). *Invisible wound of war: Psychological and cognitive injuries, their consequences, and services to assist recovery*. RAND.

Thakkar, A., Gupta, A., & De Sousa, A. (2024). Artificial intelligence in positive mental health: A narrative review. *Frontiers in Digital Health*, *6*, 1–11. DOI: 10.3389/fdgth.2024.1280235 PMID: 38562663

The Lancet Global Health. (2020). Mental health matters. *The Lancet Global health, 8*(11), *Article* 1352. https://doi.org/DOI: 10.1016/S2214-109X(20)30432-0

Tom Gruber. (2025). *Patient, know thyself: AI-powered digital brain biomarkers.* Tom Gruber. https://tomgruber.org/mindstrong-story/

Torous, J., Cerrato, P., & Halamka, J. (2019). Targeting depressive symptoms with technology. *mHealth, 5*, 19. DOI: 10.21037/mhealth.2019.06.04 PMID: 31463305

Torous, J., & Roberts, L. (2017). Needed innovation in digital health and smartphone applications for mental health: Transparency and trust. *JAMA Psychiatry, 74*(5), 437–438. DOI: 10.1001/jamapsychiatry.2017.0262 PMID: 28384700

Turing, A. M. (1950). Computing machinery and intelligence. *Mind, 59*(236), 433–460. DOI: 10.1093/mind/LIX.236.433

Turvey, B. E., & Freeman, J. L. (2012). Jury psychology. In Ramachandran, V. S. (Ed.), *Encyclopedia of human behavior* (2nd ed., pp. 495–502). Elsevier., DOI: 10.1016/B978-0-12-375000-6.00216-0

Tutun, S., Johnson, M. E., Ahmed, A., Albizri, A., Irgil, S., Yesilkaya, I., Ucar, E. N., Sengun, T., & Harfouche, A. (2022). An AI-based decision support system for predicting mental health disorders. *Information Systems Frontiers, 25*(3), 1261–1276. DOI: 10.1007/s10796-022-10282-5 PMID: 35669335

Ursin, F., Timmermann, C., Orzechowski, M., & Steger, F. (2021). Diagnosing diabetic retinopathy with artificial intelligence: What information should be included to ensure ethical informed consent? *Frontiers in Medicine, 8. Frontiers in Medicine, 695217*, 695217. Advance online publication. DOI: 10.3389/fmed.2021.695217 PMID: 34368192

Vaidyam, A. N., Wisniewski, H., Halamka, J. D., Kashavan, M. S., & Torous, J. B. (2019). Chatbots and conversational agents in mental health: A review of the psychiatric landscape. *Canadian Journal of Psychiatry, 64*(7), 456–464. DOI: 10.1177/0706743719828977 PMID: 30897957

Vallury, K., Jones, M., & Oosterbroek, C. (2015). Computerized cognitive behavior therapy for anxiety and depression in rural areas: A systematic review. *Journal of Medical Internet Research, 17(*6). *Journal of Medical Internet Research, 139*(6), e139. Advance online publication. DOI: 10.2196/jmir.4145 PMID: 26048193

Vandemeulebroucke, T., Dierckx de Casterlé, B., & Gastmans, C. (2018). The use of care robots in aged care: A systematic review of argument-based ethics literature. *Archives of Gerontology and Geriatrics, 74*, 15–25. DOI: 10.1016/j.archger.2017.08.014 PMID: 28926749

Villegas-Ch, W., & García-Ortiz, J. (2023). Toward a comprehensive framework for ensuring security and privacy in artificial intelligence. *Electronics (Basel)*, *12*(3786), 1–17. DOI: 10.3390/electronics12183786

Wager, T. D., & Woo, C. W. (2017). Imaging biomarkers and biotypes for depression. *Nature Medicine*, *23*(1), 16–17. DOI: 10.1038/nm.4264 PMID: 28060802

Wainberg, M. L., Scorza, P., Shultz, J. M., Helpman, L., Mootz, J. J., Johnson, K. A., Neria, Y., Bradford, J. E., Oquendo, M. A., & Arbuckle, M. R. (2017). Challenges and opportunities in global mental health: A research-to-practice perspective. *Current Psychiatry Reports*, *19*(5), 1–16. DOI: 10.1007/s11920-017-0780-z PMID: 28425023

Waller, R., & Gilbody, S. (2009). Barriers to the uptake of Computerized Cognitive Behavioural Therapy: A systematic review of the quantitative and qualitative evidence. *Psychological Medicine*, *39*(5), 705–712. DOI: 10.1017/S0033291708004224 PMID: 18812006

Walsh, C. G., Ribeiro, J. D., & Franklin, J. C. (2017). Predicting risk of suicide attempts over time through machine learning. *Clinical Psychological Science*, *5*(3), 457–469. DOI: 10.1177/2167702617691560

Wan, R., Wan, R., Xie, Q., Hu, A., Xie, W., Chen, J., & Liu, Y. (2025). Current status and future directions of artificial intelligence in post-traumatic stress disorder: A literature measurement analysis. *Behavioral Sciences (Basel, Switzerland)*, *15*(1), 27. DOI: 10.3390/bs15010027 PMID: 39851830

Wang, X., Hegde, S., Son, C., Keller, B., Smith, A., & Sasangohar, F. (2020). Investigating mental health of US college students during the COVID-19 pandemic: Cross-sectional survey study. *Journal of Medical Internet Research, 22*(9). *Journal of Medical Internet Research*, *22817*(9), e22817. Advance online publication. DOI: 10.2196/22817 PMID: 32897868

Westbye, H., Moltu, C., & McAleavey, A. (2024). Explainable AI for routine outcome monitoring and clinical feedback. *Counselling & Psychotherapy Research*, *25*(1), 1–8. DOI: 10.1002/capr.12764

Williams, D. R., & Cooper, L. A. (2020). COVID-19 and health equity—A new kind of "herd immunity". *Journal of the American Medical Association*, *23*(24), 2478–2480. DOI: 10.1001/jama.2020.8051 PMID: 32391852

World Health Organization. (2022a, June 17). *Mental health*. WHO. https://www.who.int/news-room/fact-sheets/detail/mental-health-strengthening-our-response

World Health Organization. (2022b). *World mental health report: Transforming mental health for all*. WHO. https://iris.who.int/bitstream/handle/10665/356119/9789240049338-eng.pdf

World Health Organization. (2025a). *Harnessing artificial intelligence for health.* WHO. https://www.who.int/teams/digital-health-and-innovation/harnessing-artificial-intelligence-for-health

World Health Organization. (2025b). *International statistical classification of diseases and related health problems (ICD)*. WHO. https://www.who.int/standards/classifications/classification-of-diseases

Wright, J., Mishkind, M., Eells, T., & Chan, S. (2019). Computer-assisted cognitive-behavior therapy and mobile apps for depression and anxiety. *Current Psychiatry Reports, 21*(62), 1–9. DOI: 10.1007/s11920-019-1031-2 PMID: 31250242

Wright, J., Owen, J., Eells, T., Antle, B., Bishop, L., Girdler, R., Harris, L., Wright, B., Wells, M., Gopalraj, R., Pendleton, M., & Ali, S. (2022). Effect of computer-assisted cognitive behavior therapy vs usual care on depression among adults in primary care: A randomized clinical trial. *JAMA Network Open, 5*(2). *JAMA Network Open, 2146716*(2), e2146716. Advance online publication. DOI: 10.1001/jamanetworkopen.2021.46716 PMID: 35142833

Xue, C., Kowshik, S. S., Lteif, D., Puducheri, S., Jasodanand, V. H., Zhou, O. T., Walia, A. S., Guney, O. B., Zhang, J. D., Pham, S. T., Kaliaev, A., Andreu-Arasa, V. C., Dwyer, B. C., Farris, C. W., Hao, H., Kedar, S., Mian, A. Z., Murman, D. L., O'Shea, S. A., & Kolachalama, V. B. (2024). AI-based differential diagnosis of dementia etiologies on multimodal data. *Nature Medicine, 30*(10), 2977–2989. DOI: 10.1038/s41591-024-03118-z PMID: 38965435

Yan, W., Ruan, Q., & Jiang, K. (2023). Challenges for artificial intelligence in recognizing mental disorders. *Diagnostics, 13*(1). *Article, 2*. Advance online publication. DOI: 10.3390/diagnostics13010002 PMID: 36611294

Yellowlees, P. (2022). Impact of COVID-19 on mental health care practitioners. *The Psychiatric Clinics of North America, 45*(1), 109–121. DOI: 10.1016/j.psc.2021.11.007 PMID: 35219432

Yoo, A., Li, F., Youn, J., Guan, J., Guyer, A. E., Hostinar, C. E., & Tagkopoulos, I. (2024). Prediction of adolescent depression from prenatal and childhood data from ALSPAC using machine learning. *Scientific Reports, 14*(1). *Scientific Reports, 23282*(1), 23282. Advance online publication. DOI: 10.1038/s41598-024-72158-9 PMID: 39375420

Younis, O., Jambi, K., Eassa, F., & Elrefaei, L. (2024). A proposal for a tokenized intelligent system: A prediction for an AI-based scheduling, secured using blockchain. *Systems*, *12*(84), 1–21. DOI: 10.3390/systems12030084

Yule, A. M., Youn, S. J., Dean, K., Woodward, D. W., Firmin, E. S., Kramer, J., Stone, M., Marques, L., & Wilens, T. E. (2024). Different factors identified by stakeholder group for barriers and facilitators to measurement-based care implementation in behavioral health clinics. *Journal of Clinical Psychology*, *80*(3), 576–590. DOI: 10.1002/jclp.23639 PMID: 38230918

Zafar, M. (2024). Enhancing university students' mental health under artificial intelligence: Principles of behaviour therapy. *OBM Neurobiology*, *8*(2). *OBM Neurobiology*, *2402225*(2), 1–5. Advance online publication. DOI: 10.21926/obm.neurobiol.2402225

Zeb, S., Nizamullah, F., Abbasi, N., & Fahad, M. (2024). AI in healthcare: Revolutionizing diagnosis and therapy. *International Journal of Multidisciplinary Sciences and Arts*, *3*(3), 118–128. DOI: 10.47709/ijmdsa.v3i3.4546

Zhang, Y., Kong, M., Zhao, T., Hong, W., Xie, D., Wang, C., Yang, R., Li, R., & Zhu, Q. (2021). Auxiliary diagnostic system for ADHD in children based on AI technology. *Frontiers of Information Technology & Electronic Engineering*, *22*(3), 400–414. DOI: 10.1631/FITEE.1900729

Zhao, G., & Li, X. (2019). Automatic micro-expression analysis: Open challenges. *Frontiers in Psychology*, *10*(1833), 1-4. https://doi.org/DOI: 10.3389/fpsyg.2019.01833

Zheng, F., Zhao, C., Usman, M., & Poulova, P. (2024). From bias to brilliance: The impact of artificial intelligence usage on recruitment biases in China. *IEEE Transactions on Engineering Management*, *71*, 14155–14167. DOI: 10.1109/TEM.2024.3442618

Zhou, S., Zhao, J., & Zhang, L. (2022). Application of artificial intelligence on psychological interventions and diagnosis: An overview. *Frontiers in Psychiatry*, *13*(811665), 1–7. DOI: 10.3389/fpsyt.2022.811665 PMID: 35370846

Zhou, T., Li, X., Pei, Y., Gao, J., & Kong, J. (2016). Internet-based cognitive behavioural therapy for subthreshold depression: A systematic review and meta-analysis. *BMC Psychiatry*, *16*(1), 356. DOI: 10.1186/s12888-016-1061-9 PMID: 27769266

Chapter 9
Artificial Intelligence and Human Mental Wellbeing:
Striking a Balance Between Innovation and Productivity

Jagneet Kour
https://orcid.org/0009-0003-0341-3636
Eternal University, Baru Sahib, India

Raino Bhatia
https://orcid.org/0000-0002-5379-3003
Eternal University, Baru Sahib, India

ABSTRACT

This research study examines how artificial intelligence is shaping ground-breaking impacts on the essence of human existence. An extensive examination reveals how artificial intelligence has transformed multiple aspects of life, ushering in a new age marked by remarkable productivity and ease of use. This study explores the complex interplay between artificial intelligence and mental well-being, analyzing its contradictory effects of positive and negative influence. Artificial intelligence (AI) technology possesses significant potential to revolutionize mental healthcare, but inherent risks. This study article provides a thorough analysis of the complexity of artificial intelligence in relation to mental well-being. This paper provides insights to use its advantages while minimizing risks, finally establishing a comprehensive plan for mental health treatment in contemporary society.

DOI: 10.4018/979-8-3373-5072-1.ch009

INTRODUCTION

Artificial intelligence is such a trans-formative force in evolving terrain of technology that is reshaping many aspects of human existence. Humans have reached a pivotal juncture in the latest industrial era, succeeding the technological, electronic, and the internet services, referred to as the "digital and web based revolution," distinguished by a convergence of several technological modalities (Pang et al.,2018; Graham et al.,2019). Artificial intelligence (AI) is a prime demonstration of an innovation that has been popularly used around since 1956(Simon, 1991). Artificial Intelligence refers to the stimulation of human intelligence in computers or machines that are programmed to think and behave like human beings it imparts a wide range of technologies and uses, including as machine learning, computer vision, natural language processing, machine learning and expert system. AI are designed to do some specific tasks that generally require human intelligence such as, understanding natural language, recognizing patterns, making decisions, and solving problems. These systems are flexible tools with applicability across various industries and domain, ability to learn from data, adapt to new inputs and enhance their efficiency` over time. The emergence of artificial intelligence (AI) has transformed the workflow, teamwork, and value creation of today's companies. Artificial intelligence has emerged as a versatile instrument used across several sectors, transforming workflows, decision-making processes, and value generation in areas including as healthcare, education, finance, and others (Dwivedi et al., 2021).

Over the past few decades, AI has emerged as a game-changing technology in a wide range of industries. It comprises several subfields, including machine learning, computer vision, natural language processing, and expert systems. These technologies facilitate systems in recognising patterns, making choices, adapting to new inputs, and enhancing over time. Artificial intelligence (AI) is a game-changer in industries as varied as medicine, teaching, and banking due to its capacity to replicate human intellect processes like learning, troubleshooting issues, and decision-making processes. Artificial Intelligence can employ advanced algorithms to extract aspects from extensive healthcare records and subsequently utilise the consequent findings to support doctors in their practice. It can additionally be outfitted with automated learning and rectifying itself capabilities to enhance its precision depending on input. An AI system can aid clinicians by supplying cutting-edge healthcare data from books, publications, and practical techniques to enhance outcomes for patients (Pearson, 2011). Realising that mental capacity is normally associated with humans, the adoption of the expression "artificial" indicates that this type of intellect is exhibited by an automated system. Artificial intelligence has become pervasive in contemporary western civilisation as the ability to access data, to manage safety measures, and to enable networking through social media (Jiang et al., 2017).

ROLE OF AI IN HEALTHCARE AND MENTAL HEALTH

Artificial Intelligence has had an enormous impact on the healthcare sector, especially in examinations, decision support systems, and handling patients. Artificial intelligence has the capability to analyse extensive health data and support practitioners by providing insights obtained from medical records, literature, and real-time analytics (Pearson, 2011). Predictive analytics, automated image analysis, and virtual health assistants are being increasingly utilised in clinical environments (Jiang et al., 2017; Murdoch & Detsky, 2013; Kolker et al., 2016). Although artificial intelligence is starting to find applications in healthcare such as DNA testing and healthcare visualisation (Jiang et al., 2017). AI has taken humans in an era of unparalleled efficiency and ease, from streamlining daily routine to revolutionary industries. However, as we delve in depth of realm of AI, it becomes an imperative to comprehend how it will profoundly impact on humankind, especially in terms of mental health. Artificial intelligence is helping the mental health sector, which has historically had little financial support. There is a greater need for effective and easily available psychological therapies due to the worldwide mental health crisis, which is driven by elements like escalating levels of stress, technological advancements, and budgetary constraints. Owing to AI's scalability and data-driven accuracy, there are alternatives that can make mental health care more feasible and democratise it. AI methods have lately prompted tremendous concern in the field of medicine, even igniting a heated debate about whether AI physicians could potentially overtake the role of genuine practitioners. Researchers assert that the skills of human doctors will not be completely supplanted by robots in the very near future; nonetheless, AI can certainly aid professionals in enhancing medical decision-making or ultimately swap discretion by humans in specific domains of medical care (e.g., radiography). The growing accessibility to health insurance information as well as the swift advancement of huge-scale analytical techniques have facilitated lately effective use of AI in the healthcare industry. Fuelled by pertinent clinical investigations, advanced AI methodologies can reveal medically vital details concealed within gigantic sets of data, hence facilitating healthcare decisions (Murdoch & Detsky, 2013; Kolker, Özdemir, & Kolker, 2016; Dilsizian & Siegel, 2014; Jiang et al.,2017).The adoption of AI in more areas, like virtual aids and algorithmic learning in psychotherapy, has changed how psychological treatment is administered. The use of AI in screening, therapy suggestions, and personalised networks of support has shown capacity. In contrast, its growing importance in interpersonal relationships and work environments raises worries about confidentiality, excessive dependency, and psychological separation.

AI and Education: A Paradigm Shift

The applications of AI in education are significantly revolutionary. It enables individualised learning, programmed evaluation, and advanced guidance platforms. These resources address various learner requirements, increase engagement, and enhance educational results to collaborate various pedagogies into education system (Bhatia, & Kaur, 2024).The notion of AI literacy, defined as the capacity to comprehend, utilise, and assess AI technologies, has emerged as a pivotal subject in policy discussions and educational curriculum design (Holmes, 2022;).Artificial intelligence can customise educational resources, monitor learner advancement, and deliver personalised constructive criticism. Additionally, its application in inclusive education can aid learners with disabilities by providing tailored settings for learning and adaptive technology. Despite this, there are problems with integrity, teacher education, technological resources, and the right way to use AI in the classroom. Also, it's important to make sure that AI tools used in education don't promote biases or get in the way of human-centred teaching.

ARTIFICIAL INTELLIGENCE (A THEME WITH MANY FACETS)

There is not a single accepted definition of AI, despite its increasing prevalence. A multifaceted interdisciplinary discipline that encompasses a variety of philosophical and empirical approaches, AI is not a singular, consistent technology, as academicians have pointed out (Holmes, 2022). Its definition frequently is contingent upon its ultimate usage, whether it be for automated processes, choice-making, anticipating, or interactivity. From a classical perspective, AI is a system that is capable of executing duties that would typically necessitate human intelligence. AI systems engage with humans and environments, occasionally operating autonomously and utilising the context of their surroundings to enhance their performance (UNICEF, 2021).

The goal of this chapter is to look at both points of view. This research paper endeavours on a journey to delve into the complex effects of AI, investigating how it has reshaped our life and society, while also including its dual impacts on mental health- both beneficial and detrimental. By comprehensive analysis spanning diverse domains like mental health, quality education is taking a huge place in our system. This article offers a detailed and sophisticated comprehension with careful consideration on AI's role in shaping our collective future. Moreover, this article seeks to highlight both its triumphs and challenges in the field of mental health. Ultimately, our focus is to contribute a comprehensive approach to mental healthcare in the digital era, where AI is used as a tool for enhancing human well-being while preserving the essence of what it means to be human. AI is a disruptive force that is evolving many aspects of human existence. AI is bringing in a new era of unmatched simplicity and efficiency, transforming industries and simplifying daily tasks. However, as AI advances, it became more crucial to understand that how will it profoundly affect human-life, particularly with regards to mental health and education. AI has become a game changer force in the field of mental health, providing innovative solutions to enduring problem. Early diagnosis of mental health issue, suicidal, and drug misuse risk early needs to be addressed on urgent basis. Artificial intelligence focused on digital treatments and virtual therapists are two intervention techniques that improve therapy accessibility and individual attention (Shah, 2022). The applicability of AI in education and the potential for learning have received a significant attention .Furthermore, debates over policy are quickly shifting toward the role of education in establishing what is now called AI literacy, or the teaching of AI in education and are quickly becoming hot topics in policy discussion (Holmes, 2022).There is no particular definition of artificial intelligence that is accepted by the majority of AI exporter, in-spite of this academic researcher' claim that it is a complex field of study with many conceptual approaches and domains of expertise. It is important to recognize that the definition of AI depends on its intended application. Academic studies sometimes underline that there is no such thing as AI and elaborate it as a complicated field of study with many difficult fields of study with many different conceptual approaches and areas of competence (Holmes, 2022). One classical definition states that AI research aims to form technology that is competent of performing tasks that would mandate human intelligence if executed by humans. AI refers to an intelligent machine that can perform various tasks like predict, suggest, or decide various work based on what human wants them to do. AI system interacts with us and acts on our environment, either directly or indirectly. Sometimes, they appear to work on their own and can learn from what's going on around them to do better (UNICEF, 2021)

BACKGROUND OF THE STUDY

AI-driven programs, such as expression analysis instruments, are utilised to evaluate psychological variations throughout communities. Mobile applications such as Mind strong monitor mental processes by analysing smartphone information on use to provide prompt therapy (Graham et al., 2019). Another instance is the application of AI in accuracy wherein personalised medication is administered based on an individual's distinct data trends (Dwyer et al., 2018).Although AI enables numerous advancements, it also produces unplanned adverse effects. Excessive reliance on AI-facilitated social connections may result in social seclusion and psychological disconnect (Ahuja, 2020). Furthermore, AI algorithms functioning autonomously may misread physiological signals, resulting in inadequate mental health services. Holmes (2020) concluded in his research article that in upcoming years AI technology will improve vastly which we can't just guess what will happen. Some people says that AI could eventually be smarter that humans. (Bhatia et al., 2023) also inculcated in their paper that AI has made mental health services more accessible and brought innovativeness in technology. On the other hand, AI has raised several social concern and privacy concern issues. Self-medication theory (Goeders, 2003) states that people whenever face depression and anxiety, they use drugs to self-medicate or prevent them self any harm, but eventually get addicted to those Drugs. Likewise, children and adolescents with AI technology dependency use smart phones, computer and tabs in order to medicate them from stress, real life problems and emotional problems (Sun et al., 2018; Joshi, Bhatia, & Kour, 2025) Graham et al.,(2019) examined twenty-eight studies on artificial intelligence and mental health that utilised digital medical records (EHRs), mental state assessment scales, neuroimaging data, innovative monitoring systems (e.g., smartphones, video), and social networking services to estimate, determine, or split mental health disorders, including depression, schizophrenia, other psychiatric conditions, and suicidal ideation and attempts. These studies combined demonstrated high accuracy and showcased AI's potential in psychological services; however, they should primarily be regarded as preliminary evidence suggesting works illustrating the feasibility of employing machine learning (ML) algorithms to tackle mental health enquiries and identifying which algorithms deliver the greatest efficiency. A theory named" Compensatory internet theory " that most of the people make busy themselves in social media or online world in order to escape them from real life problem and take some actions or receive support that helps to improve one's emotional state and reduce negative feelings, eventually growing compulsive usage of the internet or technology (Kardefelt-winther, 2014). A study found that mental-health issues can lead to relaying more on AI. Like, using AI to escape or for entertainment or for social reasons tends to be linked with anxiety and depression leading to more dependence on AI. Moreover, using AI for entertainment or practical reason doesn't to be connected to anxiety and depression leading to dependence on AI (Huang et al., 2024).

INTERSECTING REALMS: AI'S AND MENTAL HEALTH DYNAMICS

In present day world is surrounded by technology and AI (artificial intelligence) plays a vital role in every aspect of humans. AI and mental health have an intricate relationship, and AI technologies can be used to enhance mental health care through

Chabot's, virtual therapist and predictive analytics. On the other hand, concerns arise regarding privacy, ethics and the potential for AI to exacerbate biases in diagnosis or treatment. Overall, when developed and used properly and responsibly, AI has the potential to augment mental health services and support to those in need. Both directly proportional to each other one is affected by another dual phase, is that both of them have positive and negative impact on each other. Today's world is deeply surrounded by AI in various ways and affect human's personal as well as social life. It is observed that how different aspects of AI surround humans and all these are indicating in basic needs of human being life without technology human is nothing. However, all these things are time saver and helpful for humans but side by side these are making humans disabled. Human are not using their capabilities now they are just totally dependent on technology .AI helps in saving time, convenient to use, do humans all tasks, works as a source of entertainment as well as a source of education of every field. It makes home tasks easy and provides work from home services. A huge source for livelihood and earning works as a gateway for communication all over the world. Side by side there's are various cyber-crimes because of AI. It can affect life of a person in many ways. It can be also the reason of someone's entertainment but in same time it is taking a person far away from real life making them lethargic, diseased and frustrated. Now, we all know that AI works as a friend and foe to humans. Like every coin have two sides similarly AI have a positive as well as negative side. AI positive side is that it helps to monitor mental health, personalized treatment for mental health, it is very helpful in research and diagnosis. Negative aspects of AI are it has lots of privacy concerns, AI algorithm may perpetuate biases, leading to unequal access to mental health services or misdiagnosis, AI driven therapy tools may lead to lack of human connection and ethical issues such as potential for exploitation, manipulation or violation of autonomy. Overall, AI holds dual perspective negative as well as positive. It totally depends upon humans how to deal with it and how to use it. Mental health is about how our thought process works, how we think, sense and face situations in life. It's all about our emotional, psychological and social well-being. Good mental health means feeling good about you, dealing well with hard time or burden, and having healthy relationships. Moreover, it is about being able to work effectively and contribute to society. If mental health is stable then consequently the person will be able to perform tasks positively. An individual with healthy mental state will be socially adjustable and adaptable, emotionally balanced, physically fit and intellectually intelligent, he or she will be balanced in every aspect of life (Bhatia & Kaur, 2024). And on the other half a person with bad mental state will be lethargic and reluctant for every work. Although there will be sudden outburst of emotions and neither stable in society and will feel physically retarded. It is quite efficient for an individual to be mentally stable. Because it forms a positive aura of a person and they will definitely attract positive stuff. Artificial intelligence possesses the capacity to transform our way of thinking about mental well-being. The significance of chatbots providing round-the-clock care and AI-driven mental health evaluations in tackling global mental health issues is considerable (Lee et al., 2019). AI systems facilitate preventative measures by identifying early indicators of psychological trouble, so assuring prompt treatment for those in need.

AI'S ROLE IN MENTAL HEALTH DECLINE: CHALLENGES AND CONCERNS

AI's adverse effects on mental health manifest through over dependency on technology, diminished human interaction, and apprehension about privacy breaches and data security. Furthermore, there's an impending risk of magnifying biasness within algorithm, potentially resulting in misdiagnoses or unequal distribution of care. These challenges underscore the importance of addressing AI's role to ensure it enhance, rather than replace, human-centric approaches to mental health support. AI impact mental health and can lead to increased isolation, dependency on technology, compromised privacy, making people disable because on increasing dependency on AI for every work. As we see a person with stable mental state will effectively and positively use technology and he will have self-motivation and self-control on himself to use AI only for purposeful work, but at some instant if the person will get addicted to use AI tools in negative perspective than that same person might lose all his self-control and self-motivation or became mentally unstable, because using AI more will make a person to trap in the web of AI world which means to an artificial world which doesn't exist and make that individual lethargic and disorganized.

Sometime being so into in technology affects our mental health. There are various mental health programs that will help humans to use efficiently this AI tool. AI is incorporating into mental health cares and it brings up lots of ethical issue and challenges. It's really essential to keep looking at and check AI techniques. These concerns involve stuff like privacy keeping data safe, which can make people unsure about using AI tools (Fiske, 2019). It is crucial to find out what might stop some people from using AI-based mental health service, so they can get the help they need. We also need a lot of research to understand how AI and psychology are connected, and figure out the problems and limits in this era (Bhatia et al., 2023).A theory named "Attachment Theory ", initially formulated by John Bowlby in the mid of 20th century, delves to illuminate the bond between parents and children. It proposes that because children are easily influenced and lack the use of tools to handle dangers on their own, they instinctively develop behaviour to stay close to their parents. Under their parent's care, protection, affection and nurturing, hence, children enhance their chances of survival and thrive in their environment. This theory underscores the basic effectiveness of the parent-child relationship in nurturing a child's emotional and psychological development (Hazan et al., 2009). As AI works as a social actor (Kim et al., 2019). Critically, Research indicate that AI-human relationship mirror human-human relationship in many ways (Song et al., 2022).By inculcating AI in daily life, as a social actor, children and adolescent may became able to increase their social connection to technology and count on AI technology (Laestadius et al., 2022).

TWO AI EFFECTS: PROS AND CONS

Artificial intelligence functions as both a booster and a challenger. It provides remarkable rapidity, simplicity, and adaptability in the domains of mental health and education. Conversely, it poses intricate righteous, profound, and societal obstacles. The effects on social connections, emotional well-being, and intellectual sovereignty require thorough research. This chapter examines the dual aspects of AI's influence: its potential to beneficially impact lives and the challenges it poses to individuality, bonds of affection, and confidentiality.

SIGNIFICANCE

'The research article "Artificial Intelligence and Human Mental Wellbeing: Striking a balance between innovation and productivity" meticulously examines the multi faced effects of AI on mental health well-being. It navigates the terrain of both positive and negative impacts. On one hand, AI promises enhanced efficiency and accessibility in mental health services, potentially revolutionizing diagnosis, treatment, and support system. However, it also raises concerns about the potential for increased feelings of isolation, anxiety, and privacy breaches. Through a comprehensive exploration, the article aims to provide valuable insights into the complexion play between AI and mental health. This chapter delves into the many ways in which artificial intelligence (AI) affects people's mental health, looking at how it can improve mental wellness processes, solve problems, and have both good and bad effects. We will explore the intersection of innovation in productivity and mental health using the lens of artificial intelligence (AI) technology, offering examples of AI applications that improve mental health outcomes while also highlighting its possible psychological hazards. This paper is conducted to help everyone to know the impact of AI on human life and aware people to use it properly and carefully. There is no need to depend on AI completely by doing this human will became disable and one day will be replaced by AI. In this paper understanding the dual impact of AI on mental health is crucial for several reasons. First of all, it allows harnessing its potential benefits effectively while mitigating its negative consequences. And furthermore, studying this relationship fosters the development of ethical guideline and regulations to ensure responsible AI implementation in mental health care. Lastly, it empowers mental health professionals and policy makes to make informed decisions about integrating AI technologies into treatment strategies, ultimately improving patient outcomes and well-being. The incorporation of AI within medical settings must achieve equilibrium between leveraging its capacity to enhance efficiency and preventing its negative psychological consequences. The capacity of AI to deliver ongoing mental health assistance and personalized care is a significant advantage; nonetheless, ethical issues of privacy, employment displacement, and emotional detachment must be acknowledged. Human monitoring is essential in AI applications to safeguard emotional well-being. Nonetheless, akin to other technical advancements, AI's impact on mental health possesses a dual nature. Although AI-driven applications can enhance psychological achievements through continuous personalized encouragement, apprehensions about behavioral disinterest, unnecessary reliance on technology, and moral concerns about control and confidentiality remain prevalent. It is essential to examine both aspects of AI's influence on mental health, balancing its innovative potential with the emotional and social drawbacks it may entail.

FUTURE DIRECTIONS

The evolution of artificial intelligence (AI) is revealing its significant prospective to revolutionise mental health support and educational systems. Nonetheless, unlocking its complete potential necessitates tackling critical challenges and promoting collaboration across disciplines. The subsequent future directions present a strategic framework for utilising AI to improve mental wellbeing and educational results:

Human-Centered AI Design: Future AI systems should emphasise righteous and beneficial design that honours human being self-worth, ethnic backgrounds environments, and psychologically stability. This involves creating tools for explainable AI that enable educators, therapists, and patients to comprehend the reasoning behind AI-generated decisions or therapies.

AI-Enhanced Supporting Platforms: The integration of AI into psychological administration systems must prioritise personalised, responsive assistance while adhering to principles of ethics regarding security and independence. Integrating Learning Management Platforms into education sectors with facial recognition systems to facilitate a smooth experience for monitoring presence and retrieving course resources.

Tailored Approaches and Flexible Learning: Future AI tools must prioritise personalised service, delivering customised therapeutic strategies or personalised learning pathways that are motivated by instantaneously behavioural, emotional, and cognitive data. This method has the potential to assist students with learning difficulties as well as those experiencing clinical depression, anxiety, or stressful situations.

Public Consciousness and Educational Affairs: It is essential to improve societal familiarity of artificial intelligence's role in the field of psychology, highlighting its strengths and its hazards. Continuous improvements in neural networks and machine learning could enhance the quality and flexibility of facial detection algorithms. Improved algorithms could more effectively manage stressful circumstances such as fluctuations in student personalities or varied educational environments. AI technology can additionally be deployed in various educational domains, including the observation of learner, the safeguarding of venue availability, and the enhancement of personalised educational opportunities.

Partnership between AI and Behavioural Health Professionals: The creation of AI-driven emotional wellness tools must entail cooperation among doctors, experts in psychology, and artificial intelligence researchers to guarantee that the platforms deliver quality treatment.

Practical AI Learning: Governments and organisations must establish rules that protect against the adverse effects of AI on mental disorders, with a special focus on confidentiality of data, psychological wellness, and focused on humanity.

Enhancing Skills and Digital Competence: To promote equal opportunities, it is essential for educators and mental health professionals to receive training in AI tools and digital platforms. This involves incorporating AI literacy into teacher training programs and mental health courses to minimise resistance and enhance effectiveness.

Collaboration across Disciplines: Successful implementation of AI in mental health and education necessitates a partnership among technological professionals, educators, psychologists, medical professionals, and legislators. Collaborative efforts across different sectors can guarantee that AI tools are pertinent, adaptable, and rooted in practical requirements.

Longitudinal Studies and Empirical Approaches: There is a pressing need for additional longitudinal studies to assess the enduring effects of AI on educational outcomes and mental health. Thorough assessment will distinguish between exaggerated claims and genuine effectiveness, guiding policy and curriculum advancement.

Artificial Intelligence in Support of Inclusive Learning and Therapeutic Practices: Future innovations must prioritise accessibility for marginalised groups, such as children with special needs, rural populations, and individuals with limited digital access. It is essential to design AI applications with a focus on equity and inclusion to address and mitigate existing disparities.

CONCLUSION

As AI evolves, technology and human values must be balanced. Only when used carefully, ethically, and inclusively can AI improve mental health and education. This chapter encourages educators, technologists, politicians, and healthcare experts to work together to guarantee that AI enhances human nature. This research paper has investigated the intricate interplay between AI and mental health. Furthermore, AI presents exciting prospects for enhancing early detection of mental health issues and tailoring therapies to individuals. On the other side, it introduces concerns such as privacy infringements and the potential to widen social disparities AI serves as a significant resource for enhancing mental health outcomes, encompassing both diagnosis and treatment assistance. Nonetheless, its expanding influence on human relationships and effectiveness presents difficulties, especially regarding the emotional consequences of computerization and based on artificial intelligence interpersonal interactions. It is essential to advance AI technologies with a thorough understanding of their impact on psychological well-being to ensure the advantages of technological advancement do not compromise emotional health. However, admit these complexities are an opportunity for innovation and collaboration. By leveraging the positive aspects of AI while actively addressing its negative impacts, we can lay the groundwork for a future where technology serves as a powerful ally in promoting mental well-being for everyone. This calls for a mindful approach, infused with empathy and a steadfast commitment to leveraging AI's transformative potential for the betterment of society.

REFERENCES

Ahuja, V. K. (2020). Artificial Intelligence and Copyright: Issues and Challenges. ILI Law Review Winter, (2020).

Bhatia, R., & Kaur, J. (2024). Studying the Psychological Effects of Stress, Anxiety, and Depression on Secondary School Students. [IJFMR]. *International Journal for Multidisciplinary Research*, *6*(01), 1–9.

Bhatia, R., & Kaur, J. (2024). Collaborating Academia, Industry, and Government: Enhancing Business Practices Through Innovative Pedagogies. In Fostering Industry-Academia Partnerships for Innovation-Driven Trade (pp. 40-53). IGI Global.

Davenport, T. H., & Ronanki, R. (2018). Artificial intelligence for the real world. *Harvard Business Review*, *96*(1), 108–116.

Dilsizian, S. E., & Siegel, E. L. (2014). Artificial intelligence in medicine and cardiac imaging: Harnessing big data and advanced computing to provide personalized medical diagnosis and treatment. *Current Cardiology Reports*, *16*(1), 1–8. DOI: 10.1007/s11886-013-0441-8 PMID: 24338557

Dwivedi, Y. K., Hughes, L., Ismagilova, E., Aarts, G., Coombs, C., Crick, T., Duan, Y., Dwivedi, R., Edwards, J., Eirug, A., Galanos, V., Ilavarasan, P. V., Janssen, M., Jones, P., Kar, A. K., Kizgin, H., Kronemann, B., Lal, B., Lucini, B., & Williams, M. D. (2021). Artificial Intelligence (AI): Multidisciplinary perspectives on emerging challenges, opportunities, and agenda for research, practice and policy. *International Journal of Information Management*, *57*, 101994. DOI: 10.1016/j.ijinfomgt.2019.08.002

Dwyer, D. B., Falkai, P., & Koutsouleris, N. (2018). Machine learning approaches for clinical psychology and psychiatry. *Annual Review of Clinical Psychology*, *14*(1), 91–118. DOI: 10.1146/annurev-clinpsy-032816-045037 PMID: 29401044

Fiske, A. P., Henningsen, P., & Buyx, A. (2019). Your Robot Therapist Will See You Now: Ethical Implication of Embodied Artificial intelligence in Psychiatry, Psychology and Psychotherapy. *Journal of Medical Internet Research*, *5*(5), 21. DOI: 10.2196/13216

Fitzpatrick, K. K., Darcy, A., & Vierhile, M. (2017). Delivering cognitive behavior therapy to young adults with symptoms of depression and anxiety using a fully automated conversational agent (Woebot): A randomized controlled trial. *JMIR Mental Health*, *4*(2), e7785. DOI: 10.2196/mental.7785 PMID: 28588005

Goeders, N. E. (2003). The impact of stress on addiction. *European Neuropsychopharmacology, 13*(6), 435–441. DOI: 10.1016/j.euroneuro.2003.08.004 PMID: 14636959

Graham, S., Depp, C., Lee, E. E., Nebeker, C., Tu, X., Kim, H. C., & Jeste, D. V. (2019). Artificial intelligence for mental health and mental illnesses: An overview. *Current Psychiatry Reports, 21*(11), 1–18. DOI: 10.1007/s11920-019-1094-0 PMID: 31701320

Hazan, C., & Shaver, P. R. (2009). Attachment as an Organizational Framework for Research on Close Relationships. *An International Journal for the Advancement of Psychological Theory, 5*(1), 22.

Holmes, W., & Tuomi, I. (2022). State of the art and practice in AI in education. *European Journal of Education, 57*(4), 542–570. DOI: 10.1111/ejed.12533

Huang, S., Lai, X., Ke, L., Li, Y., Wang, H., Zhao, X., Dai, X., & Wang, Y. (2024). AI Technology panic—Is AI Dependence Bad for Mental Health? A Cross-Lagged Panel Model and the Mediating Roles of Motivations for AI Use among Adolescents. *Psychology Research and Behavior Management, 17*, 1087–1102. DOI: 10.2147/PRBM.S440889 PMID: 38495087

Jiang, F., Jiang, Y., Zhi, H., Dong, Y., Li, H., Ma, S., Wang, Y., Dong, Q., Shen, H., & Wang, Y. (2017). Artificial intelligence in healthcare: Past, present and future. *Stroke and Vascular Neurology, 2*(4), 230–243. DOI: 10.1136/svn-2017-000101 PMID: 29507784

Joshi, R., Bhatia, R., & Kour, J. (2025). Navigating the Mobile Learning Landscape in Education: Leadership Strategies for Success. In New Horizons in Leadership: Inclusive Explorations in Health, Technology, and Education (pp. 541-558). IGI Global Scientific Publishing.

Kardefelt-winther, D. (2014). A conceptual and methodological critique of internet addiction research: Towards a model of compensatory internet use. *Computers in Human Behavior, 31*, 351–354. DOI: 10.1016/j.chb.2013.10.059

Kim, A., Cho, M., Ahn, J., & Sung, Y. (2019). Effects of gender and relationship type on the response to artificial intelligence. *Cyberpsychology, Behavior, and Social Networking, 22*(4), 249–253. DOI: 10.1089/cyber.2018.0581 PMID: 30864826

Kim, B. J., & Lee, J. (2024). The mental health implications of artificial intelligence adoption: The crucial role of self-efficacy. *Humanities & Social Sciences Communications, 11*(1), 1–15. DOI: 10.1057/s41599-024-04018-w

Kolker, E., Özdemir, V., & Kolker, E. (2016). How healthcare can refocus on its super-customers (patients, n= 1) and customers (doctors and nurses) by leveraging lessons from Amazon, Uber, and Watson. *OMICS: A Journal of Integrative Biology*, *20*(6), 329–333. DOI: 10.1089/omi.2016.0077 PMID: 27310474

Kour, J., Bhatia, R., & Joshi, R. (2025). Artificial Intelligence in Education: Insights From Gender and Locality-Based Perspectives. In Mobo, F. (Ed.), *Impacts of AI on Students and Teachers in Education 5.0* (pp. 193–210). IGI Global Scientific Publishing., DOI: 10.4018/979-8-3693-8191-5.ch007

Laestadius, L., Bishop, A., Gonzalez, M., Illenčík, D., & Campos-Castillo, C. (2022). Too human and not human enough: A grounded theory analysis of mental health harms from emotional dependence on the social Chabot Replika. *New Media & Society*, •••, 14614448221142007.

Lee, E. E., Torous, J., De Choudhury, M., Depp, C. A., Graham, S. A., Kim, H. C., Paulus, M. P., Krystal, J. H., & Jeste, D. V. (2021). Artificial intelligence for mental health care: Clinical applications, barriers, facilitators, and artificial wisdom. *Biological Psychiatry: Cognitive Neuroscience and Neuroimaging*, *6*(9), 856–864. DOI: 10.1016/j.bpsc.2021.02.001 PMID: 33571718

Murdoch, T. B., & Detsky, A. S. (2013). The inevitable application of big data to health care. *Journal of the American Medical Association*, *309*(13), 1351–1352. DOI: 10.1001/jama.2013.393 PMID: 23549579

Pang, Z., Yuan, H., Zhang, Y. T., & Packirisamy, M. (2018). Guest editorial health engineering driven by the industry 4.0 for aging society. *IEEE Journal of Biomedical and Health Informatics*, *22*(6), 1709–1710. DOI: 10.1109/JBHI.2018.2874081

Pearson, T. (2011). *How to replicate Watson hardware and systems design for your own use in your basement*. IBM.

Raino, R., Kumari, N., Chandelkar, K., & Chetiwal, K. (2023). Role of artificial intelligence in psychological and mental well-being: A quantitative investigation. *Journal for Reattach Therapy and Developmental Diversities*, *6*(9s (2)), 149–156.

Shah, V. (2022). AI in Mental Health: Predictive Analytics and Intervention Strategies. Journal Environmental Sciences and Technology, 1(2), 55-74. *ONMENT SCIENCES AND TECHNOLOGY*, *01*(02), 20.

Simon, H. A. (1991). Artificial intelligence: Where has it been, and where is it going? *IEEE Transactions on Knowledge and Data Engineering*, *3*(2), 128–136. DOI: 10.1109/69.87993

Song, X., Xu, B., & Zhao, Z. (2022). Can people experience romantic love for artificial intelligence? An empirical study of intelligent assistants. *Information & Management*, *59*(2), 103595. DOI: 10.1016/j.im.2022.103595

Sun, J., Liu, Q., & Yu, S. (2019). Child neglect, psychological abuse and smartphone addiction among Chinese adolescents: The roles of emotional intelligence and coping style. *Computers in Human Behavior*, *90*, 74–83.

UNICEF. (2021). *Policy guidance on AI for children*. UNICEF Office of Global Insight and Policy.

Chapter 10
Artificial Intelligence in Cognitive Behavioral Therapy

Niki Tzioumaki
https://orcid.org/0009-0001-3993-0008
Hellenic Air Force, Greece

Evanthia Arvanitaki
https://orcid.org/0009-0007-3048-2847
National and Kapodistrian University of Athens, Greece

Efthimia Xirakia
https://orcid.org/0009-0002-2765-5499
European University, Cyprus

ABSTRACT

The aim of this investigation is to review the integration of Artificial Intelligence (AI) into mental health therapy, specifically in Cognitive Behavioral Therapy (CBT). AI can provide support in CBT, aiming to improve therapy accessibility. The search included scientific studies and articles indexed in the electronic databases. The results were synthesized to highlight AI's potential in CBT, while providing a detailed understanding of its capabilities. Findings indicate that the integration of AI into CBT offers a new era of more efficient and personalized mental health interventions. Additionally, conversational agents and chatbots offer effective emotional support. Overall, the relationship between cognitive psychology and artificial intelligence is a fact. We may effectively take advantage of the potential of AI to enhance the efficacy and accessibility of mental healthcare. However, challenges and limitations in current AI applications persist because the excessive reliance on AI is dangerous.

DOI: 10.4018/979-8-3373-5072-1.ch010

INTRODUCTION

In the past few years, the demand for mental health services has risen significantly, creating an urgent need for solutions that are accessible, affordable, and effective. Multiple factors have contributed to this rising, such as increased awareness around mental health issues, the post pandemic era Penninx et al 2022), which led to higher rates of depression, anxiety and suicidal ideation, some socioeconomic stressors and the growing recognition of the importance of mental health in different workplaces (Clemente-Suárez et al., 2021).

To address this increasing demand for mental health services there has been a surge in research on using AI for mental health through online therapy, digital mental health platforms, and virtual support (Chekroud et al., 2021, Thieme et al., 2020). Most of the innovation has focused on diagnosing mental health conditions and detecting symptoms, using data from sensors or text based information (Nguyen et al., 2017, Nobles et al., 2018).

COGNITIVE BEHAVIORAL THERAPY (CBT)

The most common and best studied form of psychotherapy is Cognitive behavioral therapy (CBT). Cognitive Behavioral Therapy (CBT) is a structured, time-limited psychological treatment that aims to address dysfunctional emotions, behaviors, and cognitions through a goal-oriented approach (American Psychological Association, 2017). CBT is widely recognized as an effective treatment for various mental health disorders, including anxiety, depression, and post-traumatic stress disorder (PTSD) (Petrinec et al., 2021, Liu et al., 2021; Perri et al., 2021; Twomey et al., 2015).

According to the American Psychological Association, research and clinical practice have shown that CBT can lead to noticeable improvements in a person's ability to manage daily activities and their overall well-being. In fact, many studies suggest that CBT is just as effective as, or even more effective than, other types of psychological therapies or the use of psychiatric medications (Tolin, 2010).

CBT therapists try to modify unhelpful ways of thinking, change learned patterns of unhelpful behavior, teach people better ways of coping with their psychological problems and develop better life skills. The core principle of CBT is that the psychologist and the patient work together to explore the nature of the problem and find a treatment plan, so that the individual becomes their own therapist (American Psychological Association, 2017).

Although CBT is one of the most important psychological interventions for addressing a wide range of mental health conditions (Foreman and Pollard, 2016, David et al., 2018), it is traditionally delivered face to face by a therapist, and it faces real time challenges, such as stigma and limited access to mental health services, especially in underserved areas, which makes it even more difficult for individuals to seek the help they need (Jiang et al., 2024). To overcome these barriers, technological advancements have contributed to the development of Computer-Based Cognitive Behavioral Therapy (CCBT) and Internet- Based Cognitive Behavioral Therapy (ICBT) (Webb et al., 2017).

The Integration of Artificial Intelligence (AI) in Cognitive Behavioral Therapy (CBT)

Artificial Intelligence (AI) refers to the machines that are designed to think and act like humans. They simulate human intelligence and include processes such as learning, reasoning, problem solving and language understanding. In simple terms, AI enables machines to perform tasks that typically demand human intelligence like recognizing patterns or having conversations (Russell & Norvig, 2020).

Artificial intelligence has been applied in various areas such as healthcare, transportation, finance and mental health. In the field of mental health, AI holds great potential, allowing innovative methods for early diagnosis, planning treatments, personalized interventions and tracking mental health outcomes (Torous et al., 2020). As mental health disorders continue to rise worldwide, AI could provide solutions that are scalable and accessible, and offer support beside traditional mental health services, using tools that evaluate how people are feeling, analyze data that identify behavior patterns and offer therapeutic interventions through digital platforms.

The introduction of technology in CBT began with simple programs that helped deliver therapeutic content, including self-help tools and online resources that offer psychoeducation and guided exercises (Stawarz et al., 2018). These tools include virtual therapists, mobile applications and AI systems that predict mental health risk (Firth et al., 2019). Artificial Intelligence technologies have the ability to assist clinicians to detect patterns that might be not easily visible to them. These technologies aim to make mental health care more accessible and reduce issues like stigma, high cost and difficulty reaching services.

Using Artificial Intelligence in mental health treatment includes creating chatbots and conversation based tools that can deliver psychotherapy or help people stay more engaged with mental health activities and therapeutic content, making it easier for individuals to open up and share their feelings (Fitzpatrick et al., 2017, Inkster et al., 2018, Miner et al., 2019). Early examples of these tools, include Woebot, which uses AI to offer Cognitive Behavioral Therapy (CBT) through a conversational agent (Fitzpatrick et al., 2017) and Wysa, a chatbot designed to help people dealing with depression by providing emotional support (Inkster et al., 2018).

With the improvement of technology, new platforms like mobile applications and online therapy, allowed a blended approach in which therapists and clients connect in real time, engaging in a 'face-to-face' therapy with digital interventions (Abd-Alrazaq et al., 2021). This adjustment expanded accessibility and addressed different patient needs, showing that technology could actually improve the experience of therapy (Danieli et al., 2021). Mobile health applications have been developed that use AI and can provide CBT exercises, monitor users progress and send reminders about therapeutic tasks. These applications improve patients' engagement and commitment to their treatment (Stawarz et al., 2018).

AI tools also include data analytics and Machine Learning. These systems can analyze a large amount of patients' data, identify patterns and predict treatment outcomes to help therapists customize interventions, increasing the effectiveness of CBT (Wang, 2024).

Finally, research on human- computer interaction (HCI) and human centered design can play a key role in making sure that future AI tools in the mental health domain are not only clinically effective but also ethical and easy for clients to use. These approaches help ensure that the AI platforms are in fact helpful in everyday life, in real world settings, align with the needs of the users and are likely to be successfully used in practice (Thieme et al., 2023).

ADVANTAGES OF ARTIFICIAL INTELLIGENCE IN COGNITIVE BEHAVIORAL THERAPY

Increased Accessibility

The integration of Artificial Intelligence in Cognitive Behavioral Therapy provides various advantages for therapists and clients. Initially, one of the most significant benefits of AI in CBT is that it ensures that is available and accessible to a broader range of individuals (Jiang et al.,2024). A great challenge of traditional therapy is that it requires face-to-face sessions. This can be especially difficult for clients with mobility issues, living in remote areas or dealing with busy schedules.

AI tools, such as mobile applications and online therapy platforms overcome the challenge of time and distance, by offering clients the opportunity to access therapeutic resources any time, any place (Aspvall et al., 2021).For instance, online CBT has been shown to work well for mental health conditions, including depression and anxiety and is often more convenient and affordable than traditional face-to-face therapy (Aspvall et al., 2021). This is especially important for individuals in underserved areas who may not have access to mental health professionals within reach. AI technologies offer clients timely support, which is key to effective mental health treatment.

Personalized Treatment Plans

As previously mentioned, one significant advantage of AI in CBT, for both therapists and clients is personalized treatment plans. AI tools enhance the therapy process by analyzing client data, including past treatment responses, behavioral patterns and personal preferences, to adapt the intervention to the individual. For instance, AI algorithms can help therapists identify the most effective therapeutic techniques and which of them has worked well for similar clients in the past. This allows therapists to adjust their approach to each client's needs (Harnas et al., 2021).

AI's data analysis, also shows how clients respond to different therapeutic techniques and determine which strategies work best for each individual and adjust the treatment plan based on real time feedback (Omarov et al,. 2023).

In addition, homework assignments play an important role in connecting therapy sessions, giving patients the chance to practice the skills they have learned and strengthen them, and allowing therapists to track progress and ensure the skills are being maintained over time (Beck, 1979, LeBeau et al., 2013).AI tools can help in creating more personalized homework and coping strategies, making sure that clients get the support that truly addresses their specific challenges and goals (Jiang, 2024).

Exposure Therapy

Exposure therapy is considered an effective technique of CBT and it includes the gradual exposure of patients to situations to reduce their anxiety and fear (Abramowitz, 2013). Virtual Reality provides a controllable environment for exposure therapy (Obremski et al., 2024).

By combining CBT and AI, therapists can create highly immersive environments to help clients face their anxiety and fears, such as speech anxiety. AI can enhance virtual reality (VR) scenarios, making them more tailored to each individual's specific needs and progress and help individuals learn to manage their fears by challenging their worst case beliefs and gradually exposing them in a controlled setting. This offers a personalized, dynamic approach to treatment that can adapt in real- time, providing a more supportive and effective way to address speech anxiety and build confidence in social situations (Ahs et al., 2020).

In addition, the use of digital technologies and specifically Virtual Reality (VR), which is still developing, in CBT is already showing promise that can improve the effectiveness of interventions in disorders such as ADHD. Virtual Reality tools can also be used to control emotional and behavioral disorders (Gkora & Driga, 2023).

Cognitive Restructuring

In Cognitive Behavioral Therapy therapists focus in understanding how a person thinks, behaves and feels and explore connections between these areas. By paying attention to these aspects, CBT helps individuals recognize and change cognitive and behavioral patterns (Jiang,2024).

A key part of the therapy process is Cognitive restructuring (CR). Cognitive restructuring is an intervention that focuses on helping individuals identify and challenge unhelpful thoughts and beliefs. In this process the therapist and the client work together in a supportive and goal-focused way to recognize irrational or distorted thinking patterns and aim to replace them with healthier and more realistic thoughts, which can lead to improved emotional and behavioral outcomes (Clark, 2013). Recent developments have found ways to use AI models to assist the process of Cognitive restructuring. Most of these studies focus on showing that AI language models help people shift their thinking in response to negative emotions, encouraging more positive perspectives (Jiang,2024).

Several studies have shown AI's ability to transform initial negative cognitions into more positive or realistic alternatives (de Toledo Rodriguez et al., 2021). Another study aims to understand the most effective ways to support individuals in shifting their mindset. Specifically, the study explored how negative thought patterns can be changed, how language models might help in the process and which types of restructuring people dealing with negative thoughts tend to prefer (Sharma et al., 2023a).The researchers developed a Cognitive Restructuring tool that uses human language model interactions and helps individuals by guiding them in recognizing unhelpful thought patterns and offering suggestions that are more empathetic or tailored to their specific situation, assisting in reshaping negative thoughts (Sharma et al., 2023b).

Behavioral Activation (BA)

Behavioral Activation (BA) is a significant strategy in Cognitive Behavioral Therapy (CBT), that targets specific behaviors as a way to enhance individuals manage their mood. By focusing on actions and behaviors, Behavioral Activation encourages positive changes that can lead to a reduction in negative emotional states (Petersen et al., 2016).

Many innovative interventions have been created to make BA more accessible, such as a mobile application that helps users engage with Behavioral Activation techniques. Through an application users identify their personal values and connect them with activities in five key areas of life (relationships, daily responsibilities, recreation, career and education, health) (Daphne et al., 2019).

Continuous Support and Therapy Engagement

One of the benefits of mental healthcare is that through AI applications, clients receive continuous and instant support, unlike traditional therapy sessions that are only available at certain times, which makes the treatment more effective. These AI applications and platforms are accessible 24/7 and offer CBT techniques and coping strategies at any time. This type of immediate support can be extremely valuable during a crisis, helping individuals manage their emotions (Khawaja et al., 2023).

Additionally, consistent access to these resources helps to reinforce the skills developed in therapy, making it easier for clients to use them in their everyday lives (Aspvall et al., 2021). For instance, AI chatbots can guide clients through exercises to challenge negative thinking or teach mindfulness techniques during stressful moments (Wang, 2024).

Furthermore, AI platforms are proving to be helpful in getting patients more engaged and committed to their treatment plans, as shown by a clinical trial with patients using an AI platform for behavioral therapy. This clinical trial found that the patients showed higher attendance rates and improvement in symptoms, compared to traditional methods (Sadeh- Sharvit et al., 2023). These findings indicate that AI can effectively connect the gap between therapists and clients, especially in areas where individuals have limited access to mental health resources.

Time Efficiency

A quite significant advantage of using AI in Cognitive Behavioral Therapy is its ability to help therapists refine methods, achieve better results and enhance their productivity. Many of the administrative tasks therapists have to do, such as scheduling appointments, managing client's records and handling billing can consume a lot of therapists' time and reduce time spent with clients. AI tools can automate these tasks, providing therapists with more time to focus on actually working with their clients (Omarov et al., 2023).

Administrative tasks can be completed through applications and AI systems that send appointment reminders and follow- ups, reducing the number of missed appointments and support clients to remain engaged in their treatment (Jawaid, 2023).Furthermore, AI can minimize time spending on administrative tasks by assisting therapists in data entry and management and automating the note-taking and record- keeping process. In that manner, therapists save valuable time that can be spent in therapeutic activities (Omarov et al., 2023). This increase in efficiency allows therapists to see more clients, expand their practice and provides better access in mental health care for a larger group of population (Jawaid, 2023).

Prediction of Risk Factors and Drop-Out

Additionally, AI by analyzing past data can help therapists identify risk factors and potential difficulties in commitment to therapy and predict the rate of dropping out of therapy or which clients may encounter challenges in their progress (Gutierrez, 2024). AI's capability to predict these important insights, offers therapists the opportunity to intervene in advance and customize their treatment plans and interventions to support each client meeting their specific needs.

Stigma Reduction

Finally, many people hesitate to seek mental health treatment and support because of the stigma that is associated with it. Traditional therapy settings may not always offer privacy, as opposed to AI-driven platforms that can provide a level of anonymity. This offers clients the chance to get the support they need without worrying about being judged or exposed and feel more comfortable seeking for help (Aspvall et al., 2021). Online therapy and chatbots are great tools to enhance this process, as they provide a safe space where people can explore their thoughts and emotions without the stress of human interaction (Olawade et al., 2024).

Applications of AI for Mental Health

Clinical applications of Artificial Intelligence (AI) for mental health care have experienced a spectacular growth during recent decade. In healthcare, AI has been used to aid in clinical decision-making, facilitating and monitoring disease (Gutierrez et al., 2024). It is predicted that AI-enabled technologies will offer more available and affordable approaches than the conventional mental health treatment model. Notable medical procedures have been administered by AI enabled chatbot software and applications that were previously only available from experienced healthcare professionals. So, "virtual psychiatrists" or "social robots" make an effort to improve the mental health needs of vulnerable and underserved populations. Other study revealed that nearly 70% of patients expressed interest in using mobile health (mHealth) apps to self-monitor and self-manage their mental health (Jang et al., 2021; Omarov et al., 2023; Wilhelm et al., 2024). There has been an uprising of interest in using of technological modalities such as telephone, e-mail, text, videoconferencing, mobile applications, and Web-based programs to complement conventional mental health therapy and psychological services (Omarov et al., 2023; Sadeh-Sharvit, 2023). In addition, the Covid-19 pandemic notified a lofty growth in anxiety, stress and depression, which increased a long interest in telepsychology and an increased demand for utilization of remote options for mental health treatment, including automated chatbots (Eltahawy et al., 2024).

Conversational Artificial Intelligence systems (also known as "chatbots") are among the most promising examples of the use of technology in mental health care (Grodniewicz & Hohol, 2024). An artificial intelligence (AI)–based well-being chatbot can focus on conversations with humans in an approximately natural manner, offering companionship, emotional support and guidance for emotional well-being. Therapeutic well-being chatbots develop a social relationship with the user through chatting to alleviate negative emotions (Yang et al., 2024).

Can a Chatbot Provide Therapy?

Chatbot is a digital tool type of computer program that mimics human interaction via a text- or voice-based conversational interface. It uses language to communicate like a human being and its use in the management of mental health problems has been rapidly increasing (Jang et al., 2021). Chatbots are AI-enabled software systems and innovative technologies in the field of mental health care that can communicate with people using natural language across a text or voice-based interaction. This technology has been constantly developing and is currently utilized in digital assistants such as Apples's Siri, Amazon's Alexa and other virtual assistants (Omarov et al., 2023; Yang et al., 2024). It simulates the role of a therapist and a therapeutic relationship can be formed with users to a certain degree (Jang et al., 2021). AI-based chatbots are uniquely well positioned in a middle ground between professionally provided psychotherapy and self-help apps due to the potential to simulate aspects of therapy (Eltahawy et al., 2024).

Furthermore, chatbots can be reliable tools for the screening and diagnosis of mental health disorders in α number of psychotherapeutic models, among these and Cognitive Behavioural Therapy (CBT). Also, studies have been shown that different multipurpose chatbots have significant efficacy in several psychiatric disorders, including anxiety, depression, panic disorder or autism and showed positive effects (Jang et al., 2021).

CHATBOTS IN CLINICAL PSYCHOLOGY AND PSYCHOTHERAPY

Nowadays, chatbots are created by various plain text programming languages such as RiveScript. The Language recognition relies heavily on Natural Language Processing (NLP), which is used by Google and Apple's Siri. Natural Language Understanding (NLU) and Natural Language Generation (NLG) are fundamental elements to recognize human natural language textual data and speech-based commands (Roudsari et al., 2021). Combining NLP algorithms and frame-based dialogue management into chatbots aims to simulate a conversation with another person, make the interaction more human-like and thus make a real conversation more effectively (Grodniewicz & Hohol, 2024). Today, the forefront of NLP is represented by models like ChatGPT, Gemini Advanced, and Co-pilot with their advanced text comprehension, improving patient communications (Alhur, 2024).

There are already several examples of advanced treatment, mental health virtual assistants that have been advanced to cure depression, anxiety or sadness. The earliest chatbots, which use computer vision, were ALICE and Eliza. The program Eliza was a chatbot that simulated a Rogerian psychotherapist. Their important disadvantage was that their responses were impersonal, robotic and repetitive (Carlbring et al., 2023; May & Denecke, 2022). Over the decades, the use of AI in mental healthcare has experienced a progressive extension. The most popular used chatbot applications for CBT treatment are Woebot, Wysa, Shimbot or Tess that are advertised as implementing the principles and techniques of CBT. All these applications offer treatment to patients suffering from depression, sadness, anxiety, mental well- being and mood disorders. They are based on software that can be accessed online with a computer or a smartphone, and their aim is to identify mental health problems, individualise virtual therapists, treatment plans, advances in teletherapy, and continuous monitoring (Grodniewicz & Hohol, 2024; Gual-Montolio, 2022; Olawade et al., 2024).

In addition, mobile applications, which are available on smartphone or tablet, can be used independently by the public management, assessment and treatment. Interventions can be delivered through social media platforms such as Twitter, Facebook and Instagram, email or via teleconferencing between patients and their remote healthcare provider. They can be used by the participant at any time or place without direct guidance of a healthcare provider or specialist. These mental health apps target prevention of psychological disorders, depressive disorders, post -traumatic stress disorder psychosis, attention-deficit hyperactivity disorder or sleep disorders (Magwood et al., 2023).

Wysa is a chatbot that provides therapy support for a variety of mental health conditions, including depression, anxiety, stress, and loneliness. A combination of CBT, positive psychology and mindfulness help users improve their mental health (Olawade et al., 2024; Omarov et al., 2023;).

Furthermore, two others examples of Emotional health applications are the CBT Companion that helps users practice CBT, teaches them how to identify and change negative thought patterns and behaviors (Resiliens, CBT Companion, n.d). Also, MindShift CBT is an application that helps users practice CBT techniques for anxiety and depression. A variety of interactive exercises and tools are offered to help users manage their symptoms and improve their mood (Anxiety Canada, MindShift CBT, n.d.).

Especially, the AI-driven mental health app Woebot provides CBT-based therapy for depression and anxiety. Woebot developed in 2017 to offer a structured cognitive-behavioral therapy for people experiencing depression, anxiety, or other mental health difficulties (Alhur, 2024; Eltahawy et al., 2024).

Findings indicated that dividuals, who used Woebot, showed a considerable decline in depression after two weeks of its use (Eltahawy et al., 2024; Olawade et al., 2024; Omarov et al., 2023;).

The main ways in which producers of mental health chatbots implement the principles of CBT show in an exemplary conversation with "Woedot":

«Woebot: Can you say more about what's going on?

User: I'm feeling nervous.

Woebot: If I've understood you correctly, this sounds like an issue with stress or anxiety, is that right?

User: [picking one of the available continuations] Yes, you got it.

Woebot: I'm sorry to hear you're dealing with this [user's name]. That can be difficult.

User: [picking the only available continuation] Yeah....

Woebot: Let's start by challenging the thoughts that are creating this feeling.» (Grodniewicz & Hohol, 2024, p. 797).

In the most conversations with Woebot, the main therapeutic strategy is cognitive restructuring. If the user decides to go on, Woebot asks them to input three thoughts that are particularly troubling for the user and then helps the user to analyze them one by one. At each stage, Woebot shares psychoeducation and explains the terms it uses. (Grodniewicz & Hohol, 2024).

The mental health chatbots help their clients to obtain positive therapeutic effects through cognitive and affective change. This cognitive work takes place by notice, assessment and development their maladaptive thinking patterns. Several patient's ccharacteristics and needs can be analyzed by AI algorithms, such as genetic predispositions or behavioural patterns. This overall analysis allows AI to customize treatment plans remarkably. AI-driven personalization enables therapists to design more effective treatments and shorter recovery, virtual therapists and chatbots provide stigma-free platform for individuals to engage with mental health support and seek help whenever needed (Grodniewicz & Hohol, 2024).

ChatGPT is a chatbot that simulates human-like conversation and based on a large language model developed by OpenAI called GPT (Generative Pre-trained Transformer). Every person only needs to create an account and log in and then you can ask ChatGPT any question you want answered. The simplicity of its use is the main reason why chatbots like ChatGPT will be used for questions about difficult life challenges and different psychological issues. In psychotherapy, it can be useful for screening and diagnosis, emotional support and guidance to patients during treatment. Although ChatGPT is a very young phenomenon, the number of scientific texts it creates is growing rapidly (Raile, 2024).

ChatGPT and Psychotherapy

In the context of psychotherapy, psychotherapists and care professionals, patients suffering from mental illness and their relatives could apply the chatbot. Anyone with internet access may as well use ChatGPT. In psychotherapy, ChatGPT can be used by 1) psychotherapists during an active psychotherapy session as an AI assistant or supervision tool 2) patients suffering mentally who does not consult a psychotherapist, 3) patients regularly consult a psychotherapist but, there is an interruption in psychotherapy sessions due to numerous possible reasons (vacations, the next session is not scheduled until after a longer period of time or has not yet been scheduled) (Raile, 2024).

ChatGPT could become a supportive tool for psychotherapists. Asked ChatGPT help them in diagnosing, suggestion on treatment adequately as a second opinion and a successful approach in treating their patients. ChatGPT received a detailed description of the patients and their symptoms and then it promptly responded and suggested diagnoses and each brief explanation. (Raile, 2024). Furthermore, there are combinations of different internet-based treatments available such as real time video therapy or digital self-help programs with or without human guidance. According to a recent meta-analysis, therapist-guided internet-based cognitive behavior therapy yields similar effects as face-to-face therapy for psychiatric and somatic disorders. Among others, one possible solution could be the AI integration into the platforms either as a virtual psychoeducational coach or psychotherapist, giving constructive feedback (Carlbring et al., 2023).

Numerous studies have indicated that perfectionism has been increasing over the last decades. Different facets of perfectionism are the excessively high personal standards, social context to be demanding or imposing demanding and unrealistic standards on others. Perfectionism is associated with poorer mental health disorders, eating disorders and symptoms of depression and anxiety. All these symptoms can be improved by cognitive behavior therapy for perfectionism (ICBT-P) (Galloway et al., 2022; Johnson et al., 2024; Robinson & Wade, 2021).

According to one study, Cognitive- Behavior Therapy for perfectionism (CBT-P) sets high standards or concerns over mistakes and its acceptability of a co-designed CBT-P intervention with guidance provided through an AI tool, such as ChatGPT. Young people mostly expressed positive statements about AI, for example:

"I like AI because it is reassuring to have one output, it appears accurate, professional and informative. I really like the interactive nature, it gives me a nice starting point, I use it every day".

"Initially I was skeptical, but now every question I have, I ask ChatGPT. It's very detailed, I like it, it's interesting. I like its honesty and accuracy".

Also, it was expressed the opinion that an AI tool was preferable to seeing a person face-to-face when experiencing social anxiety or it would be comfortable, low cost, lack of stigma, acceptable asking questions about their mental health to an AI tool like ChatGPT, rather than seeing a person (Carlbring et al., 2023; Lindqvist, 2024; Johnson et al., 2024; Sarah & Egan Roz Shafran, 2024;)

The AI algorithms provide opportunities for the best treatments according to particular patients' needs and making current interventions more flexible. AI methods focus on idiosyncratic/idiographic information of patients at the right time as a result of improving psychotherapy (Gual-Montolio, 2022).

According to a study with therapy interfering in adults with diagnosed muscle dysmorphia (MD), it was found evidence that an 8-week individual CBT program (delivered via telehealth) can reduce MD symptoms. Participants, who expressed interest in participating in the study, booked a clinician-led diagnostic assessment interview using automated scheduling software (Calendly). All diagnostic interviews were carried out on a secure video-conferencing platform (Zoom). The results indicate that a telehealth program can deliver meaningful psychotherapy outcomes in adults with MD. If patients are unable to commit regularly to face-to-face sessions due to many reasons such as location or unavoidable work commitments, clinicians may consider offering telehealth sessions in such cases as a complement to in-person sessions (Martenstyn, 2024).

Future studies may as well focus on development and validation of AI-augmented interventions. But, it is valuable to examine the possibility of growing large open-source datasets in mental health that could serve as benchmarks for AI algorithm development. Furthermore, it is significant to acknowledge that use of these encouraging interventions may be limited to those without a reliable level of technology literacy or access to the internet and internet-enabled devices. So, all these systemic barriers can border the intended profit of these interventions. It is important to support all communities with internet-enabled devices or supporting technology literacy to overcome these barriers (Gutierrez et al., 2024).

Cognitive Behavioral Therapy, or CBT, is an evidence-based psychotherapeutic treatment mainly used for treating a wide range of psychological abnormalities, such as anxiety, depression, and post-traumatic stress disorder, by changing the pathological emotions, behaviors, and cognitions. The astounding effectiveness of CBT considerably depends upon an interactional relationship between the therapist and the patient, where individual therapy along with empathy and understanding is crucially involved. In recent years, the integration of artificial intelligence into CBT has been a promising augmentation in furthering the cause of accessibility and efficiency of the therapeutic services on offer (Hofmann et al., 2012). AI applications in CBT have ranged from automated chatbots to sophisticated algorithms analyzing patient data with the aim of optimizing treatment plans and have shown promise in supporting standard therapeutic practices (Hofmann et al., 2012).

However, with this implementation of AI in CBT also comes the serious loss of needed human touches that exist within a therapeutic relationship. It is true that AI can provide consistency, at times offering elements of personalized engagement, yet by its nature, it intrinsically cannot attain the human level of perception and reaction to nonverbal cues—everything necessary for good therapy (Darcy et al., 2021).While AI does represent a remarkable development in the terms of access and administration of CBT, this paper will contend that it cannot—and should not—replace human therapists but be used as an adjunctive tool to complement traditional techniques. Nuanced insight and empathetic interaction by human therapists are irreplaceable and integral to the deep, personalized engagement necessary in CBT (Weizenbaum, 1976).

Lying at the heart of the success of CBT therapy is something that cannot be emulated fully by AI technologies: the therapeutic alliance, or the collaborative bond between the therapist and the patient (Luxton, 2014). The integration of AI into CBT needs to be done with caution so as not to compromise the therapist-patient relationship but rather enhance it. Ongoing research on AI in CBT is needed regarding advantages and disadvantages, so a balance comes whereby technology supplements psychological healing caused by humans (Martin et al., 2000).

The Therapist-Patient Relationship in CBT

The therapeutic alliance is central to CBT, and as discussed above, it highly contributes to treatment outcomes, underlining the human contact that is important in psychological therapies (Norcross & Lambert, 2019). Human interaction in CBT is not just a question of delivery of the therapeutic content but involves the building of trust, empathetic understanding, and the subtle interpretation of non-verbal cues that are so important for adapting interventions to the client's emotional state and needs. For many years, researchers have emphasized the importance of the relationship between the therapist and patient; the quality of the interaction appears to be strongly related to therapeutic success on a number of psychological disorders (Norcross & Lambert, 2019).

From a psychological point of view, there are numerous theories emphasizing the importance of human-led therapy. Humanistic psychology, for instance, maintains that relationship-based therapeutic settings form the bedrock of presumed personal growth and healing. According to Rogers (1961), some of the core conditions required at the heart of therapy include empathy, congruence, and unconditional positive regard—all of which AI-driven interventions still lack. These human-specific qualities enable therapists to connect with their patients on a human level, thus allowing for deeper involvement in the process and more long-lasting change.

The psychodynamic approach further elucidates why human interaction in therapy is irreplaceable. It postulates that the therapeutic relationship may, in itself, be a corrective emotional experience for the patients. Interactions with the therapist will help the patients to work out unresolved conflicts and dysfunctional interpersonal patterns that are at the core of psychological distress (Shedler, 2010). This requires an intuitive and responsive understanding from a therapist, which AI has yet to successfully mimic.

Behavioral activation also necessitates the capacity of motivational and engaging expertise of the CBT therapist-developing skills, thus essentially requiring an ingenious perception of being human, which is very well beyond achievable by AI devices. The way a therapist develops treatment approaches considering the patient's values and priorities and modifies that treatment approach throughout the course considering the patient's response is very crucial in giving rise to adequate interventions (Shedler, 2010).

Empirical research points toward the importance of human contact in treatment (Flückiger et al., 2018). Therapeutic efficacy is deeply influenced by the therapeutic relationship; therefore, it becomes crucial that this human contact must be important to cause healing. There is an increasing amount of evidence to show that while AI can support aspects of therapy, such as data collection and preliminary diagnoses, it cannot replace the empathetic, adaptive, intuitive interactions with a human therapist.

It is therefore an irreplaceable and central role of the human therapist, though AI may support and enhance some logistical aspects of therapy. It is these nuanced and empathetic human interactions that form the heart of the therapeutic relationship in CBT and are basic to its success. As such, AI should be thought of as a tool designed to augment human-driven psychological interventions, but not to replace them (Dimidjian et al., 2011).

The Role of Artificial Intelligence in CBT

In modern times, CBT has progressively combined with artificial intelligence, with various new ideas aiming to help therapeutic treatment. Further development in this integration of AI ranges from purely symptomatic assessments through automation to apps designed for therapies that are developed to widen the reach of therapy and improve treatment outcomes. These technologies capitalize on the capabilities of AI for data processing and pattern recognition to make recommendations on treatment, monitor patient improvement, and intervene with CBT consonant with human therapist delivery that human therapists cannot reasonably achieve on a continuous basis (Fitzpatrick et al., 2017).

A very popular application of AI in CBT is through virtual therapists or chatbots. These AI-driven platforms, including the likes of Woebot and Wysa, can interact with the user either through text or voice by providing CBT-based guidance in an effort to keep symptoms of anxiety and depression at bay. These bots apply natural language processing and machine learning to provide interventions at any moment in time. This can greatly increase access for people who either feel stigmatized or have logistical issues that prevent them from getting conventional therapy (Inkster et al., 2018).

Another significant benefit of AI in CBT is that it can offer continuous monitoring and feedback. Wearable devices and mobile apps track physiological data, such as heart rate and sleep patterns, which are analyzed by AI algorithms to assess the status of a user's emotional and physical health. In fact, real-time data collection could enable an AI system to tailor its interventions to current needs, which may serve to enhance the timeliness and relevance of therapeutic interventions. AI-enhanced CBT apps, for example, may prompt users to engage in specific behavioral activities designed to improve mood or reduce anxiety, based on data collected (Luxton, 2014).

AI also increases the scalability of CBT. By automating less human-intensive parts of therapy, like initial screenings or routine follow-ups, AI frees human therapists to take on more complex cases or stages in therapy where human judgement may prove more salient. This can be particularly useful in areas that lack sufficient trained mental health professionals and provide some level of care that may otherwise not be accessible (Torous & Roberts, 2017).

Furthermore, AI-powered data analysis offers deep insights into treatment outcomes that may even go unnoticed by a human therapist. In so doing, this grants the therapist the capability to optimize CBT techniques in developing personalized treatment plans that, over time, adapt to the patient's needs and responses to therapy. Such data-driven approaches may also foster the development of more effective and efficient therapeutic processes that reduce the aforementioned time and cost of traditional modalities of therapy.

However, even without taking the place of human therapists, AI clearly has a very important role to play in the support and augmentation of CBT. Applications of AI increase the access to CBT, offer tailored interventions, provide 24/7 support, and also optimize interventions using the continuous stream of data being analyzed. From these advantages, there seems to be an immense opportunity for AI to alter CBT regarding accessibility, efficiency, and personalization to needs (Bickmore et al., 2010).

Risks of Over-Reliance on AI in CBT

While the integration of AI in CBT offers several benefits, over-reliance on such technologies creates significant risks that may undermine the effectiveness of treatment and the core values of therapeutic practice. A major concern is that it might weaken the relationship between a therapist and a patient, which is one of the most essential components of successful CBT. No AI applications can logistically support a level of interaction comparable to the deep, human empathy of a human therapist. This is actually the relational component in therapy, and not an added ingredient but the heart, enabling trust, motivation, and emotional insight—all very important in any patient's growth and improvement process (Norcross & Wampold, 2018).

Empirical research has underlined the therapeutic alliance as a predictive of treatment outcomes across a wide range of psychotherapies, including CBT. Empathic connection, mutual understanding, and collaboration from therapist to patient are some aspects that AI alone can hardly replicate. This is the risk: if over-reliance on such methods occurs, then these essential human elements may get lost, accompanied by the possibility of poorer treatment outcomes (Flückiger et al., 2018).

However, there are considerable ethical and practical limitations, too. First, there are several ethical issues related to confidentiality, data security, and provided informed consent regarding the use of AI in therapy. The use of AI systems collecting, storing, and analyzing patient data creates risks of data breaches and unauthorized access, raising serious confidentiality issues. The informed consent aspect complicates dynamics further because one may not know how far his or her data are used or shared when interacting with AI-driven therapeutic tools (Luxton, 2014).

On a practical level, one limitation to this is that in the process of managing such transiently complicated human behaviors, often ambiguous and deeply contextual, AI will not do particularly well in most instances where patients answer non-standardly or when nuanced interpretation of emotional states requires performance. Such situations would require therapeutic intuition and adaptive decision-making skills, which AI currently lacks. Furthermore, overgeneralization may also occur, where AI deploys generalized treatment protocols that do not effectively address the needs of individual patients, leading to disengagement or suboptimal therapy outcomes (Bickmore et al., 2010).

This could further be compounded by the impersonality of the AI itself, which might lead to further feelings of isolation or stigma among the patients. To patients dealing with mental health problems, the so-called therapeutic relationship reflects understanding and respect not conveyed without human touch: therapy would thus be less affirming and less supportive; the underpinning for effectiveness would, therefore, be fully undermined.

Lat but not least, although AI holds great promise for the administrative and analytical levels of CBT, there will be the need for being careful with the limitations and risks associated with it. Over-reliance on AI threatens the salience of this relationship between a therapist and their patient, one so important for effective therapy to occur. Further ethical and practical considerations may also ensue that weaken the care for the patients. It is thus best if there exists a balanced approach whereby AI plays a supplementary rather than substitutional role with human therapists to further complement human touch in clinical practice (Vandekerckhove & Cluydts, 2010).

Necessity for Ongoing Research and Improvement Areas

The integration of artificial intelligence into cognitive behavioral therapy is a field just burgeoning, with huge potential to transform therapeutic practices. However, the rapid advancement and application of AI technologies in this arena necessitate ongoing research and careful scrutiny to optimize benefits and mitigate risks. Critical areas that still need further investigation include the development of AI systems that can more accurately mimic human emotional intelligence, the ethical implications of AI in therapy, and the long-term effects of AI-assisted therapy on patient outcomes (Darcy et al., 2021).

First, there is a need to improve the emotional intelligence of AI. The current systems lack the complete understanding and interpretation of complex human emotions and social cues, which form the basis of effective CBT. Current research should also aim at ensuring that the ability of AI to recognize and respond to subtle emotional expression is enhanced, a development that could lead to empathetic and more personalized AI therapists.

The ethical dimensions regarding the use of AI in therapy also need exhaustive exploration: data security, privacy, and informed consent. Since AI systems are going to collect and process sensitive personal data, strong safeguards and frankness in communication with the patients will be needed to preserve ethics and assure confidence (Luxton, 2014).

In addition, methods should be devised for studying AI impact in CBT in the long run. Such research would give information on the sustainability of the therapeutic gain made with the use of AI and would reveal potential adverse effects in the long term as well.

The future of AI in enhancing CBT is bright. With continued development, AI has the potential to create increasingly personalized, accessible, and effective mental health interventions. However, to realize the full potential of AI in this domain, continuous research, ethical consideration, and technological improvement are required. Ensuring that AI supports rather than supplants the human elements of therapy will be crucial in maintaining the efficacy and integrity of CBT (Bickmore et al., 2010).

CONCLUSION

The integration of artificial intelligence into cognitive behavioral therapy is a field just burgeoning, with huge potential to transform therapeutic practices. However, the rapid advancement and application of AI technologies in this area necessitates ongoing research and careful scrutiny to optimize benefits and mitigate risks. Critical areas that still need further investigation include the development of AI systems that can more accurately mimic human emotional intelligence, the ethical implications of AI in therapy, and the long-term effects of AI-assisted therapy on patient outcomes.

First, there is a need to improve the emotional intelligence of AI. The current systems lack the complete understanding and interpretation of complex human emotions and social cues, which form the basis of effective CBT. Current research should also aim at ensuring that the ability of AI to recognize and respond to subtle emotional expression is enhanced, a development that could lead to empathetic and more personalized AI therapists.

The ethical dimensions regarding the use of AI in therapy also need exhaustive exploration: data security, privacy, and informed consent. Since AI systems are going to collect and process sensitive personal data, strong safeguards and frankness in communication with the patients will be needed to preserve ethics and assure confidence.

In addition, methods should be devised for studying AI impact in CBT in the long run. Such research would give information on the sustainability of the therapeutic gain made with the use of AI and would reveal potential adverse effects in the long term as well.

The future of AI in enhancing CBT is bright. With continued development, AI has the potential to create increasingly personalized, accessible, and effective mental health interventions. However, to realize the full potential of AI in this domain, continuous research, ethical consideration, and technological improvement are required. Ensuring that AI supports rather than supplants the human elements of therapy will be crucial in maintaining the efficacy and integrity of CBT.

REFERENCES

Abd-Alrazaq, A., Alajlani, M., Ali, N., Denecke, K., Bewick, B., & Househ, M. (2021). Perceptions and opinions of patients about mental health chatbots: Scoping review. *Journal of Medical Internet Research*, *23*(1), e17828. DOI: 10.2196/17828 PMID: 33439133

Abramowitz, J. S. (2013). The practice of exposure therapy: Relevance of cognitive behavioral theory and extinction theory. *Behavior Therapy*, *44*(4), 548–558. DOI: 10.1016/j.beth.2013.03.003 PMID: 24094780

Adnan, J. S. (2023). AI and Its Application on Human Health. *Journal of Advances in Artificial Intelligence*, *1*(1), 57–66. DOI: 10.18178/JAAI.2023.1.1.57-66

Åhs, F., Mozelius, P., & Dobslaw, F. (2020). Artificial Intelligence Supported Cognitive Behavioral Therapy for Treatment of Speech Anxiety in Virtual Reality Environments. *Proceedings of the European Conference on the Impact of Artificial Intelligence and Robotics*, 2. https://doi.org/DOI: 10.34190/EAIR.20.030

Alhur, A. (2024). Redefining Healthcare With Artificial Intelligence (AI): The Contributions of ChatGPT, Gemini, and Co-pilot. *Cureus*, *16*(4), 1–9. DOI: 10.7759/cureus.57795 PMID: 38721180

American Psychological Association. (2017) *What is Cognitive Behavioral Therapy?*https://www.apa.org/ptsd-guideline/patients-and-families/cognitive-behavioral

Anxiety Canada. MindShift CBT, Anxiety Canada. (n.d.). https://www.anxietycanada.com/resources/mindshift-cbt/", (Accessed 06 January 2024).

Aspvall, K., Sampaio, F., Lenhard, F., Melin, K., Norlin, L., Serlachius, E., Mataix-Cols, D., & Andersson, E. (2021). Cost-effectiveness of internet-delivered vs in-person cognitive behavioral therapy for children and adolescents with obsessive-compulsive disorder. *JAMA Network Open*, *4*(7), e2118516. DOI: 10.1001/jamanetworkopen.2021.18516 PMID: 34328501

Beck, A. T. (1979). *Cognitive therapy and the emotional disorders*. Penguin.

Bickmore, T. W., Mitchell, S. E., Jack, B. W., Paasche-Orlow, M. K., Pfeifer, L. M., & Odonnell, J. (2010). Response to a relational agent by hospital patients with depressive symptoms. *Interacting with Computers*, *22*(4), 289–298. DOI: 10.1016/j.intcom.2009.12.001 PMID: 20628581

Carlbring, P., Hadjistavropoulos, H., Kleiboer, A., & Andersson, A. (2023). A new era in Internet interventions: The advent of Chat-GPT and AI-assisted therapist guidance. *Internet Interventions : the Application of Information Technology in Mental and Behavioural Health*, *32*, 1–3. DOI: 10.1016/j.invent.2023.100621 PMID: 37273936

Chekroud, A. M., Bondar, J., Delgadillo, J., Doherty, G., Wasil, A., Fokkema, M., Cohen, Z., Belgrave, D., DeRubeis, R., Iniesta, R., Dwyer, D., & Choi, K. (2021). The promise of machine learning in predicting treatment outcomes in psychiatry. *World Psychiatry; Official Journal of the World Psychiatric Association (WPA)*, *20*(2), 154–170. DOI: 10.1002/wps.20882 PMID: 34002503

Clark, D. A. (2013) Cognitive restructuring. The Wiley handbook of cognitive behavioral therapy pp 1–22 DOI: 10.1002/9781118528563.wbcbt02

Clemente-Suárez, V. J., Martínez-González, M. B., Benitez-Agudelo, J. C., Navarro-Jiménez, E., Beltran-Velasco, A. I., Ruisoto, P., Diaz Arroyo, E., Laborde-Cárdenas, C. C., & Tornero-Aguilera, J. F. (2021, September 24). The Impact of the COVID-19 Pandemic on Mental Disorders. A Critical Review. *International Journal of Environmental Research and Public Health*, *18*(19), 10041. DOI: 10.3390/ijerph181910041 PMID: 34639341

Dahne, J., Collado, A., Lejuez, C., Risco, C. M., Diaz, V. A., Coles, L., Kustanowitz, J., Zvolensky, M. J., & Carpenter, M. J. (2019). Pilot randomized controlled trial of a spanish-language behavioral activation mobile app (activate) for the treatment of depressive symptoms among united states latinx adults with limited english proficiency. *Journal of Affective Disorders*, *250*, 210–217. DOI: 10.1016/j.jad.2019.03.009 PMID: 30870770

Danieli, M., Ciulli, T., Mousavi, S., & Riccardi, G. (2021). A conversational artificial intelligence agent for a mental health care app: Evaluation study of its participatory design. *JMIR Formative Research*, *5*(12), e30053. DOI: 10.2196/30053 PMID: 34855607

Darcy, A., Daniels, J., Salinger, D., Wicks, P., & Robinson, A. (2021). Evidence of human-level bonds established with a digital conversational agent: Cross-sectional, retrospective observational study. *JMIR Mental Health*, *5*(5). https://preprints.jmir.org/preprint/27868 PMID: 33973854

David, D., Cristea, I., & Hofmann, S. G. (2018). Why cognitive behavioral therapy is the current gold standard of psychotherapy. *Frontiers in Psychiatry*, *9*, 333730. DOI: 10.3389/fpsyt.2018.00004 PMID: 29434552 de Toledo Rodriguez, I., Salton, G., & Ross, R. (2021) Formulating automated responses to cognitive distortions for cbt interactions. In: *Proceedings of the 4th International Conference on Natural Language and Speech Processing (ICNLSP 2021)*, 108– 116

Dimidjian, S., Barrera, M.Jr, Martell, C., Muñoz, R. F., & Lewinsohn, P. M. (2011). The origins and current status of behavioral activation treatments for depression. *Annual Review of Clinical Psychology*, *7*(1), 1–38. DOI: 10.1146/annurev-clinpsy-032210-104535 PMID: 21275642

Eltahawy, L., Essig, T., Myszkowski, N., & Trub, L. (2024). Can robots do therapy?: Examining the efficacy of a CBT bot in comparison with other behavioral intervention technologies in alleviating mental health symptoms. *Computers in Human Behavior: Artificial Humans*, *2*, 1–14.

Firth, J., Torous, J., Stubbs, B., Firth, J. A., Steiner, G. Z., Smith, L., Alvarez-Jimenez, M., Gleeson, J., Vancampfort, D., Armitage, C. J., & Sarris, J. (2019). The "online brain": How the Internet may be changing our cognition. *World Psychiatry; Official Journal of the World Psychiatric Association (WPA)*, *18*(2), 119–129. DOI: 10.1002/wps.20617 PMID: 31059635

Fitzpatrick KK, Darcy A, Vierhile M, (2017) Delivering Cognitive Behavior Therapy to Young Adults With Symptoms of Depression and Anxiety Using a Fully Automated Conversational Agent (Woebot): A Randomized Controlled Trial JMIR Ment Health 2017;4(2):e19 doi: PMID: 28588005PMCID: 5478797 DOI: 10.2196/mental.7785

Flückiger, C., Del Re, A. C., Wampold, B. E., & Horvath, A. O. (2018). The alliance in adult psychotherapy: A meta-analytic synthesis. *Psychotherapy (Chicago, Ill.)*, *55*(4), 316–340. DOI: 10.1037/pst0000172

Foreman, E. I., & Pollard, C. (2016). *Cognitive Behavioural Therapy (CBT)*. Your Toolkit to Modify Mood, Overcome Obstructions and Improve Your Life. Icon Books, Limited.

Fulmer, R., Joerin, A., Gentile, B., Lakerink, L., & Rauws, M. (2018). Using Psychological Artificial Intelligence (Tess) to Relieve Symptoms of Depression and Anxiety: Randomized Controlled Trial. *JMIR Mental Health*, *5*(4), 1. DOI: 10.2196/mental.9782 PMID: 30545815

Gkora, V. and Driga, A. (2023). Virtual reality, digital technologies and brain rewiring techniques for intervention in attention-deficit/hyperactivity disorder (adhd). Journal Health and Technology - JHT, 2(2), e2237. https://doi.org/DOI: 10.47820/jht.v2i2.37

Greer, J., Jacobs, J., Pensak, N., MacDonald, J., Fuh, C., Perez, G., Ward, A., Tallen, C., Muzikansky, A., Traeger, L., Penedo, F. J., El-Jawahri, A., Safren, S. A., Pirl, W. F., & Temel, J. (2019). Randomized trial of a tailored cognitive-behavioral therapy mobile application for anxiety in patients with incurable cancer. *The Oncologist, 24*(8), 1111–1120. DOI: 10.1634/theoncologist.2018-0536 PMID: 30683710

Grodniewicz, J. P., & Hohol, M. (2024). Therapeutic Chatbots as Cognitive-Affective Artifacts. *Topoi, 43*(3), 795–807. DOI: 10.1007/s11245-024-10018-x

Gual-Montolio, P., Jaén, I., Martínez-Borba, V., Castilla, D., & Suso-Ribera, C. (2022). Using Artificial Intelligence to Enhance Ongoing Psychological Interventions for Emotional Problems in Real- or Close to Real-Time: A Systematic Review. [MDPI]. *International Journal of Environmental Research and Public Health, 19*(13), 7737. DOI: 10.3390/ijerph19137737 PMID: 35805395

Gutierrez, G., Stephenson, C., Eadie, J., Asadpour, K., & Alavi, N. (2024). Examining the role of AI technology in online mental healthcare: Opportunities, challenges, and implications, a mixed-methods review. *Frontiers in Psychiatry, 15*, 1356773. DOI: 10.3389/fpsyt.2024.1356773 PMID: 38774435

Harnas, S., Knoop, H., Evertsz, F., Booij, S., Dekker, J., Laarhoven, H., & Braamse, A. (2021). Personalized versus standard cognitive behavioral therapy for fear of cancer recurrence,depressive symptoms or cancer-related fatigue in cancer survivors: Study protocol of a randomized controlled trial (match-study). *Trials, 22*(1), 696. Advance online publication. DOI: 10.1186/s13063-021-05657-z PMID: 34641961

Held, P. (2024). A novel cognitive behavioral therapy–based generative ai tool (socrates 2.0) to facilitate socratic dialogue: protocol for a mixed methods feasibility study (preprint). https://doi.org/DOI: 10.2196/preprints.58195

Hofmann, S. G., Asnaani, A., Vonk, I. J., Sawyer, A. T., & Fang, A. (2012). The efficacy of cognitive behavioral therapy: A review of meta-analyses. *Cognitive Therapy and Research, 36*(5), 427–440. DOI: 10.1007/s10608-012-9476-1 PMID: 23459093

Inkster, B., & Sarda, S. (2018). Subramanian VAn Empathy-Driven, (2016) Conversational Artificial Intelligence Agent (Wysa) for Digital Mental Well-Being. *Real-World Data Evaluation Mixed-Methods Study JMIR Mhealth Uhealth, 6*(11), e12106. DOI: 10.2196/12106 PMID: 30470676

Jang, S., Kim, J. J., Kim, S. J., Hong, J., Kim, S., & Kim, E. (2021). Mobile app-based chatbot to deliver cognitive behavioral therapy and psychoeducation for adults with attention deficit: A evelopment and feasibility/usability study. *International Journal of Medical Informatics*, *150*, 104440. Advance online publication. DOI: 10.1016/j.ijmedinf.2021.104440 PMID: 33799055

Jiang, M., Zhao, Q., Li, J., Wang, F., He, T., Cheng, X., Yang, B.X., Ho, G.W., & Fu, G. (2024). A Generic Review of Integrating Artificial Intelligence in Cognitive Behavioral Therapy. *ArXiv, abs/2407.19422.*

Johnson, C., Egan, S. J., Carlbring, P., Shafran, R., & Wade, T. D. (2024). Artificial intelligence as a virtual coach in a cognitive behavioural intervention for perfectionism in young people: A randomised feasibility trial. *Internet Interventions : the Application of Information Technology in Mental and Behavioural Health*, *38*, 1–9. DOI: 10.1016/j.invent.2024.100795 PMID: 39717697

Khawaja, Z., & Bélisle-Pipon, J. C. (2023). Your robot therapist is not your therapist: Understanding the role of AI-powered mental health chatbots. *Frontiers in Digital Health*, *5*, 1278186. DOI: 10.3389/fdgth.2023.1278186 PMID: 38026836

LeBeau, R. T., Davies, C. D., Culver, N. C., & Craske, M. G. (2013). Homework compliance counts in cognitive-behavioral therapy. *Cognitive Behaviour Therapy*, *42*(3), 171–179. DOI: 10.1080/16506073.2013.763286 PMID: 23419077

Lindqvist, K., Mechler, J., Midgley, N., Carlbring, P., Carstrop, K., Neikter, H. K., Strid, T., VonBelow, C., & Philips, B. (2024). I didn't have to look her in the eyes: Participants experiences of the therapeutic relationship in internet-based psychodynamic therapy for adolescent depression. *Psychotherapy Research*, *34*(5), 648–662. DOI: 10.1080/10503307.2022.2150583 PMID: 36473231

Liu, W., Li, G., Wang, C., Wang, X., & Yang, L. (2021). Efficacy of Sertraline Combined with Cognitive Behavioral Therapy for Adolescent Depression: A Systematic Review and Meta-Analysis. *Computational and mathematical methods in medicine, 2021*, 5309588. (Retraction published Comput Math Methods Med. 2023 Dec 6;2023:9896050.).DOI: 10.1155/2021/5309588

Luxton, D. D. (2014). Artificial intelligence in psychological practice: Current and future applications and implications. *Professional Psychology, Research and Practice*, *45*(5), 332–339. DOI: 10.1037/a0034559

Magwood, O., Saad, A., Ranger, D., Volpini, K., Rukikamirera, F., Haridas, R., Sayfi, S., Alexander, L., Tan, Y., & Pottie, K. (2023). Mobile apps to reduce depressive symptoms and alcohol use in youth: A systematic review and meta-analysis: A systematic review. *Campbell Systematic Reviews*, *20*, 1–50. PMID: 38680950

Martenstyn, J. A., Russell, J., Tran, C., Griffiths, S., & Maguire, S. (2024). Evaluation of an 8-week telehealth cognitive-behavioural therapy (CBT) program for adults with muscle dysmorphia: A pilot and feasibility study. *Body Image*, *52*, 101842. Advance online publication. DOI: 10.1016/j.bodyim.2024.101842 PMID: 39721449

Martin, D. J., Garske, J. P., & Davis, M. K. (2000). Relation of the therapeutic alliance with outcome and other variables: A meta-analytic review. *Journal of Consulting and Clinical Psychology*, *68*(3), 438–450. DOI: 10.1037/0022-006X.68.3.438 PMID: 10883561

May, R., & Denecke, K. (2022). Security, privacy, and healthcare-related conversational agents: A scoping review. *Informatics for Health & Social Care*, *47*(2), 194–210. DOI: 10.1080/17538157.2021.1983578 PMID: 34617857

Miner, A. S., Shah, N., Bullock, K. D., Arnow, B. A., Bailenson, J., & Hancock, J. (2019). Key Considerations for Incorporating Conversational AI in Psychotherapy. *Frontiers in Psychiatry*, *10*, 746. DOI: 10.3389/fpsyt.2019.00746 PMID: 31681047

Nguyen, T., O'Dea, B., Larsen, M., Phung, D., Venkatesh, S., & Christensen, H. (2017). Using linguistic and topic analysis to classify sub-groups of online depression communities. *Multimedia Tools and Applications*, *76*(8), 10653–10676. DOI: 10.1007/s11042-015-3128-x

Nobles, A. L., Glenn, J. J., Kowsari, K., Teachman, B. A., & Barnes, L. E. (2018). Identification of Imminent Suicide Risk Among Young Adults using Text Messages. *Proceedings of the SIGCHI conference on human factors in computing systems. CHI Conference, 2018*, 413. https://doi.org/DOI: 10.1145/3173574.3173987

Norcross, J. C., & Lambert, M. J. (2019). Evidence-based psychotherapy relationships: The third task force. In Norcross, J. C., & Lambert, M. J. (Eds.), *Psychotherapy relationships that work: Evidence-based therapist contributions* (3rd ed., pp. 1–23). Oxford University Press., DOI: 10.1093/med-psych/9780190843953.003.0001

Obremski, D., & Wienrich, C. (2024). Autonomous VR Exposure Therapy for Anxiety Disorders Using Conversational AI—Ethical and Technical Implications and Preliminary Results. *Journal of Computer and Communications*, *12*(4), 111–138. DOI: 10.4236/jcc.2024.124010

Olawade, D., Wada, O., Odetayo, A., David-Olawade, C., Asaolu, F., & Eberhardt, J. (2024). Enhancing Mental Health with Artificial Intelligence: Current Trends and Future Prospects. *Journal of Medicine, Surgery, and Public Health, 100099*, 100099. Advance online publication. DOI: 10.1016/j.glmedi.2024.100099

Omarov, B., Zhumanov, Z., Gumar, A., & Kuntunova, L. (2023). Artificial intelligence enabled mobile chatbot psychologist using aiml and cognitive behavioral therapy. *International Journal of Advanced Computer Science and Applications, 14*(6). Advance online publication. DOI: 10.14569/IJACSA.2023.0140616

Penninx, B. W., Benros, M. E., Klein, R. S., & Vinkers, C. H. (2022). How covid-19 shaped mental health: From infection to pandemic effects. *Nature Medicine, 28*(10), 2027–2037. DOI: 10.1038/s41591-022-02028-2 PMID: 36192553

Perri, R. L., Castelli, P., La Rosa, C., Zucchi, T., & Onofri, A. (2021). COVID-19, Isolation, Quarantine: On the Efficacy of Internet-Based Eye Movement Desensitization and Reprocessing (EMDR) and Cognitive-Behavioral Therapy (CBT) for Ongoing Trauma. *Brain Sciences, 11*(5), 579. DOI: 10.3390/brainsci11050579 PMID: 33946179

Petersen, T. J., Sprich, S. E., & Wilhelm, S.. (2016). *The Massachusetts general hospital handbook of cognitive behavioral therapy. Tech. rep*. Springer. DOI: 10.1007/978-1-4939-2605-3

Petrinec, A., Hughes, J., Zullo, M., Wilk, C., & George, R. (2021). Smartphone delivery of cognitive behavioral therapy for post intensive care syndrome-family: Protocol for a pilot study. *JMIR Research Protocols, 10*(8), e30813. DOI: 10.2196/30813 PMID: 34346900

Raile, P. (2024). The usefulness of ChatGPT for psychotherapists and patients. *Humanities & Social Sciences Communications, 11*(47), 1–8. DOI: 10.1057/s41599-023-02567-0

Resiliens, C. B. T. Companion – a comprehensive app for cognitive behavioral therapy, Resiliens. (n.d.). “https://resiliens.com/cbt-companion/”, (Accessed 06 January 2024).

Rogers, C. R. (1961). *On becoming a person: A therapist’s view of psychotherapy*. Constable.

Roudsari, A. H., Afshar, J., Lee, W., & Lee, S. (2021). PatentNet: Multi-label classification of patent documents using deep learning based language understanding. *Scientometrics, 127*(1), 207–231. DOI: 10.1007/s11192-021-04179-4

Russell, S., & Norvig, P. (2021). *Artificial Intelligence* (Global Edition). Pearson Education., https://elibrary.pearson.de/book/99.150005/9781292401171

Sadeh-Sharvit, S., Camp, D., Horton, S., Hefner, J., Berry, J., Grossman, E., & Hollon, S. (2023). Effects of an artificial intelligence platform for behavioral interventions on depression and anxiety symptoms: Randomized clinical trial. *Journal of Medical Internet Research*, *25*, e46781. DOI: 10.2196/46781 PMID: 37428547

Sarah, J., & Egan Roz Shafran, A. (2024). A pilot study of the perceptions and acceptability of guidance using artificial intelligence in internet cognitive behaviour therapy for perfectionism in young people. *Internet Interventions : the Application of Information Technology in Mental and Behavioural Health*, ●●●, 35.

Sharma, A., Rushton, K., Lin, I. W., ... (2023a) Cognitive reframing of negative thoughts through human-language model interaction. arXiv preprint arXiv:230502466 DOI: 10.18653/v1/2023.acl-long.555

Sharma, A., Rushton, K., Lin, I. W., ... (2023b) Facilitating self-guided mental health interventions through human-language model interaction: A case study of cognitive restructuring. arXiv preprint arXiv:231015461

Shedler, J. (2010). The efficacy of psychodynamic psychotherapy. *The American Psychologist*, *65*(2), 98–109. DOI: 10.1037/a0018378 PMID: 20141265

Stawarz, K., Preist, C., Tallon, D., Wiles, N., & Coyle, D. (2018). User experience of cognitive behavioral therapy apps for depression: An analysis of app functionality and user reviews. *Journal of Medical Internet Research*, *20*(6), e10120. DOI: 10.2196/10120 PMID: 29875087

Thieme, A., Belgrave, D., & Doherty, G. (2020). Machine Learning in Mental Health: A Systematic Review of the HCI Literature to Support the Development of Effective and Implementable ML Systems. *ACM Transactions on Computer-Human Interaction*, *27*(5), 1–53. DOI: 10.1145/3398069

Thieme, A., Hanratty, M., Lyons, M., Palacios, J., Marques, R. F., Morrison, C., & Doherty, G. (2023). Designing human-centered AI for mental health: Developing clinically relevant applications for online CBT treatment. *ACM Transactions on Computer-Human Interaction*, *30*(2), 1–50. DOI: 10.1145/3564752

Tolin, D. F. (2010). Is cognitive-behavioral therapy more effective than other therapies? A meta-analytic review. *Clinical Psychology Review*, *30*(6), 710–720. DOI: 10.1016/j.cpr.2010.05.003 PMID: 20547435

Torous, J., Jän Myrick, K., Rauseo-Ricupero, N., & Firth, J. (2020). Digital Mental Health and COVID-19. *Using Technology Today to Accelerate the Curve on Access and Quality Tomorrow JMIR Ment Health*, *7*(3), e18848. DOI: 10.2196/18848

Torous, J., & Roberts, L. W. (2017). Needed innovation in digital health and smartphone applications for mental health: Transparency and trust. *JAMA Psychiatry, 74*(5), 437–438. DOI: 10.1001/jamapsychiatry.2017.0262

Twomey C, O'Reilly G, Byrne M., (2014) Effectiveness of cognitive behavioural therapy for anxiety and depression in primary care: a meta-analysis. Fam Pract. 2015 Feb;32(1):3-15.. Epub 2014 Sep 22. PMID: 25248976.DOI: 10.1093/fampra/cmu060

Vaidyam, A. N., Wisniewski, H., Halamka, J. D., Kashavan, M. S., & Torous, J. B. (2019). Chatbots and conversational agents in mental health: A review of the psychiatric landscape. *Canadian Journal of Psychiatry, 64*(7), 456–464. DOI: 10.1177/0706743719828977 PMID: 30897957

Vandekerckhove, M., & Cluydts, R. (2010). The emotional brain and sleep: An intimate relationship. *Sleep Medicine Reviews, 14*(4), 219–226. DOI: 10.1016/j.smrv.2010.01.002 PMID: 20363166

Wang, B. (2024). Psychological ai: A critical analysis of capabilities, limitations, and ramifications. *Applied and Computational Engineering, 53*(1), 205–212. DOI: 10.54254/2755-2721/53/20241373

Webb, C. A., Rosso, I. M., & Rauch, S. L. (2017). Internet-based cognitive-behavioral therapy for depression: Current progress and future directions. *Harvard Review of Psychiatry, 25*(3), 114–122. DOI: 10.1097/HRP.0000000000000139 PMID: 28475503

Weizenbaum, J. (1976). *Computer power and human reason: From judgment to calculation*. W. H. Freeman.

Wilhelm, S., Bernstein, E. E., Bentley, K. H., Snorrason, I., Hoeppner, S., Klare, D., Greenberg, J. L., Weingarden, H., McCoy, T. H., & Harrison, O. (2024). Feasibility, Acceptability, and Preliminary Efficacy of a Smartphone App–Led Cognitive Behavioral Therapy for Depression Under Therapist Supervision: Open Trial. *JMIR Mental Health, 11*, 1–16. DOI: 10.2196/53998 PMID: 38592771

Yang, Y., Tavares, J., & Oliveira, T. (2024). A New Research Model for Artificial Intelligence–Based Well-Being Chatbot Engagement: Survey Study. *JMIR Human Factors, 11*, 1–21. DOI: 10.2196/59908 PMID: 39527812

Chapter 11
Approaches to AI Integration in Education and Healthcare

S. Ida Evangeline
https://orcid.org/0000-0003-2997-7897
Government College of Engineering, Tirunelveli, India

ABSTRACT

This chapter explores the integration of artificial intelligence (AI) into education and healthcare through a multidisciplinary lens, emphasizing both the transformative potential and the complex ethical, infrastructural, and contextual challenges of implementation. While AI promises personalized learning, advanced diagnostics, and administrative efficiency, real-world applications often reveal limitations—including algorithmic bias, infrastructural inequities, and stakeholder resistance. The chapter argues that successful AI deployment demands collaborative engagement among technologists, educators, clinicians, ethicists, and policymakers. Drawing from foundational literature and global case studies, it highlights the need for ethical safeguards, inclusive design, and responsive governance. Ultimately, the chapter advocates for an approach to AI integration that is both innovative and grounded in social equity, aiming to guide future applications toward sustainable, just, and context-sensitive outcomes in human-centered systems.

INTRODUCTION

Artificial intelligence (AI) is revolutionizing various domains, significantly transforming education and healthcare systems, two sectors intrinsically tied to human well-being. The integration of AI in these fields presents a unique opportunity to

DOI: 10.4018/979-8-3373-5072-1.ch011

enhance accessibility, personalize services, and improve decision-making processes (Dave & Patel, 2023). However, the complexity of these sectors, each deeply rooted in diverse societal, ethical, and practical dimensions, demands a multidisciplinary approach for AI integration to be effective and sustainable (Charow et al. 2021).

This chapter examines the pivotal role of multidisciplinary strategies in addressing the challenges and maximizing the potential of AI in education and healthcare. It highlights how collaborative efforts among experts in technology, pedagogy, medicine, ethics, sociology, and policy-making are critical for creating AI solutions that are not only innovative but also equitable and ethical. The chapter underscores that the success of AI in these domains is contingent upon the ability to transcend traditional disciplinary boundaries and integrate insights from a broad spectrum of expertise.

Education and healthcare systems are deeply interconnected with the social fabric, influencing individuals and communities in profound ways. AI's ability to adapt learning experiences to individual needs, automate complex administrative tasks, and provide real-time feedback has the potential to transform educational outcomes (Chen et al. 2020). Similarly, in healthcare, AI offers advanced diagnostic capabilities, personalized treatment options, and streamlined patient management (Jiang et al. 2017). However, alongside these opportunities come significant challenges, including concerns over data privacy, algorithmic bias, and the equitable distribution of AI-driven benefits. These concerns are amplified by the ethical implications of deploying AI in contexts that directly impact vulnerable populations, where the stakes for fairness and accountability are high.

The purpose of this chapter is to provide a comprehensive analysis of how multidisciplinary approaches can guide the integration of AI into education and healthcare in ways that prioritize inclusivity, ethics, and systemic improvement. By exploring the intersections of technology with social, ethical, and policy considerations, the chapter aims to provide a robust framework for understanding the collaborative efforts required to address these challenges. It also delves into the opportunities presented by AI, demonstrating how diverse perspectives can contribute to designing systems that align with societal values and objectives.

Ultimately, this chapter serves as a call to action for researchers, practitioners, and policymakers to embrace interdisciplinary collaboration in shaping the future of AI in education and healthcare. By fostering an integrated approach, it seeks to pave the way for systems that are not only technologically advanced but also equitable, ethical, and sustainable.

THE ROLE OF AI IN EDUCATION AND HEALTHCARE

Artificial intelligence (AI) is fundamentally reshaping the landscapes of education and healthcare, driving innovations that promise to revolutionize both sectors. In education, AI has introduced personalized learning systems capable of adapting to individual student needs, fostering more engaging and effective learning experiences (Hashim et al. 2022). These systems leverage algorithms to analyze student performance, identify gaps in understanding, and suggest tailored interventions that enhance comprehension and retention. AI is also transforming administrative processes by automating repetitive tasks such as grading, attendance tracking, and scheduling, allowing educators to focus more on teaching and mentorship. Real-time feedback mechanisms powered by AI provide students and educators with actionable insights, facilitating a dynamic and responsive learning environment (Pratama et al. 2023).

In healthcare, AI innovations have opened new frontiers in diagnostics, treatment planning, and patient management. Machine learning algorithms are now capable of analyzing vast amounts of medical data to detect diseases earlier and with greater accuracy than traditional methods (Prabhod, 2024). For instance, AI-driven imaging tools can identify anomalies in radiographs or scans, enabling faster and more precise diagnoses. Treatment planning has also seen significant advancements, with AI assisting clinicians in developing personalized care strategies based on patient data and predictive analytics. Furthermore, virtual health assistants and robotic systems are improving patient management by enhancing accessibility to care, reducing administrative burdens, and providing continuous monitoring and support (Strika et al. 2025).

The opportunities presented by AI in these sectors are vast, particularly in enhancing access and equity. By automating processes and providing scalable solutions, AI can extend educational and healthcare services to underserved populations, bridging gaps in resource-limited settings. In education, AI-powered platforms can reach rural and remote areas, offering high-quality learning materials to students who may otherwise lack access to well-equipped schools or skilled educators (Murari & Parmar, 2025). Similarly, in healthcare, AI can improve outcomes for patients in regions with limited access to specialists, enabling remote diagnostics and telemedicine services (Chaturvedi et al. 2025). The ability of AI to analyze complex datasets and identify patterns also holds the potential to improve outcomes by offering personalized solutions that cater to the specific needs of learners and patients alike.

Despite these benefits, the integration of AI into education and healthcare is not without challenges. Algorithmic bias poses a significant risk, as AI systems trained on unrepresentative data can perpetuate existing inequalities or introduce new forms of discrimination (Strika et al. 2025). For example, in education, biased algorithms may disproportionately disadvantage students from marginalized communities, while in healthcare, they could lead to misdiagnoses or unequal access to care (Rashidi et al. 2025a). Data privacy concerns also emerge as a critical issue, given the sensitive nature of educational and medical information. Ensuring the security of this data and maintaining the trust of users is paramount. Systemic inequities, such as disparities in infrastructure and digital literacy, further complicate the adoption of AI, particularly in resource-constrained environments (Arar et al. 2025).

AI's role in education and healthcare is marked by a duality of immense promise and significant responsibility. As these sectors increasingly rely on AI, the need for thoughtful integration becomes essential. Addressing the challenges of bias, privacy, and equity requires not only technological solutions but also a multidisciplinary approach that incorporates ethical, social, and policy considerations.

MULTIDISCIPLINARY COLLABORATION: THE FOUNDATION OF AI INTEGRATION

The successful integration of artificial intelligence (AI) into education and healthcare systems is deeply reliant on multidisciplinary collaboration. The complexity of these sectors demands expertise that spans pedagogy, medicine, computer science, ethics, sociology, and policy-making. Each discipline brings a unique perspective and set of skills essential for addressing the multifaceted challenges and opportunities posed by AI (Fan et al. 2025). Pedagogy provides insights into effective teaching and learning processes, ensuring that AI aligns with educational goals and fosters meaningful engagement. Medicine contributes clinical expertise, guiding the development of AI systems that support accurate diagnoses and patient care (Srivastava et al. 2025). Computer science drives technological innovation, crafting the algorithms and infrastructure that underpin AI applications. Ethics addresses critical questions about fairness, accountability, and the societal impact of AI. Sociology examines the broader societal implications, such as equity and cultural factors, while policy establishes the regulatory frameworks needed to govern AI's deployment responsibly (Rezaev & Tregubova, 2025).

The interplay among these disciplines creates the foundation for interdisciplinary synergies, enabling the development of AI solutions that are both effective and ethical. Successful projects illustrate the power of collaboration across fields. For instance, in education, interdisciplinary teams have developed adaptive learning platforms that integrate pedagogical theory, psychological insights, and machine learning algorithms to enhance student outcomes (Lin et al. 2025). In healthcare, partnerships between clinicians, data scientists, and ethicists have led to AI systems capable of early disease detection while addressing ethical considerations related to data use and patient consent. These synergies are achieved through a combination of mutual respect, clear communication, and shared goals, which foster a culture of cooperation and innovation (Zabaleta et al. 2025). Strategies for encouraging such collaboration include cross-disciplinary training programs, joint research initiatives, and platforms for ongoing dialogue between technical and non-technical stakeholders.

However, fostering effective interdisciplinary collaboration is not without its challenges. One of the most significant barriers is the existence of silos between disciplines, where experts operate in isolation, limiting the flow of knowledge and ideas (Hai & Tien, 2025). These silos are often reinforced by differences in professional jargon, methodologies, and priorities, which can impede understanding and collaboration. Overcoming these barriers requires deliberate effort and institutional support (Asrifan et al. 2025). Creating shared spaces for interdisciplinary interaction, such as conferences, workshops, and collaborative research centers, can help break down these silos. Additionally, fostering a culture of curiosity and mutual respect among professionals from diverse backgrounds is essential for building trust and encouraging the exchange of ideas.

Collaboration across disciplines is not merely a practical necessity; it is the foundation for addressing the ethical, technical, and societal dimensions of AI integration. By bringing together diverse perspectives, interdisciplinary teams can anticipate and mitigate potential risks while maximizing the benefits of AI in education and healthcare (Akpan et al. 2025).

ETHICAL CONSIDERATIONS IN AI INTEGRATION

The integration of artificial intelligence (AI) into education and healthcare presents profound ethical challenges that require careful consideration and proactive strategies (Miyake et al. 2025). Both sectors involve vulnerable populations whose lives and futures can be directly shaped by AI-driven decisions. In education, students, particularly those from marginalized backgrounds, face risks associated with algorithmic bias that can perpetuate systemic inequities (Rashidi et al. 2025b). Similarly, in healthcare, patients may encounter challenges stemming from opaque AI systems, where a lack of algorithmic accountability can lead to mistrust or adverse outcomes. The question of equity and inclusivity in AI design emerges as a critical concern, as algorithms trained on biased datasets risk excluding or disadvantaging specific groups, further widening existing disparities (Schmidt et al. 2025).

Addressing these challenges demands the development of robust ethical frameworks that guide the responsible use of AI. Such frameworks must be built upon foundational principles, including fairness, transparency, accountability, and respect for privacy (Shiferaw et al. 2025). Responsible AI development requires the inclusion of diverse perspectives to ensure that systems are designed with an awareness of cultural, social, and ethical nuances. For instance, case studies in education have demonstrated the importance of embedding equity-focused principles into AI systems to prevent biases in student assessment and resource allocation (Miller et al. 2025). In healthcare, examples such as AI-driven diagnostic tools underscore the need for systems that prioritize patient safety and consent, illustrating the value of ethical guidelines in mitigating risks and maximizing benefits (Ajmal et al. 2025).

Participatory approaches play a crucial role in fostering ethical AI integration, emphasizing the importance of stakeholder engagement in the design and implementation of AI systems (Salimi et al. 2025). By involving educators, healthcare providers, patients, students, and community representatives, participatory methods ensure that AI solutions are not only technologically sound but also socially and ethically aligned with the needs of those they serve. These approaches create opportunities for feedback and co-creation, enabling the identification and resolution of potential issues before they escalate. For example, engaging teachers and students in the development of AI-powered learning platforms has been shown to enhance their relevance and accessibility, while involving patients in healthcare AI projects builds trust and ensures alignment with patient priorities (El-Sayed et al. 2025).

Ethical considerations are not an ancillary concern but a central pillar of AI integration in education and healthcare. As these technologies continue to evolve, the need for ethical vigilance will only grow, requiring a sustained commitment to fairness, accountability, and inclusivity (Cascella et al. 2025).

POLICY AND GOVERNANCE

The integration of artificial intelligence (AI) into education and healthcare necessitates a robust policy and governance framework to address the unique challenges posed by these critical sectors. Effective regulation is essential to balance the promotion of innovation with the protection of individual rights and societal values. In both education and healthcare, data privacy laws and standards form the cornerstone of regulatory efforts (Ashraf & Mustafa, 2025). The sensitive nature of data in these domains—whether it involves student learning records or patient health information—demands stringent safeguards to prevent misuse and ensure confidentiality. In healthcare, guidelines for clinical AI applications must establish criteria for safety, accuracy, and ethical deployment, ensuring that AI tools align with medical standards. Similarly, in education, policies must govern the use of AI in teaching and administration, ensuring equitable access while safeguarding student data (Kothari et al. 2025).

Promoting responsible AI use involves a careful balancing act between encouraging innovation and mitigating risks. Policies must be designed to foster an environment where AI can thrive while ensuring that its development and deployment remain ethically grounded and socially beneficial. Examples of effective policy interventions illustrate how this balance can be achieved. For instance, regulatory frameworks in some regions have implemented mandatory bias audits for AI systems used in education, ensuring that algorithms do not perpetuate systemic inequalities (Sasseville et al. 2025). In healthcare, initiatives such as the FDA's guidelines for AI-based medical devices have emphasized transparency and ongoing evaluation, fostering trust in AI-driven technologies while enabling their adoption (Alderman et al. 2025).

Data governance is another critical aspect of policy and governance in AI integration. Issues of consent, data ownership, and interoperability present complex challenges that require nuanced solutions (Sanchini et al. 2025). In education, students and parents must retain agency over how their data is collected and used, with policies ensuring informed consent and clear guidelines on data sharing (Venkata, 2025). In healthcare, patient data ownership is a contentious issue, particularly when AI systems rely on large datasets for training (Aman & Qidwai, 2025). Policymakers must establish frameworks that respect patient autonomy while enabling the data sharing necessary for innovation. Interoperability, or the ability of AI systems to communicate and function across different platforms and institutions, is equally vital (Bobade et al. 2025). Policies that promote open standards and collaboration can enhance the effectiveness of AI systems while preventing fragmentation and inefficiency.

The development of comprehensive policy and governance frameworks is essential to harnessing the transformative potential of AI in education and healthcare. These frameworks must address regulatory needs, promote responsible innovation, and navigate the complexities of data governance, creating an environment where AI can flourish without compromising ethical and societal priorities (Jiao et al. 2025).

WORKFORCE DEVELOPMENT AND CAPACITY BUILDING

The integration of artificial intelligence (AI) into education and healthcare systems requires deliberate efforts in workforce development and capacity building (Chau et al. 2025). These efforts must ensure that professionals in both sectors are equipped with the skills, knowledge, and cultural readiness to harness AI effectively and responsibly. The growing prevalence of AI technologies introduces a demand for specialized competencies that extend beyond technical proficiency to encompass a deep understanding of ethical considerations and interdisciplinary collaboration (Prabhakar, 2025).

A key aspect of workforce development is fostering skills essential for AI integration. Professionals in education and healthcare must possess data literacy, enabling them to interpret and utilize the vast datasets that power AI systems. Understanding algorithmic transparency is equally critical, as it ensures that users can assess how AI systems make decisions and identify potential biases or errors (Gupta et al. 2025). Ethical awareness is perhaps the most vital skill, given the significant implications of AI for vulnerable populations and the societal impact of its deployment. Developing a workforce that can critically evaluate AI's ethical dimensions is fundamental to ensuring its responsible use (Nnorom, 2025).

Multidisciplinary training programs play a pivotal role in building this skill set. Successful examples from both education and healthcare illustrate how tailored training initiatives can prepare professionals for the complexities of AI integration (Hai et al. 2025). For instance, programs that combine technical training with courses in ethics, sociology, and policy provide participants with a holistic understanding of AI's multifaceted challenges. In healthcare, cross-disciplinary workshops involving clinicians, data scientists, and ethicists have demonstrated the value of collaborative learning environments where diverse perspectives are shared. Professional development initiatives should prioritize flexibility and accessibility, offering modular courses, certifications, and hands-on workshops that cater to varied professional needs. Such programs must also emphasize real-world applications, enabling participants to engage directly with AI tools and systems relevant to their domains (King, 2025).

Beyond individual skills and training, cultivating a collaborative culture is essential for the successful adoption of AI. Cross-disciplinary communication and teamwork are vital for addressing the intersectional challenges that AI integration presents (Imjai et al. 2025). Strategies to foster such a culture include creating interdisciplinary working groups, organizing collaborative projects, and establishing platforms for ongoing dialogue between professionals from diverse backgrounds (Kasinidou et al. 2025). These initiatives can help break down silos, build mutual respect, and encourage the co-creation of solutions that are both innovative and inclusive.

Workforce development and capacity building are foundational to the transformative potential of AI in education and healthcare. By equipping professionals with the necessary skills, fostering multidisciplinary training programs, and cultivating a culture of collaboration, these efforts ensure that AI integration is both effective and ethically sound.

BRIDGING THE DIGITAL DIVIDE

The integration of artificial intelligence (AI) in education and healthcare has the potential to revolutionize these sectors, but this promise remains elusive for many communities due to the persistent digital divide. In resource-limited settings, challenges such as inadequate infrastructure, low digital literacy, and funding constraints create significant barriers to adopting and benefiting from AI technologies. Schools and clinics in rural areas often lack reliable internet connectivity, sufficient hardware, and skilled personnel, making it difficult to implement and sustain AI-driven solutions. These limitations are compounded by a lack of awareness and understanding of AI's capabilities, leading to skepticism or underutilization of its potential (Kalantzis & Cope, 2025).

Addressing these challenges requires the development of inclusive AI solutions that are specifically designed to meet the needs of underserved populations. AI technologies must be tailored to function effectively in environments with limited resources, ensuring that they are not overly dependent on high-speed internet or expensive hardware (Zhang et al. 2025). For instance, lightweight AI models capable of operating on low-cost devices can expand access to critical tools in education and healthcare. Moreover, these solutions must be culturally and contextually relevant, aligning with the specific needs, languages, and practices of the communities they serve. Inclusivity also entails active engagement with local stakeholders, involving them in the design, implementation, and evaluation of AI systems to ensure that these technologies are both accessible and impactful (Fong et al. 2025).

Case studies highlight the transformative potential of inclusive AI initiatives in bridging the digital divide. In rural schools, AI-powered learning platforms have been deployed to provide personalized education despite limited teacher resources (Çela et al. 2025). For example, adaptive learning tools have enabled students in remote areas to receive tailored instruction that aligns with their individual needs and progress (Singh et al. 2025). Similarly, in rural healthcare settings, AI has facilitated significant advancements in diagnostics and patient care. Mobile-based AI tools have been used to screen for diseases such as tuberculosis and cervical cancer, delivering accurate results even in locations with minimal infrastructure (Asanza, 2025). These initiatives demonstrate how thoughtful design, and implementation can overcome resource constraints and deliver tangible benefits to underserved communities.

Bridging the digital divide is essential to ensuring that the benefits of AI are distributed equitably and that its transformative potential is realized for all. By addressing the unique challenges faced by resource-limited settings, designing inclusive solutions, and learning from successful case studies, stakeholders can create pathways for equitable AI adoption in education and healthcare (Nong et al. 2025).

EMERGING TRENDS AND FUTURE DIRECTIONS

The landscape of artificial intelligence (AI) in education and healthcare is rapidly evolving, shaped by the emergence of new technologies that promise to amplify its capabilities. Innovations such as the Internet of Things (IoT), blockchain, and augmented reality (AR) are converging with AI to create novel solutions that enhance outcomes in both sectors (Khan et al. 2025). IoT devices, for instance, enable real-time data collection and monitoring, offering new possibilities for personalized care in healthcare and tailored instruction in education (Shruti Rani & Boulila, 2025). In healthcare, wearable IoT devices track patient metrics such as heart rate and blood pressure, providing continuous data that AI systems analyze to identify risks and recommend interventions (Bhamidipaty et al. 2025). In education, IoT-enabled classrooms can gather information on student engagement and learning patterns, allowing AI algorithms to adapt lessons dynamically. Blockchain technology further complements AI by addressing critical issues of data security and interoperability, ensuring that sensitive educational and medical data can be shared and stored securely while maintaining transparency and trust. Meanwhile, AR combines AI with immersive experiences, enabling applications such as virtual anatomy lessons for medical students or interactive simulations for skill development (Rathore et al. 2025).

While these advancements offer significant opportunities, they also introduce new challenges and risks that must be carefully managed. The integration of emerging technologies with AI raises questions about scalability, ethical use, and the potential for unintended consequences. For example, IoT devices generate vast amounts of data, raising concerns about privacy and the security of sensitive information. Blockchain, though secure, requires substantial computational resources, which may limit its feasibility in resource-constrained settings. AR applications demand high levels of accuracy and realism, and any failure in these systems could undermine their educational or clinical efficacy. Balancing innovation with these challenges requires a proactive approach that incorporates robust governance, ethical frameworks, and collaborative strategies to ensure that emerging technologies enhance rather than compromise the effectiveness of AI systems (Gill et al. 2025).

Looking toward the future, the integration of AI with emerging technologies will depend on the cultivation of collaborative pathways that bring together stakeholders from diverse disciplines and sectors. Researchers, policymakers, technologists, educators, and healthcare professionals must work in concert to develop solutions that address real-world needs while remaining adaptable to technological advancements. This vision for the future emphasizes the importance of inclusivity and equity, ensuring that the benefits of AI and its associated technologies are accessible to all communities. Strategic investments in research and development, along with the creation of interdisciplinary platforms for collaboration, will be critical in driving innovation while safeguarding against potential risks (Cui et al. 2025).

The future of AI in education and healthcare is one of immense potential, defined by its ability to harness emerging technologies to address pressing challenges and improve outcomes. By balancing innovation with thoughtful planning and fostering collaboration across disciplines, stakeholders can ensure that AI continues to evolve as a tool for equity, sustainability, and progress. This chapter examines these trends and their implications, offering a forward-looking perspective on how AI can shape the future of education and healthcare in transformative ways.

CONCLUSION

The integration of artificial intelligence (AI) into education and healthcare represents a profound opportunity to transform these essential sectors, enhancing outcomes for individuals and communities alike. However, realizing this potential requires a commitment to multidisciplinary approaches that blend expertise from diverse fields such as technology, pedagogy, medicine, ethics, sociology, and policy. These collaborative efforts are essential for navigating the complex landscape of AI integration, addressing challenges such as algorithmic bias, data privacy, and equitable access. Throughout this chapter, the importance of balancing technological advancements with ethical and practical considerations has been emphasized, highlighting the need for a holistic perspective that prioritizes both innovation and societal well-being.

The success of AI in education and healthcare hinges on fostering interdisciplinary research and collaboration. By bringing together diverse stakeholders, from technical experts to policymakers and community representatives, it becomes possible to design and implement AI solutions that are not only effective but also inclusive and ethical. These collaborative efforts must focus on creating systems that address the unique needs of different populations, particularly those in underserved or resource-limited settings. Equally important is the promotion of equitable and sustainable AI adoption, ensuring that the benefits of these technologies reach all communities while mitigating risks and preventing the exacerbation of existing disparities.

As AI continues to evolve, so too must our approaches to its integration. This chapter calls on researchers, practitioners, and policymakers to embrace a shared vision for the future of AI in education and healthcare—one that is rooted in collaboration, inclusivity, and a steadfast commitment to ethical principles. By working together across disciplines and sectors, stakeholders can harness the transformative power of AI to build systems that are not only innovative but also just, equitable, and sustainable for generations to come.

REFERENCES

Ajmal, C. S., Yerram, S., Abishek, V., Nizam, V. M., Aglave, G., Patnam, J. D., Raghuvanshi, R. S., & Srivastava, S. (2025). Innovative Approaches in Regulatory Affairs: Leveraging Artificial Intelligence and Machine Learning for Efficient Compliance and Decision-Making. *The AAPS Journal*, *27*(1), 22. DOI: 10.1208/s12248-024-01006-5 PMID: 39776314

Akpan, I. J., Kobara, Y. M., Owolabi, J., Akpan, A. A., & Offodile, O. F. (2025). Conversational and generative artificial intelligence and human–chatbot interaction in education and research. *International Transactions in Operational Research*, *32*(3), 1251–1281. DOI: 10.1111/itor.13522

Alderman, J. E., Palmer, J., Laws, E., McCradden, M. D., Ordish, J., Ghassemi, M., Pfohl, S. R., Rostamzadeh, N., Cole-Lewis, H., Glocker, B., Calvert, M., Pollard, T. J., Gill, J., Gath, J., Adebajo, A., Beng, J., Leung, C. H., Kuku, S., Farmer, L.-A., & Liu, X. (2025). Tackling algorithmic bias and promoting transparency in health datasets: The STANDING Together consensus recommendations. *The Lancet. Digital Health*, *7*(1), e64–e88. DOI: 10.1016/S2589-7500(24)00224-3 PMID: 39701919

Aman, Z., & Qidwai, M. A. (2025). Role of Artificial Intelligence in Strengthening Healthcare Systems. In *Intersection of Human Rights and AI in Healthcare* (pp. 253–282). IGI Global Scientific Publishing.

Arar, K., Tlili, A., Schunka, L., Salha, S., & Saiti, A. (2025). Reimagining Educational Leadership and Management Through Artificial Intelligence: An Integrative Systematic Review. *Leadership and Policy in Schools*, 1–23. DOI: 10.1080/15700763.2025.2451982

Asanza, D. M. (2025). Emerging Trends and Future Perspectives in Digital Dentistry for Rural Areas: An Update. *Transforming Dental Health in Rural Communities: Digital Dentistry*, 1-20.

Ashraf, Z. A., & Mustafa, N. (2025). AI Standards and Regulations. *Intersection of Human Rights and AI in Healthcare*, 325-352.

Asrifan, A., Rusmayadi, R., Hasmawaty, H., Nirwana, N., Sivaraja, S., & Dewi, A. C. (2025). Synergizing Human and Machine: Innovations in Knowledge Discovery and Management. In *AI and Green Technology Applications in Society* (pp. 249-282). IGI Global Scientific Publishing.

Bhamidipaty, V., Bhamidipaty, D. L., Guntoory, I., Bhamidipaty, K. D. P., Iyengar, K. P., Botchu, B., & Botchu, R. (2025). Revolutionizing Healthcare: The Impact of AI-Powered Sensors. *Generative Artificial Intelligence for Biomedical and Smart Health Informatics*, 355-373.

Bobade, S., Asutkar, S., Nagpure, D., & Kadav, A. (2025). A brief review of practical use of artificial intelligence in surgery in the current era. *Multidisciplinary Reviews*, *8*(3), 2025085–2025085. DOI: 10.31893/multirev.2025085

Cascella, M., Shariff, M. N., Viswanath, O., Leoni, M. L. G., & Varrassi, G. (2025). Ethical Considerations in the Use of Artificial Intelligence in Pain Medicine. *Current Pain and Headache Reports*, *29*(1), 10. DOI: 10.1007/s11916-024-01330-7 PMID: 39760779

Çela, E., Vajjhala, N. R., Eappen, P., & Vedishchev, A. (2025). Artificial Intelligence in Vocational Education and Training. In *Transforming Vocational Education and Training Using AI* (pp. 1–16). IGI Global Scientific Publishing.

Charow, R., Jeyakumar, T., Younus, S., Dolatabadi, E., Salhia, M., Al-Mouaswas, D., Anderson, M., Balakumar, S., Clare, M., Dhalla, A., Gillan, C., Haghzare, S., Jackson, E., Lalani, N., Mattson, J., Peteanu, W., Tripp, T., Waldorf, J., Williams, S., & Wiljer, D. (2021). Artificial intelligence education programs for health care professionals: Scoping review. *JMIR Medical Education*, *7*(4), e31043. DOI: 10.2196/31043 PMID: 34898458

Chaturvedi, U., Chauhan, S. B., & Singh, I. (2025). *The Impact of Artificial Intelligence on Remote Healthcare: Enhancing Patient Engagement, Connectivity, and Overcoming Challenges*. Intelligent Pharmacy.

Chau, M., Arruzza, E., Spuur, K., & Ofori-Manteaw, B. (2025). From classroom to global impact: How radiography education advances the sustainable development goals. *Radiography*, *31*(1), 224–230. DOI: 10.1016/j.radi.2024.11.015 PMID: 39616979

Chen, L., Chen, P., & Lin, Z. (2020). Artificial intelligence in education: A review. *IEEE Access : Practical Innovations, Open Solutions*, *8*, 75264–75278. DOI: 10.1109/ACCESS.2020.2988510

Cui, Z., Qi, C., Zhou, T., Yu, Y., Wang, Y., Zhang, Z., Zhang, Y., Wang, W., & Liu, Y. (2025). Artificial intelligence and food flavor: How AI models are shaping the future and revolutionary technologies for flavor food development. *Comprehensive Reviews in Food Science and Food Safety*, *24*(1), e70068. DOI: 10.1111/1541-4337.70068 PMID: 39783879

Dave, M., & Patel, N. (2023). Artificial intelligence in healthcare and education. *British Dental Journal, 234*(10), 761–764. DOI: 10.1038/s41415-023-5845-2 PMID: 37237212

El-Sayed, B. K. M., El-Sayed, A. A. I., Alsenany, S. A., & Asal, M. G. R. (2025). The role of artificial intelligence literacy and innovation mindset in shaping nursing students' career and talent self-efficacy. *Nurse Education in Practice, 82*, 104208. DOI: 10.1016/j.nepr.2024.104208 PMID: 39637623

Fan, Y., Zhao, C., & Fan, S. (2025). Bridging the Rural-Urban Healthcare Gap: A Multidisciplinary Approach Leveraging Artificial Intelligence and Sociological Analysis in Sepsis Survivorship. *Critical Care Medicine, 53*(1), e254–e255. DOI: 10.1097/CCM.0000000000006471 PMID: 39774238

Fong, Y., Melstrom, L., & Evans, H. L. (2025). Practical guide to remote patient monitoring in surgical patients. *JAMA Surgery, 160*(4), 457. DOI: 10.1001/jamasurg.2024.6015 PMID: 39776114

Gill, S. S., Golec, M., Hu, J., Xu, M., Du, J., Wu, H., Walia, G. K., Murugesan, S. S., Ali, B., Kumar, M., Ye, K., Verma, P., Kumar, S., Cuadrado, F., & Uhlig, S. (2025). Edge AI: A taxonomy, systematic review and future directions. *Cluster Computing, 28*(1), 1–53. DOI: 10.1007/s10586-024-04686-y

Gupta, S., Kumar, V., & Gupta, P. (2025). Role of artificial intelligence in health sector. In *Challenges in Information, Communication and Computing Technology* (pp. 690-695). CRC Press.

Hai, D. M., & Tien, N. H. (2025). Analysis of the Potential of Artificial Intelligence in Medicine. *International Journal of Advanced Multidisciplinary Research and Studies, 5*(1), 64–73.

Hashim, S., Omar, M. K., Ab Jalil, H., & Sharef, N. M. (2022). Trends on technologies and artificial intelligence in education for personalized learning: Systematic literature. *Journal of Academic Research in Progressive Education and Development, 12*(1), 884–903. DOI: 10.6007/IJARPED/v11-i1/12230

Imjai, N., Yordudom, T., Yaacob, Z., Saad, N. H. M., & Aujirapongpan, S. (2025). Impact of AI literacy and adaptability on financial analyst skills among prospective Thai accountants: The role of critical thinking. *Technological Forecasting and Social Change, 210*, 123889. DOI: 10.1016/j.techfore.2024.123889

Jiang, F., Jiang, Y., Zhi, H., Dong, Y., Li, H., Ma, S., Wang, Y., Dong, Q., Shen, H., & Wang, Y. (2017). Artificial intelligence in healthcare: Past, present and future. *Stroke and Vascular Neurology*, *2*(4), 230–243. DOI: 10.1136/svn-2017-000101 PMID: 29507784

Jiao, J., Afroogh, S., Chen, K., Atkinson, D., & Dhurandhar, A. (2025). Generative AI and LLMs in Industry: A text-mining Analysis and Critical Evaluation of Guidelines and Policy Statements Across Fourteen Industrial Sectors. *arXiv preprint arXiv:2501.00957*.

Kalantzis, M., & Cope, B. (2025). Literacy in the Time of Artificial Intelligence. *Reading Research Quarterly*, *60*(1), e591. DOI: 10.1002/rrq.591

Kasinidou, M., Kleanthoys, S., & Otterbacher, J. (2025). Cypriot Teachers' digital skills and attitudes towards AI. *Discover Education*, *4*(1), 1–23. DOI: 10.1007/s44217-024-00390-6

Khan, A. A. R., Ilyas, R. M., & Meeral, M. N. (2025). Applications of Artificial Intelligence and Internet of Things in Healthcare Industries. In *Evolution of Machine Learning and Internet of Things Applications in Biomedical Engineering* (pp. 1–17). CRC Press.

King, S. A. (2025). Reflections on AI-augmented professional development in special education: Promises and pitfalls. In *Transforming Special Education Through Artificial Intelligence* (pp. 431–458). IGI Global.

Kothari, A. N., Kaji, A. H., & Melton, G. B. (2025). Practical guide to the use of AI-enabled analytics in research. *JAMA Surgery*, *160*(5), 590. DOI: 10.1001/jamasurg.2024.6028 PMID: 39777455

Lin, X. F., Shen, W., Huang, S., Wang, Y., Zhou, W., Ling, X., & Li, W. (2025). Exploring Chinese teachers' concerns about teaching artificial intelligence: The role of knowledge and perceived social good. *Asia Pacific Education Review*, •••, 1–20. DOI: 10.1007/s12564-024-10034-x

Miller, J. C., Miranda, J. P. P., & Tolentino, J. C. G. (2025). Artificial Intelligence in Physical Education: A Review. *Global Innovations in Physical Education and Health*, 37-60.

Miyake, Y., Retrosi, G., & Keijzer, R. (2025). Artificial intelligence and pediatric surgery: Where are we? *Pediatric Surgery International*, *41*(1), 1–8. PMID: 39625492

Murari, U. K., & Parmar, H. (2025). Leveraging Artificial Intelligence for Rural Development: Opportunities and Challenges in the Indian Context. *AI Strategies for Social Entrepreneurship and Sustainable Economic Development*, 265-284.

Nnorom, I. C. (2025). Ethical Considerations in Artificial Intelligence and Academic Integrity: Balancing Technology and Human Values. *AI and Ethics, Academic Integrity and the Future of Quality Assurance in Higher Education, 15.*

Nong, P., Adler-Milstein, J., Apathy, N. C., Holmgren, A. J., & Everson, J. (2025). Current Use And Evaluation Of Artificial Intelligence And Predictive Models In US Hospitals: Article examines uses and evaluation of artificial intelligence and predictive models in US hospitals. *Health Affairs*, *44*(1), 90–98. DOI: 10.1377/hlthaff.2024.00842 PMID: 39761454

Prabhakar, A. C. (2025). AI Strategies for Sustainable Development Goals: Collective Action for Poverty Alleviation. In *AI Strategies for Social Entrepreneurship and Sustainable Economic Development* (pp. 393-442). IGI Global Scientific Publishing.

Prabhod, K. J. (2024). The Role of Artificial Intelligence in Reducing Healthcare Costs and Improving Operational Efficiency. *Quarterly Journal of Emerging Technologies and Innovations*, *9*(2), 47–59.

Pratama, M. P., Sampelolo, R., & Lura, H. (2023). Revolutionizing education: harnessing the power of artificial intelligence for personalized learning. *Klasikal: Journal of education, language teaching and science, 5*(2), 350-357.

Rashidi, H. H., Hu, B., Pantanowitz, J., Tran, N., Liu, S., Chamanzar, A., Gur, M., Chang, C.-C. H., Wang, Y., Tafti, A., Pantanowitz, L., & Hanna, M. G. (2025a). Statistics of Generative Artificial Intelligence and Nongenerative Predictive Analytics Machine Learning in Medicine. *Modern Pathology*, *38*(3), 100663. DOI: 10.1016/j.modpat.2024.100663 PMID: 39579984

Rashidi, H. H., Pantanowitz, J., Hanna, M., Tafti, A. P., Sanghani, P., Buchinsky, A., & Pantanowitz, L. (2025b). Introduction to Artificial Intelligence (AI) and Machine Learning (ML) in Pathology & Medicine: Generative & Non-Generative AI Basics. *Modern Pathology*, •••, 100688. DOI: 10.1016/j.modpat.2024.100688 PMID: 39755237

Rathore, N., Kumari, A., Patel, M., Chudasama, A., Bhalani, D., Tanwar, S., & Al-abdulatif, A. (2025). Synergy of AI and Blockchain to Secure Electronic Healthcare Records. *Security and Privacy*, *8*(1), e463. DOI: 10.1002/spy2.463

Rezaev, A. V., & Tregubova, N. D. (2025). Looking at human-centered artificial intelligence as a problem and prospect for sociology: An analytic review. *Current Sociology*, *73*(1), 120–138. DOI: 10.1177/00113921231211580

Salimi, H., Bahramjerdi, S. F. N., & Tootoonchi, R. (2025). The Role of Geographic Information Systems (GIS) in Participatory Conservation of Heritage Areas. *European Journal of Geography*, s1-s11.

Sanchini, V., Marelli, L., Monturano, M., Bonizzi, G., Peruzzotti, G., Orecchia, R., & Pravettoni, G. (2025). A comprehensive ethics and data governance framework for data-intensive health research: Lessons from an Italian cancer research institute. *Accountability in Research*, *32*(1), 59–76. DOI: 10.1080/08989621.2023.2248884 PMID: 37608751

Sasseville, M., Ouellet, S., Rhéaume, C., Sahlia, M., Couture, V., Després, P., Paquette, J.-S., Darmon, D., Bergeron, F., & Gagnon, M. P. (2025). Bias Mitigation in Primary Health Care Artificial Intelligence Models: Scoping Review. *Journal of Medical Internet Research*, *27*, e60269. DOI: 10.2196/60269 PMID: 39773888

Schmidt, E., Putora, P. M., & Fijten, R. (2025). The Epistemic Cost of Opacity: How the Use of Artificial Intelligence Undermines the Knowledge of Medical Doctors in High-Stakes Contexts. *Philosophy & Technology*, *38*(1), 5. DOI: 10.1007/s13347-024-00834-9

Shiferaw, K. B., Roloff, M., Balaur, I., Welter, D., Waltemath, D., & Zeleke, A. A. (2025). Guidelines and standard frameworks for artificial intelligence in medicine: A systematic review. *JAMIA Open*, *8*(1), ooae155. DOI: 10.1093/jamiaopen/ooae155 PMID: 39759773

Shruti, R., Rani, S., & Boulila, W. (2025). Securing internet of things device data: An ABE approach using fog computing and generative AI. *Expert Systems: International Journal of Knowledge Engineering and Neural Networks*, *42*(2), e13691. DOI: 10.1111/exsy.13691

Singh, B., Kaunert, C., Lal, S., & Arora, M. K. (2025). Enhancing AI-Augmented Classrooms: Teacher-Centric Integration of Intelligent Tutoring Systems and Adaptive Learning Environments. In *Fostering Inclusive Education With AI and Emerging Technologies* (pp. 99-130). IGI Global.

Srivastava, V., Kumar, R., Wani, M. Y., Robinson, K., & Ahmad, A. (2025). Role of artificial intelligence in early diagnosis and treatment of infectious diseases. *Infectious Diseases*, *57*(1), 1–26. DOI: 10.1080/23744235.2024.2425712 PMID: 39540872

Strika, Z., Petkovic, K., Likic, R., & Batenburg, R. (2025). Bridging healthcare gaps: A scoping review on the role of artificial intelligence, deep learning, and large language models in alleviating problems in medical deserts. *Postgraduate Medical Journal*, *101*(1191), 4–16. DOI: 10.1093/postmj/qgae122 PMID: 39323384

Venkata, N. S. V. S. (2025). AI Model Deployment in Healthcare: MLOps Innovations and Challenges. *Journal ID*, *9471*, 1297.

Zabaleta, J., Aguinagalde, B., Lopez, I., Fernandez-Monge, A., Lizarbe, J. A., Mainer, M., Ferrer-Bonsoms, J. A., & de Assas, M. (2025). Utility of Artificial Intelligence for Decision Making in Thoracic Multidisciplinary Tumor Boards. *Journal of Clinical Medicine*, *14*(2), 399. DOI: 10.3390/jcm14020399 PMID: 39860405

Zhang, K., Li, L., & Yu, H. C. (2025). Analysis on Concept of AI Literacy According and Future Education to the Result of Systematic Review. *Journal of Lifestyle and SDGs Review*, *5*(1), e03293–e03293. DOI: 10.47172/2965-730X.SDGsReview.v5.n01.pe03293

Chapter 12
Brain-Computer Interface Technology for Emotion Recognition and Social Cue Analysis in Individuals With Neurological and Mental Health Disorders

Avantika Jain
https://orcid.org/0009-0008-8948-7439
PES University, India

V. Shantha
PES University, India

N. Veena
https://orcid.org/0000-0001-8446-9401
PES University, India

ABSTRACT

This chapter examines how Brain-Computer Interfaces (BCIs) are transforming communication and emotion recognition for individuals with conditions like Locked-In Syndrome (LIS), Autism Spectrum Disorder (ASD), and Amyotrophic Lateral Sclerosis (ALS). By translating brain signals into actionable outputs, BCIs bypass traditional pathways, enabling non-muscular communication. The chapter

DOI: 10.4018/979-8-3373-5072-1.ch012

highlights the role of non-invasive methods like EEG, which, alongside machine learning advancements, have improved BCI accuracy and accessibility. Despite their promise, BCIs face ethical challenges, including consent, data privacy, and limited affordability. This chapter also explores innovations such as wireless, AI-driven BCIs designed for home use, offering solutions to these barriers. By addressing these issues, BCIs can significantly enhance social interaction and quality of life for individuals with neurological disorders.

INTRODUCTION

Emotions are the different types of cognitive experiences one is subjected to, based on how one perceives their environment and surroundings. In other words, they are the psychological states that are generated due to the different feelings, thoughts, and actions one is going through. People convey these feelings and emotions through different modes of communication, may it be verbal or non-verbal gestures (He, Z., & Li, Z. (2020)). Thus, this makes it imperative and extremely crucial to learn how to recognize emotions correctly. This is especially important for patients with neurological disorders such as locked-in syndrome, amyotrophic lateral sclerosis and emotional expression disorders, etc. Therefore, emotion recognition is critical to improving health and providing them with correct medications. To better assist this goal brain-computer interfaces are used to understand and transcribe the cognitive and neural messages being shot in the patient's brain. It is one of the best creations made to bridge the gap between professionals and the patient. (He & Li. (2020)). Brain-computer interface which is also known as brain-machine interface helps people suffering from different kinds of neurological disorders. It is a software and hardware interface between the brain and artificial intelligence. It observes and interprets the neural messages being transmitted and translates them into electrical signals Many research laboratories around the world, as well as a handful of companies, are now focused on BCI development and research (Hochberg, L. R., & Anderson, (2012)). This phenomenon stands in sharp contrast to the very small number of people using BCIs outside of a research environment. If we define a BCI as a system that provides brain control of an external device, BCIs are currently in daily use by fewer than 10 people (primarily people with advanced amyotrophic lateral sclerosis). The public, scientific, and media interest in BCI research results not from its widespread achievements, then, but rather from promising early demonstrations of the remarkable potential for BCIs to help people replace or restore functions that have been compromised by illness or injury (Hochberg et al., (2006)).

The messages being recorded are based on the user's intentions and the process is completely non-muscular. EEG, as a non-invasive method, has become a foundation in BCI research due to its ability to monitor neurophysiological signals in real time. Though less accurate than invasive methods, EEG's accessibility and cost-effectiveness have pushed its adoption in various applications, from emotion recognition to neurofeedback training (Yike Sun & Xiaogang Chen, 2024). Recent advancements in signal preprocessing and machine learning have enhanced the accuracy of EEG-based BCIs, making them increasingly reliable for capturing nuanced emotional and cognitive states (He et al., (2020)).

TYPES OF BRAIN-COMPUTER INTERFACE (BCI)

In general, there are two types of BCI: invasive and non-invasive.

Invasive BCIs require electrodes to be implanted directly into the individual's brain. While invasive BCI devices produce higher-quality signals, their use (the same as any neurosurgery) involves considerable risks (Wolpaw et al, (2000)). Non-invasive BCI systems capture brain signals externally, usually through electroencephalogram (EEG) electrodes. Although non-invasive BCI devices are susceptible to noise, they are cheaper to set up, easier to use, and, unlike invasive systems, they do not require a surgical procedure and therefore pose an inherently lower risk to the user (Wolpaw et al, (2000)). For these reasons, it is thought that non-invasive BCI systems are likely to show significant promise as practical assistive technology medical devices for use in neurological rehabilitation.

We need BCI as the increasing incidence and prevalence of patients with chronic brain injury and current financial constraints have led to a need for a more effective way to implement the current neurorehabilitation service provision.

There are five main stages to this whole process and the first one is the signal acquisition stage. There are two ways of attaining neural information, one being invasive and the other being a non-invasive technique. The invasive method involves surgically implanting electrodes into the cerebral cortex (the outermost layer of the brain) and gathering information directly from the brain. By doing so, the machine can read the brain and the neural signals better and thus translate these messages into electric signals in the most accurate way. In the non-invasive technique, the machine relies solely on the recordings of neural signals over the skull (Nicolas-Alonso, L. F., & Gomez-Gil, (2012)). This type of signal acquisition is slightly more complicated due to the limited electrical conductivity of the skull. Thus, the skull acts as a barrier that does not allow for smooth conductivity which in turn hampers the translation of the signals. One of the most commonly used non-invasive techniques involves using Electroencephalogram or EEG-based systems. These systems have electrodes that are connected to the scalp and record the neural messages being transmitted (Yike Sun & Xiaogang Chen (2024)).

Next comes the preprocessing or signal enhancement stage. Here, the neural signals or the messages are prepared to be processed in a more suitable form. Next is the feature extraction stage which facilitates the extraction of the data that needs to be read and translated thereby enhancing the signal characteristics and features. (Signal Preprocessing Techniques, Brain-Computer Interfaces Class Notes, Fiveable, n.d.). In this stage, the signal-to-noise ratio (SNR) is improved thereby allowing no stray messages to interfere in the translations. All of the unwanted neural messages such as blinking of an eye or twitch of a muscle are removed. The signal is not at rest and is constantly being fired from one neuron to another, moreover, it can sometimes get distorted by the machines being used such as electroencephalogram, electromyography, and others. Therefore, by using good discriminative features we can achieve effective pattern recognition which in turn helps us in figuring out the intentions of the user. This is an extremely challenging and complicated task as many of the brain signals are intertwined. Therefore, the main message that needs to be translated needs to be extracted and that is what happens in this stage.

The fourth stage is the classification stage. In this stage, the electric signals being shot are classified by keeping the feature vectors in focus. This helps us in the process of distinguishing jargon from meaningful and important data. The final stage is called the control interface stage. This is the stage where the classified neural messages get translated into electric signals so that the connected device can interpret and perform the required action (Nicolas-Alonso, L. F., & Gomez-Gil, ((2012)). Six basic emotions that are frequently specified in research papers are happiness, sadness, anger, disgust, fear, and surprise. Many studies have shown that combinations of systems can significantly enhance emotion recognition accuracy in comparison to a single system. For example, combining eye movements, which are measured using an eye-tracking method, and EEG can considerably improve the performance of emotion recognition systems (He et al., (2020)).

Thus, these five stages work together to help in translating and predicting neural and cognitive patterns. This helps in breaking through physical barriers that confine the patient from being unable to express themselves the way they want. It helps promote emotion recognition and good intercommunication between those who are suffering from neural conditions and their loved ones. The brain-computer interface models are being currently used as a functional communicative assistant technology for various neural conditions such as locked-in syndrome, Parkinson's Disease, amyotrophic lateral sclerosis (ALS), and autism spectrum disorder (ASD). In the next subtopic, we delve more into this in detail.

APPLICATIONS OF BCI

There are multiple applications of BCI in different neurological, and mental disorders in individuals, some of which will be explored in this chapter.

BCI technology has the potential to have a substantial influence on those with severe communication difficulties despite having intact cognition. One clinical ailment, locked-in syndrome (LIS), is often regarded as the most immediate priority for BCI research. Plum and Posner described LIS in 1966 as "a state in which selective supranuclear motor de-differentiation causes paralysis of all four limbs and the last cranial nerves without interfering with consciousness." Voluntary motor paralysis hinders people from communicating by speech or body movement. (Plum & Posner (1966)).

Bauer (Bauer et al 1979) (c.f. (Laureys et al 2005) provided a useful advance in the definition by distinguishing between:

- Classical LIS (with intact vertical eye movements or blinking, using eye blinks alone),
- Total LIS (with the absence of all voluntary movement, including eye movements), and
- Incomplete LIS (with retention of remnants of voluntary movement, for example, finger twitch).

In summary, locked-in syndrome is an extremely rare neurological condition that leaves the entire body paralyzed except for the ability to blink and move their eyes vertically. They are essentially trapped in their body with no way of communicating with the outside world. Thus, BCI acts as a beacon of hope by transcribing their inner thoughts and translating them into readable text that is visible on the preferred screen. This way we can make sure that all their needs are met and the medications being prescribed have the required effect on the patient. One of the biggest barriers these people are faced with is social exclusion and the stigmatization is often more difficult and painful than compared to the physical barriers. Therefore, allowing them to share their experiences and thoughts while being paralyzed helps them overcome these barriers gradually. A functional communicative assistant technology such as BCI comes of use to help maintain the patient's relationships with their spouses, parents, friends, and other family relatives. It should be their right to have access to BCI models so they can communicate and break free from the confinement of their thoughts and turmoil (Johansson, V. & Soekadar, (2017)). The Wyss Center is an independent, non-profit, research organization, that aims to develop a unique fully implantable Brain-Computer Interface (BCI) system for people with locked-in syndrome (LIS) – a condition in which paralysis severely limits communication, caused by a progressive neurodegenerative disease, which involves the gradual loss of motor control. This chapter will delve more into the application of BCI on different neurological and mental disorders in detail (Scott-Admin, (2024)).

On the other hand, in the case of patients suffering from Parkinson's Disease, it is extremely difficult to control their movement as a result of a progressive brain disorder. It also causes a plethora of mental health issues and other health concerns. As the brain disorder gets worse, so does their ability to control their motor senses causing major difficulty in talking and walking. Here through motor imagery, the patient is trained to produce task-appropriate actions. This is based on the theory that the neurons that are associated with motor imagery are also the ones that assist in the actual movement as well. Therefore, BCI helps provide feedback and predictions on the motor imagery based on the sensorimotor rhythms observed in the brain pathways of the patient. In this process, the patient undergoes cognitive training, with the help of a brain-computer interface, and is made to imagine the affected body part to move in a required way causing the neurons associated with the same to be fired. This therapeutic approach facilitates better motor performance. This only comes with more practice and usage of motor imagery and the subsequent uptake of task-appropriate preparedness and actions.

For individuals with neurological conditions such as Amyotrophic Lateral Sclerosis (ALS) or Autism Spectrum Disorder (ASD), BCIs offer a lifeline for communication and emotional expression (Kashihara, 2014). Passive BCIs, in particular, have shown promise in emotion recognition, enabling machines to adapt to a user's emotional and cognitive states without conscious input (Vlek, R. J. (2012)). This is crucial for populations that struggle with conventional modes of communication, such as those with locked-in syndrome or severe motor impairments. In affective computing, BCIs have been integrated with modalities like eye tracking to enhance emotion recognition, improving human-computer interactions and enabling the development of adaptive systems that respond to user needs (He et al., (2020)). People suffering with these neurological conditions are unable to express emotions and feelings properly as they lack the cognitive capabilities for it. Even though emotions can be inferred by observing the person's nonverbal gestures such as facial expressions, body posture, and the way they are portraying themselves, emotion recognition and prediction for neutral faces requires a higher level of intelligence and judgment (Kashihara, K. (2014)).

For people with incomplete or classical LIS, early BCIs using induced potentials to choose among items in a matrix, or to provide one-directional or unidimensional cursor control, have already been shown to enable the selection of letters or words on a screen. BCIs of this kind are currently used by a small number of people with advanced ALS. In addition, BCIs provide two-dimensional point-and-click interfaces that have already been demonstrated (Kim et al (2007)) which could enable significant and intuitive control over standard software. When combined with text-to-speech programs and word-prediction algorithms, and are made generally available, these first-generation BCIs are expected to restore basic communication to people with incomplete or classical LIS. For people with total LIS, such as some people with advanced ALS and chronic mechanical ventilation, there has not yet been a successful demonstration of BCI use. The use of BCIs to maintain communication for people with ALS raises critical questions for both clinical decisions and technology development. Though most individuals with ALS in the U.S. currently decline mechanical ventilation, BCIs enabling continued communication may influence this choice (Hochberg & Cochrane 2011). Additionally, ALS-related cognitive impairments, like those linked to frontotemporal degeneration, pose challenges for the brain signals BCIs can use and the concentration required from users (Geser et al. 2010; Merrilees et al. (2010)).

BCI has many other applications and uses outside of the healthcare sector as well. It has made quite a development in the entertainment business in the form of cognitive neuro-games. Thus, instead of using the traditional gaming equipment which is controlled by the person's hands, it uses their physiological functions such as neural signals, facial expressions, heartbeat beat, and so on. There have been quite a few games that have been developed such as "The Mind Balance video game", "NeuroMage", and "NeuroRacer" among others. You play these games by imagining the desired movements. This is then picked up by the EEG headsets which record all the neural signals being shot across the brain's surface (Umair, A. & Ashfaq (2017)).

IMPAIRED COMMUNICATION

Impaired mobility, as a result of diseases or injuries, significantly affects the mental health of the individual and quality of life, particularly for people with conditions like tetraplegia. The loss of their ability to perform basic and simple activities of daily living (ADLs), such as eating, dressing themselves, or even engaging in professional and social interactions, can lead to feelings of dependency, social isolation, and psychological distress (Anderson, 2004). Restoring even limited mobility, such as hand grasp function, can dramatically enhance a person's autonomy and self-esteem, reducing the mental health burden associated with such disabilities (Anderson, (2004)).

Tetraplegia, characterized by the total or partial loss of function in the arms, trunk, legs, and pelvic organs, often is a result of conditions like cervical spinal cord injury, brainstem stroke, ALS (amyotrophic lateral sclerosis), cerebral palsy, and multiple sclerosis among others (Maynard et al., (1997)). These conditions do not just disrupt physical function but also have profound psychological impacts.

Chronic dependence on their caregivers, limited access to assistive technologies, or rehabilitative therapies, and restricted participation in meaningful activities are common contributors to anxiety, depression, and feelings of helplessness (Hitzig et al., (2008)).

THE ROLE OF BCIS IN ADDRESSING MENTAL HEALTH NEEDS

Brain-computer interfaces (BCIs) are upcoming technologies that aim to restore functions that are lost due to neurological conditions. For those individuals with tetraplegia, BCIs could help restore some necessary capabilities for example, arm and hand function, which is a priority for almost half of the individuals that were surveyed to have this condition (Anderson, 2004). This restoration is not merely a physical gain—it can ease psychological stress by increasing independence and enabling greater participation in daily life and social interactions (Anderson, (2004)).

BCIs also hold promise in modifying the mental health impacts of disability by enabling computer-based communication and environmental control. These tools allow users to regain a sense of agency in the digital world, accessing entertainment, education, and work opportunities, or simply communicating more effectively (Hochberg et al., (2006)). Such advancements can help people combat isolation and improve psychological well-being.

While the potential of BCIs is immense, designing them requires careful reflection of users' needs and mental health consequences. Surveys reveal that individuals with tetraplegia prioritize functional gains without necessarily having an understanding of how BCIs might achieve them, underscoring the importance of clear communication and realistic goal-setting (Anderson, 2004). Moreover, introducing novel neurotechnologies involves working through psychological barriers, as the risks and uncertainties of invasive procedures like implanted BCIs might deter users. Previous historical examples, such as the adoption of deep brain stimulation for Parkinson's disease, show that widespread acceptance often follows clear evidence of safety and efficacy (Pahwa et al., (2006)).

Paraplegia, characterized by the complete or partial loss of movement in the lower extremities, often includes impairments in bladder, bowel, and sexual functions due to autonomic dysfunction. It most commonly is a result of spinal cord injuries but it can also arise from conditions such as post-polio syndrome, multiple sclerosis, cerebral palsy, and vascular complications (e.g., artery of Adamkiewicz ischemia). These impairments can significantly affect an individual's quality of life and mental health, as they impede independence and social integration (Maynard et al., (1997)).

A survey by Anderson (2004) of individuals with paraplegia found that their priorities for functional restoration were different from those with tetraplegia. Sexual function was ranked as the top priority for 26.7% of respondents, which was followed by bladder and bowel function for 18%. This preference emphasizes the significance of the psychological and social impact of these autonomic impairments, which often overshadows some visible disabilities like their ability to walk. The social stigma and the logistical challenges associated with bladder and bowel dysfunction, for instance, could lead to anxiety, depression, and social withdrawal. Similarly, the loss of sexual function affects an individual's self-esteem and interpersonal relationships, further exacerbating mental health struggles (Anderson (2004)).

BCIs also offer a unique opportunity to address these critical needs by possibly restoring certain autonomic functions like bladder and bowel control and enhancing mobility through advanced assistive devices. Technologies integrating BCIs with functional electrical stimulation (FES) systems could provide highly functional solutions, such as activating paralyzed muscles to restore mobility with improved speed and control (Donoghue et al., 2007a; (2007)). This restoration would not only address physical disabilities but also alleviate mental health challenges by fostering independence and reducing the stigma associated with autonomic dysfunctions.

The emphasis on restoring bladder, bowel, and sexual functions reflects the deeply personal and social nature of these needs. For instance, bladder and bowel control significantly influence one's ability to engage in public life and maintain a sense of dignity. These priorities often surpass regaining walking ability, underlining the disconnect between able-bodied perceptions of disability and the lived experiences of those affected. BCIs could play a transformative role by providing precise control over these functions, offering users the ability to regain autonomy in socially and physically demanding situations (Donnelly et al (2004)).

For people who have experienced amputation or have reduced ability to manipulate their environment, BCIs can enhance prosthetic functionality. Traditional prosthetic limb controllers are often slow and require significant cognitive effort, limiting their usability. BCIs, by contrast, could enable more rapid, complex, and intuitive control, providing a higher degree of dexterity and independence (Aaron et al., (2006)). This development could significantly impact mental health by improving self-reliance and reducing frustration associated with limited prosthetic functionality.

They may also supplement neurorehabilitation therapies for people recovering from a stroke or other brain injuries. By leveraging the brain's capacity for plasticity, BCIs can help facilitate in restorating of normal brain activity and movements during therapeutic exercises (Bolognini et al., (2009)). This could improve mental health outcomes by increasing the efficacy of rehabilitation and reducing the psychological toll of having a long-term disability. For BCIs to achieve widespread adoption in rehabilitation, they should be user-friendly, suitable for home use, and require minimal professional intervention, making them more accessible to a larger population (Buntin, (2007)).

BCIs offer transformative potential in addressing neurological and psychiatric illnesses by detecting and intervening in abnormal brain activity. One prominent example is their application in managing epilepsy, where cortical surface recordings detect the onset of seizures. By integrating BCIs with neural stimulators, these systems could suppress such abnormal activity before seizures become clinically evident, as demonstrated by Sun et al. (2008)). This closed-loop approach not only offers the possibility of preventing seizures but also provides early warnings, significantly enhancing patient autonomy and mental well-being. BCIs could also tackle broader neuropsychiatric challenges, such as those associated with behaviours linked to neural processing deficits. For example, in cases of morbid obesity caused by inadequate satiety processing, a BCI could detect moderate signals to enforce satiation after appropriate caloric intake. This application highlights the potential for BCIs to address mental health and behavioural conditions beyond traditional psychiatric disorders, contributing to overall well-being (Sun et al. (2008)).

Similar to responsive neural stimulators for epilepsy, BCIs are being explored in the treatment of cognitive and mood disorders. Deep brain stimulation (DBS) has shown promise in managing obsessive-compulsive disorder (OCD) and major depression, where stimulation of specific brain regions lessens symptoms (Greenberg et al., 2010; Lozano et al., 2008; Malone et al., 2009). Combining BCIs with neural stimulation technologies could enable real-time detection of neurophysiological changes related to mood disorders. For instance, BCIs could identify early markers of mania or depression in bipolar disorder and deliver targeted neurostimulation to stabilize mood, offering a proactive approach to mental health management (Malone et al., (2009)).

In critical care settings, BCIs could play an essential role in managing life-threatening conditions like traumatic brain injuries, status epilepticus, and cerebral vasospasm. By detecting early indicators of these conditions, BCIs could provide apt warnings on time and enable rapid interventions, improving patient outcomes. For example, a BCI system could monitor brain activity in patients with traumatic brain injuries, predicting secondary complications and triggering preventive treatments. This real-time capability could reduce the psychological toll on both patients and caregivers during the recovery process (Sun et al (2008)).

As the number of patients with neurological diseases has increased over the past decades, new rehabilitation techniques that enable recovery and improve brain-body links are needed. The BCI and VR technology provide a new and promising way of rehabilitation for neurological diseases. As compared with the simple BCI system, the BCI-VR system does not need too many external devices for the rehabilitation environment as VR can better replace various complex real rehabilitation environments and offer individuals a rich rehabilitation environment and real experience. In addition, with the rich and vivid information and feedback that VR offers, individuals can now go on with the training process in a small physical space while increasing their enthusiastic engagement for more active training given a virtual and immersive environment. By combining both BCI and VR techniques, the neurorehabilitation process can improve performance and reduce learning and training time. The BCI-VR systems might play an increasingly important role in the development and application of neural engineering and rehabilitation medicine (Wen et al., (2020)).

However, when using the BCI-VR system for rehabilitation, there are still some challenges.

Currently, the information transfer rate is not ideal. This refers to how efficiently and precisely it can detect the brain signals which are to be translated into electric signals. Whereas past research has revealed that BCI systems can enable fairly quick communication when combined with VR headsets, upcoming BCI-VR systems must take into account real-world metrics like how responsive the user experience is in VR. Not only that but also the variety of interactions or commands users can provide. Enhancing the transmission speed of EEG signals (electrical brain activity recorded via electrodes on the scalp) is thus a prime objective to guarantee smoother and more interactive communication between users and virtual environments. EEG signals in the BCI system are weak in nature and are susceptible to external noise.

This includes signals from movement of the body (motor interference), muscle contractions (electromyography or EMG), and movement of the eyes (electrooculography or EOG). When people wander around within the VR space, these external signals can confuse or interfere with the brain signals so that it's hard for the system to interpret what the person is attempting to do. Therefore, future studies must emphasize enhancing real-time preprocessing, which is better filtering and cleansing of the EEG data while it is being gathered, so that the system will better recognize brain commands even in the case of active VR use.

In Motor Imagery (MI) paradigm BCI-VR systems, systems in which the user controls them by imagining specific body movements, a lot of training is typically necessary before people are able to work the system well. The training consists of imaging movements without producing them, engaging corresponding brain regions. But both the quality of the training and the fidelity of brain control (how accurately users' thoughts translate into desired actions) differ widely from individual to individual. To further add, the capacity of the system to perform well in a generalizable manner across different individuals (generalization performance) remains to be improved greatly. Improving the underlying algorithms that translate EEG signals is crucial to making this happen.

In P300 (a positive deflection occurring 300 milliseconds after an unusual stimulus occurs) and SSVEP (a communication channel that connects the brain and external devices based on visual stimuli response) paradigm-based BCI-VR systems, the user is less active. They have to concentrate intently on flickering lights or particular visual stimuli in the VR world to initiate commands. This approach can decrease the naturalness and immersion of the interaction since it involves conscious and usually exhausting concentration to manipulate the virtual world. Thus, more natural and intuitive modes of brain-machine interaction need to be developed utilizing these paradigms in order to enhance usability and user experience.

To finish, although BCI, VR, and BCI-VR hold great hope for neurological rehabilitation, the mitigation of these current limitations, such as low signal velocity, external disturbances, extensive training requirements for the user, and unnatural interaction style, will prove crucial. Ongoing technological development, BCI-VR systems may have the potential to have a strong positive impact on enhancing the lives of people with neurological disorders, such that rehabilitation would be more engaging, personalized, and efficient (Wen et al., 2020).

As most neurological diseases become more prevalent with advancing age, the global trend toward an aging population is anticipated to increase the incidence of these conditions due to population growth and aging (Sundquist et al., (2004)). The ramifications of neurological diseases are extensive and multifaceted. Patients often endure significant lifestyle disruptions, resulting in social isolation and psychological distress, while their caregivers face considerable familial and economic burdens (Feigin et al., (2019)). The socio-economic impacts include high medical resource utilization, productivity losses, and financial strains associated with long-term care. Neurological impairments significantly reduce the quality of life; stroke survivors may struggle with mobility, comatose patients suffer cognitive deficits, and individuals with motor dysfunction experience severe physical limitations. Furthermore, neurological and psychiatric disorders such as depression and schizophrenia cause mood instability, cognitive impairments, and social difficulties. Traditional treatment methods often fail to address the complexities of neurological dysfunction adequately, highlighting the urgent need for innovative treatment strategies. In this context, brain-computer interface (BCI) technology has emerged as a key area of contemporary medical research due to its potential for groundbreaking applications (Santhanam et al., (2006)).

Depression is a common and serious mental health condition. Many people do not respond well to traditional treatments like medication or therapy. BCI technology offers a new approach by directly interacting with the brain's processes. Two key methods for treating depression with brain-based technologies are deep brain stimulation (DBS) and EEG-based BCIs.

In the domain of depression treatment, BCI technology and DBS represent two different but potentially balancing approaches. While BCI usually involves non-invasive or minimally invasive methods to interpret along with modulating brain activity DBS is an invasive technique that includes the implantation of electrodes into targeted brain regions such as the amygdala or the subgenual cingulate cortex, presenting potential benefits for individuals suffering from treatment-resistant depression. Despite the surgical risks linked to DBS, it represents an important alternative for those unresponsive to traditional treatments.

SEVERAL KEY STUDIES ARE MENTIONED BELOW

A significant investigation into this area involved a multi-centre, randomized, sham-controlled trial assessing the safety and efficacy of DBS within the subcallosal cingulate region for treatment-resistant depression. The findings revealed that improvements were observed in both the actively stimulated and sham groups over 6 months, and yet no significant differences in response rates were detected. The trial also confirmed the safety and possibility of subcallosal cingulate DBS, encouraging the need for further research to establish its antidepressant effectiveness (Holtzheimer, P. E. & Husain, (2017)).

Another study on habenula (a pea sized brain region that helps in connecting areas involved in decision making, motivation and emotion processing) DBS involved seven patients with treatment-resistant depression. Over 12 months, it showed a 49% reduction in depressive symptoms, correlating habenula activity with the severity of symptoms (Zhang & C.(2022)).

EEG-based BCI systems have been progressively recognized for their adjunctive role in the treatment of depression. These systems function by monitoring and interpreting specific brainwave patterns, offering feedback that assists patients in managing their emotional and cognitive symptoms, thereby extenuating depressive manifestations. Additionally, EEG-based BCIs are capable of categorizing and evaluating depression in patients by real-time analysis of particular frequency bands and electrodes 139 This technology not only facilitates the detection of depression but also offers a quantitative scoring of symptoms, enhancing personalized treatment approaches and monitoring of patient progress (Paquette & V. (2009)).

Emotion Recognition/Regulation

Emotion regulation plays an important role in human beings' daily lives by helping them deal with social problems and protecting their mental and physical health. However, objective assessment of the effectiveness of emotion regulation and assessment of the improvement in emotion regulation ability at the individual level remain challenging. Neurofeedback is an innovative tool for emotion regulation and has become the topic of broad study in recent years. Real-time feedback based on both EEG and fMRI was shown to be efficient in improving emotion regulation. Twenty healthy subjects performed 10 BCI-based neurofeedback training sessions to regulate their emotion toward a specific emotional state (positive, negative, or neutral), while their EEG signals were analysed in real-time via machine learning to predict their emotional states. In neurofeedback training, neural biomarkers can be measured and presented back to subjects to help them take more active roles in performing self-controlling activities in specific brain regions. In this study, the researchers developed a novel method to help subjects regulate their emotional states through neurofeedback training with an EEG-based BCI. Compared with the control group without feedback, the experimental group achieved better performance as the experiment proceeded, especially for sessions without video stimulus. These results suggested that neurofeedback played an important role in enabling subjects to improve emotion regulation ability. Moreover, the decoding accuracies of each binary classifier also increased as the experiments progressed. In addition, TPRs of each emotional state for each frequency band were also increased relative to the first session and the last several sessions. These results demonstrated that EEG-based BCI neurofeedback training is an effective way to help subjects regulate their emotional states and has potential as a form of emotion regulation therapy (Huang et al., (2021)).

The Physiological and Behavioural Markers

In a person's day-to-day life, they are constantly experiencing emotional experiences, which may be bad or good. These experiences are jointly created with multiple sensory channels that trigger the different parts of the brain, specifically the amygdala. So, for example when a person sees an emotional facial expression or hears a familiar voice in an emotional tone, these two combine to create a much more holistic emotional experience. This experience where the auditory aspect combines with the visual input related to social communication and emotion recognition has become a topic of interest to many researchers across the globe. Thus in addition to behaviour, one should focus on the stimuli created by neuroimaging, electro-, and peripheral-physiological findings. According to studies conducted, the combined audiovisual integration can facilitate and improve the perception and emotional recognition of a person with a neurological condition more than an unimodal face-voice stimulus. On a much more neurological level, the face and voice integration may happen even at the earlier stages of perception of stimulus. Moreover, particular areas of the brain such as the Superior and Inferior Temporal structures, as well as parts of the emotion processing network including the Amygdala, Thalamus, Fusiform Gyrus, Basal ganglia, and so on are all working together continuously in the integration of emotional face-voice recognition. Thus, by looking at the bigger picture we realize the importance and significance of swift and correct emotion recognition and the role it plays as a part of social interaction and social cues. Thus, the early integration of these two components and the conditioning that comes with it plays a big role in the ability of the individual to be socially cognisant and emotionally intelligent (Gerdes, A. B., Wieser, (2014)).

Sounds when compared to pictures, that elicit a visual response, are somewhat less amenable to experimental designs in the laboratory. However, sounds can very clearly prompt a much more emotional response out of a person than compared to a visual cue as observed in a large internet-based survey. It was also noticed that emotionally arousing sounds had a much better effect than neutral sounds in a free recall task. On a physiological level, the emotionally stimulating sounds give out a much larger electrodermal activity as it is known to react to the arousal of emotional stimuli. This all entails that, for an individual cues and sounds that are emotionally stimulated create much faster and deeper influences on their brain as it has been personalized. A recently done research study focused on investigating the relationship between affective representations and the sensory modality. Thus, the emotionally stimulating picture and the sound stimuli were then presented in an event that was related to an fMRI experiment. The results of this research study said that a specific part of the brain responded to emotionally stimulating pictures while the other part of the brain reacted to the emotions that were generated from sounds. However, the fMRI did not reveal anything regarding parts of the brain that responded to both the emotions elicited from the pictures and sounds. This could indicate that the brain processes the emotions from these stimuli in separate areas rather than letting one singular brain part control both aspects (Gerdes, A. B. & Wieser, (2014)).

ETHICAL ISSUES

Issues such as consent, data privacy, and the potential for unauthorized access to sensitive information pose significant challenges. Misuse or exposure of sensitive data can be detrimental to the patient's mental health. It goes against the confidentiality guidelines set between the patient and the professionals. Not only that but it can cause unnecessary stress and frustration to the patient as this is their only means of communication. (Vlek, 2012). For individuals with locked-in syndrome, getting informed consent for invasive procedures is particularly complex. Additionally, the high cost and limited availability of BCIs hinder accessibility for many in need (Vlek, 2012). Ensuring equitable access and robust safeguards is vital for the responsible development and deployment of BCI technologies (Nicolas-Alonso & Gomez-Gil, (2012)).

Though the Brain-Computer Interface has several exceptional aspects to it, it does have a few limitations or things of concern that need to be addressed. Locked-in syndrome is an extremely rare neurological disorder that leaves the patient with almost full body paralysis except for the ability to move their eyes and blink. Having an invasive surgery done on such a patient will certainly be extremely helpful as it could help us have two-way communication that could be entirely non-muscular. However, in such cases, the ethicality and consent of the situation are brought into question. Without an understanding and trustworthy guardian, circumstances can go wrong very quickly (Vlek, R & J. (2012)).

Brain-computer interface (BCI) is also something that is not available to everyone in need. It is not something that can be found easily in the market which makes it rather inaccessible. This poses a major problem because a lot of people with neurological diseases may not be financially stable or well-to-do. Another thing to take into consideration is that it could access certain thoughts and emotions that the client is unwilling to reveal. This could lead to unauthorized access to information that the client did not consent to giving. For instance, if the machine were to fall into the wrong person's hands or were to get hacked then it could pose an extremely serious problem (Vlek, R & J. (2012)).

The patient must be completely informed on all the different scenarios and of what to expect when it comes to use BCI technology. This is extremely necessary to ensure complete trust on this communicative assistant technology. This is highly required to be able to manage the expectations of the client and their relatives. Oftentimes, the brain-computer interface's effectiveness may reduce due to the everchanging neuroplasticity of the brain. Since it is constantly changing and evolving, it becomes ever so difficult to be able to accurately transcribe and translate the cognitive thoughts of the patient. The other concern that may arise is the misinterpretation of the neural signals and thought processes. Due to the multiple physical barriers, such as the skull and cerebrospinal fluid, and the inaccuracy of the system, the transcribed messages may not be as accurate and thus lead to miscommunication and misunderstandings. (Vlek, R & J. (2012)).

CHALLENGES AND LIMITATIONS

While creating brain-computer interface- controlled prosthetics the engineer needs to understand the functioning of the brain. Brain is an extremely complex organ and needs to be studied thoroughly to be able to connect the outside world to it using technology. The engineer needs to take the key brain regions that are involved in this process into consideration. This is incredibly important for the prosthetics to function flawlessly. This is a very challenging task and needs multiple trials and experimentation to ensure complete safety of the patient (Umair, A. & Ashfaq (2017)).

Another challenge that has been often observed is that patients expect BCI to be extremely user-friendly and easy to handle. Unfortunately, this is not the case as the brain-computer interface is a very complex system which makes it look intimidating to its users. Thus, to make such a machine interface easier for the patient to use is a very difficult task. To curb this barrier, they are required to receive training to ensure improved ability of using it. Therefore, the professionals must guide and detach the patient on how to use BCI based prosthetics or the communication tools for a much smoother functioning. Prior training and clarity can help remove much of the stigma and the intimidation that comes with this system (Umair, A. & Ashfaq (2017)).

There are a lot of issues associated with the electroencephalographic headsets. The first issue encountered by the patients was that the EEG headsets required a gel or some sort of liquid to be applied to the electrodes. This was deemed to be extremely uncomfortable for them and thus for practicality purposes, the patients would usually opt to not use the conductive gel, which was applied between the scalp and the electrode pad, as it was not mandatory. Many studies claim that both the dry and the wet methods have similar signal-capturing properties whereas some say that the dry EEG headsets may contain a significantly higher amount of noise-to-signal ratio and artifacts. This aspect of BCI needs to be further investigated and also look into much more user-friendly systems and machine models as well as those that give the best results (Rashid, M. & Sulaiman (2020)).

The next issue with them is that the EEG Headsets with dry electrodes do not have a standardized number of electrodes. There have been many different models of EEG headsets that have been released into the market but unfortunately due to the non-uniformity of the number of electrodes, these headsets are not compatible with each other. The electrode count ranges from 1 to 64 which is a huge margin to work with, making inter-communication very difficult. Therefore, we desperately require a standardization of the number of electrodes to allow for communication and bridge the gap between the patient and their loved ones (Rashid, M. & Sulaiman (2020)).

Over the past few years, extensive research has been conducted scaling across the various physiological and psychological factors involved in this interface system. Yet not much research has been carried out in how the linguistic and cultural barriers may affect the language and signal processing as well as the BCI efficiency. A user's language and culture deeply impact and modulate the way they form their cognitive thoughts. It also shapes their emotions, human behaviour, and views on the world's social issues and societal standards. It also affects their personal experiences concerning their health issues and surgical experiences and how they feel toward technological devices. Cultural backgrounds set people apart in terms of norms, beliefs, practices, values, childhood upbringing, morals, and so on. All this together helps in creating a sense of identity and outlook that is very different from that of people from other cultural backgrounds. These differences may prove to be a barrier to communication when using the BCI. Therefore, these barriers play a very important role and heavily impact the signal identification and transcription process of the brain-computer interface system. Despite that, not much research has been conducted to address this problem. Every BCI user needs to be able to comprehend the oral or written instructions provided by the machine for communication purposes such as the well-known EEG—P300-spellers. Thus, is it critical for the patient to at least have some basic linguistic understanding. Thus, for future research and experimentations of BCI, it is very important to include language and cultural differences as part of human factors. Based on the other papers and research studies that have been conducted, it has become quite clear that we require a systematic study of the BCI user's language understanding capabilities, their mental and neural representation of cognitive thoughts, and cultural differences to be able to create a much more culturally and linguistically sensitive BCI system. Hence, focusing on the perception, processing, and evaluation of information in a cultural context can help make it more acceptable and easier to use for a larger group of people (Herbert & C. (2024)).

SUCCESS STORIES OF PEOPLE USING BCI

- Casey Harrell, is a 45-year-old man with amyotrophic lateral sclerosis (ALS), who experienced severe speech impairment due to the advancement of his condition. To address this, researchers at UC Davis Health developed a brain-computer interface (BCI) designed to translate brain signals into speech. They implanted sensors in the region of Harrell's brain responsible for coordinating speech. When activated, the system enabled Harrell to communicate his intended speech with an accuracy of up to 97%. This technological advancement has the potential to significantly enhance the quality of life for individuals who have lost their ability to speak due to paralysis or neurodegenerative disease (*UC Davis Health-Developed Technology Translates Brain Signals Into Speech With 97% Accuracy* | *AHA*, n.d.-b).
- Holland Bloorview Kids Rehabilitation Hospital's Clinical BCI Program has been incorporating BCI technology into clinical practice since 2019, primarily serving children with severe neuromotor conditions. Recently, there has been growing interest from families of autistic children, leading to their inclusion in both individual occupational therapy (OT) BCI sessions and therapeutic recreation (TR) BCI group programs. The subject of this case report is

an autistic male adolescent with co-occurring Attention Deficit Hyperactivity Disorder (ADHD). With parental consent, a retrospective chart review was conducted to assess his experiences with BCI technology in recreational settings. Their findings are as follows:

a. **Enjoyment and Engagement:** The participant expressed significant enjoyment during BCI sessions and actively sought continued participation in BCI programming.
b. **Performance Improvement:** Enhanced scores on the Canadian Occupational Performance Measure (COPM) were observed in BCI programming, surpassing those from other recreational programs.
c. **Social Communication and Self-Advocacy:** Clinicians noted improvements in the participant's social communication efforts and self-advocacy during BCI sessions(Van Damme et al.,(2024)).

- Mark, a 64-year-old man with amyotrophic lateral sclerosis (ALS), has become the first person to control an Amazon Alexa device using only his thoughts, thanks to an implanted brain-computer interface (BCI) developed by Synchron. The BCI uses Synchron's Stentrode technology, a minimally invasive device implanted in a blood vessel near the motor cortex—the brain region responsible for voluntary movement. This device records neural activity connected with movement intentions and wirelessly transmits these signals to external devices. By integrating the BCI with Amazon's Tap to Alexa feature on a Fire tablet, Mark can control smart home devices without the need for physical movement or speech. This capability allows him to perform tasks such as streaming shows, making video calls, and controlling smart home devices, thereby enhancing his independence and quality of life. This advancement represents a significant step forward in assistive technologies for individuals with severe paralysis, demonstrating the potential of BCIs to restore autonomy and improve daily living.
- In the year 2015, there was a 73-year-old female patient who was suffering from amyotrophic lateral sclerosis. She was in complete locked in state except for being able to move her eyes to communicate and blink. When she was much healthier and mobile, painting had been one of her favourite hobbies which she was unable to pursue after being paralysed. Unable to express or apply this passion physically, brain painting piqued her interest to explore her hobby once more. The patient had about one session a day and finished up to 200 sessions according to the date at which the data analysis was done. This spanned over the course of 14 months. By the end of this timeline the patient was able to paint several times a week. These brain computer interface

sessions were then evaluated based on time, efficiency, comfort and satisfaction. To have a good efficient functioning the compatibility between the machine and patient is very important (Holz, E. & M. (2015)).

- Catalin Voss, in association with Stanford University, created the Autism Glass Project—a wearable AI system based on Google Glass to help children with Autism Spectrum Disorder (ASD) identify emotions. The system utilizes machine learning algorithms to examine facial expressions and offer real-time visual and audio feedback to the wearer. Clinical tests at Stanford Medical School proved that children who were using the device had remarkable advancements in socialization and emotion understanding. In 2018, the technology was licensed to paediatric behavioural health firm Cognoa Voss, C. (n.d.).
- In 2024, Synchron made headlines with its minimally invasive BCI implant, which uses a stent-like device to interpret brain signals. "Before Synchron, I couldn't speak or move. Now, I can text my family and browse the web just by thinking," says John Smith, a 42-year-old ALS patient participating in Synchron's trials. The system translates neural signals into commands, allowing users like John to regain autonomy Wiz and Wiz (2025).

These actual cases vividly illustrate the life-changing power of Brain-Computer Interface technology. Whether restoring speech for those with ALS, improving emotional understanding in autism, or enabling paralyzed patients to regain autonomy, BCIs are not only enhancing quality of life but also bringing hope and independence where it was previously lost.

FUTURE DIRECTIONS

The latest developments observed in research studies and experiments in Brain-computer interface systems have contributed a lot to emotion detection and classification. Thus, this is used in all sorts of settings such as communication, entertainment, education, medicine, and so on. Thus, to fulfil the requirements of these different types of settings, BCI researchers have been conducting various experiments such as in several frequency bands, different methods of provoking and processing emotions, and various models of affective states. These different types of approaches mentioned above are being employed in studies to help gauge the emotional states of the participants or patients from the BCI signals that were recognized and acquired (Al-Nafjan & A. (2017)).

Several research studies have been conducted in the recent past due to the creation and marketing of brain-computer interface systems that are affordable and easy to use for patients. This is an incredibly important step when it comes to the future directions the BCI model should go towards. Taking notice of whether patients can use the device without too much difficulty is of incredible importance. The majority of the known Electroencephalography datasets were collected by using visual elicitation tools in strict laboratory settings. Thus, initially, in the earlier stages, the emotional condition of the subjects was not taken into account before the experiment was taken. These individual differences and limitations could cause the dataset to be highly variable and inconsistent. Thus, now slowly and gradually researchers have started considering this aspect of BCI as well (Houssein, E. H. & Hammad (2022)).

BCI has come to be extremely useful in aiding cognitively and physically impaired individuals. It assists them in multiple ways such as in controlling their movements, locomotion, emotion recognition, perception, social adjustment, and involvement, etc. this assistance opens up a channel of communication between the human brain and the machine which allows the individual to comprehend and function better in the outside world. The three requirements of neurologically challenged individuals are mobility, autonomic function, and communication. Very shortly, BCI could take over the medicinal field by dominating the rehabilitation and recovery centre. It has the potential to become one of the most crucial parts of recovery as well as daily life assistance for these people. As mentioned earlier this is only possible if the target users, who are the people with neurological conditions, are constantly involved and asked to participate in the tests and trials of the experimental stage of this research project. This is important to focus on producing systems that help in addressing their problems rather than just looking at the minor deficits of the able-bodied population. BCI's potential may eventually serve people of other populations and backgrounds as well. The bigger picture, however, will always entail that BCI was initially created to be a safe, affordable, aesthetically pleasing to the eyes, and user-friendly system (Hochberg, L. R. (2012)).

BCI systems have an immense amount of potential to grow specifically in the areas of treatment, diagnosis, and rehabilitation for people with neurological conditions, yet their practical and clinical applications seem highly unstable, experimental and have several barriers that restrict their smooth functioning. One extremely crucial aspect of these challenges is developing biocompatibility and the long-term stability of the technical aspect of it. This is highly important to ensure the safety of the patients as well as for the sustenance of the device's performance. Advancing electrodes and sensor technologies are both equally and highly crucial for the improvement in the performance of the BCI systems. They are specifically important in forming the foundation for accurate signal acquisition and reliable operation. Researchers also need to work on making compact and portable BCI systems. This would allow its technology to be both easier for its users to access and convenient both in clinical and personal usage. Furthermore, it is important to focus on the first stage of the BCI systems which is signal acquisition. It is crucial to enhance the signal decoding accuracy and reliability and to allow for seamless real-time performance. The machine needs to also be able to decode and understand the context of what the patient is thinking to be able to transcribe accurately. For this, the technology needs to be more adaptable to incorporate the needs of its diverse users including culture, religion, racial, geographical, etc aspects of it (Zhang & Hongyu, (2024)).

The other challenge that has been observed over the years in BCI research is that it lies heavily on the reliance on its pilot studies. Pilot studies are usually small-scale studies or designs that help in improving the larger much more complete scale studies. Although this is relatively indispensable in laying the foundational work for future advancements, it often leads to results in data that is neither very reliable nor confirmable. This constant reliance can cause non-replicable data to gradually diminish the overall credibility and quality of its research in the neurological field. As mentioned earlier, pilot studies are very important in the initial stages of the development of the BCI system as they give crucial insight into the potential problems or changes one needs to make to refine the technological aspect of it for flawless functioning. However, these studies still lack overall clarity and have a lot of limitations in their scope and scale, specifically when the system's protocols are relatively novel and have been only talked about briefly in a paper or two. The next issue with these studies is that researchers have noticed a lack of control groups. This unfortunately makes it almost impossible to isolate the factors and variables that play into this study and the effects of the interventions from other external and unrelated factors. For example, the severity of the fast-paced changes of seasonal depression has been observed to significantly influence the results yet these factors and variables remain unaccounted for due to the lack of a rigorous experimental design (Vladimir Khorev (2024)).

Another concern regarding the BCI system is that there is a noticeable lack of large-scale, repeated, and rigorous studies in this research field. Independent replication is the key step to progress in the scientific field. This is to ensure that the results and findings always remain robust, up to date with the current world's requirements, generalizable, and not a result of some coincidence or complicated and intricate experimental conditions. Addressing these weaknesses is imperative in realizing its potential and advancing the reliability and practical use of BCI technologies (Vladimir Khorev (2024)).

The development of BCIs tailored to restore mobility must integrate mental health considerations into their design and implementation. Restoring arm and hand function, for instance, could significantly enhance functional independence, while innovations in computer interface control could foster greater engagement in work and social activities. As research advances, addressing mental health directly through BCIs—such as interventions targeting anxiety, depression, or neurocognitive rehabilitation—may become a complementary focus, further enhancing the quality of life for individuals with severe disabilities (Donoghue et al. (2007)).

In conclusion, BCIs have the potential not only to restore physical capabilities but also to improve mental health outcomes for individuals with impaired mobility. By addressing both the physical and psychological impacts of disability, these technologies could transform lives and expand opportunities for meaningful participation in society.

CONCLUSION

Brain-computer interfaces (BCIs) are a game-changing technology for solving the issues that people with neurological and mental health disorders confront. This chapter examined the revolutionary uses of BCIs, which ranged from restoring communication in people with amyotrophic lateral sclerosis (ALS) and locked-in syndrome (LIS) to enabling mobility in people with paraplegia and tetraplegia. BCIs provide an important link between cerebral activity and external devices, allowing freedom and improving the quality of life for persons who suffer substantial physical and neurological limitations.

Beyond treating physical limitations, BCIs have shown great promise in improving mental health outcomes. Neurofeedback and emotion recognition systems can help to alleviate conditions including depression, anxiety, and emotional dysregulation, which frequently accompany neurological illnesses or develop on their own. EEG-based brain-computer interfaces can monitor and modulate emotional states in real-time, providing therapeutic advantages to people suffering from mood disorders. For example, neurofeedback training allows users to alter brain activity, promoting improved emotional regulation and minimizing psychological suffering.

The incorporation of BCIs into virtual reality (VR) systems emphasizes their importance in mental health and social rehabilitation. These technologies enable immersive settings for skill development, emotional control, and social interaction, which can help people with autism spectrum disorder (ASD), post-stroke emotional deficits, and other disorders. The capacity of BCIs to battle loneliness, boost self-esteem, and restore a sense of agency tackles not just physical constraints, but also emotional and social issues for users.

While BCIs show great potential, numerous challenges remain. Ethical factors such as data protection, informed permission, and fair access are essential for responsible deployment. Technical obstacles, such as increasing signal processing accuracy and creating user-friendly interfaces, necessitate continued study. Nonetheless, an increasing amount of data shows their potential to revolutionize both mental and physical health care.

In conclusion, BCIs offer an innovative and interdisciplinary solution to the multifaceted challenges posed by neurological and mental health conditions. By restoring autonomy, enhancing communication, and improving emotional well-being, BCIs are poised to transform lives. Continued advancements in this field, alongside efforts to address existing challenges, will ensure that these technologies become accessible, effective, and ethically sound tools for those in need.

REFERENCES

Aaron, R. K., Herr, H. M., Ciombor, D. M., Hochberg, L. R., Donoghue, J. P., Briant, C. L., Morgan, J. R., & Ehrlich, M. G. (2006). Horizons in prosthesis development for the restoration of limb function. *The Journal of the American Academy of Orthopaedic Surgeons*, *14*(Supplement), S198–S204. DOI: 10.5435/00124635-200600001-00043 PMID: 17003199

Al-Nafjan, A., Hosny, M., Al-Ohali, Y., & Al-Wabil, A. (2017). Review and classification of emotion recognition based on EEG brain-computer interface system research: A systematic review. *Applied Sciences (Basel, Switzerland)*, *7*(12), 1239. DOI: 10.3390/app7121239

Anderson, K. D. (2004). Targeting recovery: Priorities of the spinal cord-injured population. *Journal of Neurotrauma*, *21*(10), 1371–1383. DOI: 10.1089/neu.2004.21.1371 PMID: 15672628

Bauer, G., Gerstenbrand, F., & Rumpl, E. (1979). Varieties of the locked-in syndrome. *Journal of Neurology*, *221*, 77–91.

Bolognini, N., Pascual-Leone, A., & Fregni, F. (2009). Using non-invasive brain stimulation to augment motor training-induced plasticity. *Journal of Neuroengineering and Rehabilitation*, *6*(1), 8. DOI: 10.1186/1743-0003-6-8 PMID: 19292910

Chaudhary, U., Xia, B., Silvoni, S., Cohen, L. G., & Birbaumer, N. (2017). Brain-Computer Interface–Based Communication in the Completely Locked-In State. *PLoS Biology*, *15*(1), e1002593. DOI: 10.1371/journal.pbio.1002593 PMID: 28141803

Donnelly, C., Eng, J. J., Hall, J., Alford, L., Giachino, R., Norton, K., & Kerr, D. S. (2004). Client-centered assessment and the identification of meaningful treatment goals for individuals with a spinal cord injury. *Spinal Cord*, *42*(5), 302–307. DOI: 10.1038/sj.sc.3101589 PMID: 14993893

Donoghue, J. P., Hochberg, L. R., Nurmikko, A. V., Black, M. J., Simeral, J. D., & Friehs, G. (2007a). Neuromotor prosthesis development. *Medicine and Health, Rhode Island*, *90*, 12–15. PMID: 17487029

Donoghue, J. P., Nurmikko, A., Black, M., & Hochberg, L. R. (2007b). Assistive technology and robotic control using motor cortex ensemble-based neural interface systems in humans with tetraplegia. *The Journal of Physiology*, *579*(3), 603–611. DOI: 10.1113/jphysiol.2006.127209 PMID: 17272345

Feigin, V. L., Nichols, E., Alam, T., Bannick, M. S., Beghi, E., Blake, N., Culpepper, W. J., Dorsey, E. R., Elbaz, A., Ellenbogen, R. G., Fisher, J. L., Fitzmaurice, C., Giussani, G., Glennie, L., James, S. L., Johnson, C. O., Kassebaum, N. J., Logroscino, G., Marin, B., & Vos, T. (2019). Global, regional, and national burden of neurological disorders, 1990–2016: A systematic analysis for the Global Burden of Disease Study 2016. *Lancet Neurology*, *18*(5), 459–480. DOI: 10.1016/S1474-4422(18)30499-X PMID: 30879893

Gerdes, A. B., Wieser, M. J., & Alpers, G. W. (2014). Emotional pictures and sounds: A review of multimodal interactions of emotion cues in multiple domains. *Frontiers in Psychology*, *5*, 1351. DOI: 10.3389/fpsyg.2014.01351 PMID: 25520679

Geser, F., Lee, V. M., & Trojanowski, J. Q. (2010). Amyotrophic lateral sclerosis and frontotemporal lobar degeneration: A spectrum of TDP-43 proteinopathies. *Neuropathology*, *30*(2), 103–112. DOI: 10.1111/j.1440-1789.2009.01091.x PMID: 20102519

Greenberg, B. D., Gabriels, L. A., Malone, D. A.Jr, Rezai, A. R., Friehs, G. M., Okun, M. S., Shapira, N. A., Foote, K. D., Cosyns, P. R., Kubu, C. S., Malloy, P. F., Salloway, S. P., Giftakis, J. E., Rise, M. T., Machado, A. G., Baker, K. B., Stypulkowski, P. H., Goodman, W. K., Rasmussen, S. A., & Nuttin, B. J. (2010). Deep brain stimulation of the ventral internal capsule/ventral striatum for obsessive-compulsive disorder: Worldwide experience. *Molecular Psychiatry*, *15*(1), 64–79. DOI: 10.1038/mp.2008.55 PMID: 18490925

He, Z., Li, Z., Yang, F., Wang, L., Li, J., Zhou, C., & Pan, J. (2020). Advances in multimodal emotion recognition based on Brain-Computer interfaces. *Brain Sciences*, *10*(10), 687. DOI: 10.3390/brainsci10100687 PMID: 33003397

Herbert, C. (2024). Brain-computer interfaces and human factors: The role of language and cultural differences—Still a missing gap? *Frontiers in Human Neuroscience*, *18*, 1305445. DOI: 10.3389/fnhum.2024.1305445 PMID: 38665897

Hitzig, S. L., Tonack, M., Campbell, K. A., McGillivray, C. F., Boschen, K. A., Richards, K., & Craven, B. C. (2008). Secondary health complications in an aging Canadian spinal cord injury sample. *American Journal of Physical Medicine & Rehabilitation*, *87*(7), 545–555. DOI: 10.1097/PHM.0b013e31817c16d6 PMID: 18574346

Hochberg, L. R., & Anderson, K. D. (2012). BCI users and their needs. *Brain-computer interfaces: Principles and practice*, 317-324.

Hochberg, L. R., & Cochrane, T. I. (2011 in press). Implanted Neural Interfaces: Ethics in Research and Treatment. In Farah, M., & Chatterjee, A. (Eds.), *Neuroethics in Practice*. Dana Press.

Holtzheimer, P. E., Husain, M. M., Lisanby, S. H., Taylor, S. F., Whitworth, L. A., McClintock, S., Slavin, K. V., Berman, J., McKhann, G. M., Patil, P. G., Rittberg, B. R., Abosch, A., Pandurangi, A. K., Holloway, K. L., Lam, R. W., Honey, C. R., Neimat, J. S., Henderson, J. M., DeBattista, C., & Mayberg, H. S. (2017). Subcallosal cingulate deep brain stimulation for treatment-resistant depression: A multisite, randomized, sham-controlled trial. *The Lancet. Psychiatry*, *4*(11), 839–849. DOI: 10.1016/S2215-0366(17)30371-1 PMID: 28988904

Holz, E. M., Botrel, L., Kaufmann, T., & Kübler, A. (2015). Long-term independent brain-computer interface home use improves quality of life of a patient in the locked-in state: A case study. *Archives of Physical Medicine and Rehabilitation*, *96*(3), S16–S26. DOI: 10.1016/j.apmr.2014.03.035 PMID: 25721543

Houssein, E. H., Hammad, A., & Ali, A. A. (2022). Human emotion recognition from EEG-based brain-computer interface using machine learning: A comprehensive review. *Neural Computing & Applications*, *34*(15), 12527–12557. DOI: 10.1007/s00521-022-07292-4

Johansson, V., Soekadar, S. R., & Clausen, J. (2017). Locked out: Ignorance and responsibility in brain-computer interface communication in locked-in syndrome. *Cambridge Quarterly of Healthcare Ethics*, *26*(4), 555–576. DOI: 10.1017/S0963180117000081 PMID: 28937339

Kashihara, K. (2014a). A brain-computer interface for potential non-verbal facial communication based on EEG signals related to specific emotions. *Frontiers in Neuroscience*, *8*. Advance online publication. DOI: 10.3389/fnins.2014.00244 PMID: 25206321

Khorev, V., Kurkin, S., Badarin, A., Antipov, V., Pitsik, E., Andreev, A., Grubov, V., Drapkina, O., Kiselev, A., & Hramov, A. (2024). Review on the Use of Brain-Computer Interface Rehabilitation Methods for Treating Mental and Neurological Conditions. *Journal of Integrative Neuroscience*, *23*(7), 125. DOI: 10.31083/j.jin2307125 PMID: 39082285

Kim, S. P., Simeral, J. D., Hochberg, L. R., Donoghue, J. P., Friehs, G. M., & Black, M. J. (2007). Multistate decoding of point-and-click control signals from motor cortical activity in a human with tetraplegia. Neural Engineering, 2007. CNE '07. 3rd International IEEE/EMBS Conference on, pp. 486-9

Lozano, A. M., Mayberg, H. S., Giacobbe, P., Hamani, C., Craddock, R. C., & Kennedy, S. H. (2008). Subcallosal cingulate gyrus deep brain stimulation for treatment-resistant depression. *Biological Psychiatry*, *64*(6), 461–467. DOI: 10.1016/j.biopsych.2008.05.034 PMID: 18639234

Malone, D. A.Jr, Dougherty, D. D., Rezai, A. R., Carpenter, L. L., Friehs, G. M., Eskandar, E. N., Rauch, S. L., Rasmussen, S. A., Machado, A. G., Kubu, C. S., Tyrka, A. R., Price, L. H., Stypulkowski, P. H., Giftakis, J. E., Rise, M. T., Malloy, P. F., Salloway, S. P., & Greenberg, B. D. (2009). Deep brain stimulation of the ventral capsule/ventral striatum for treatment-resistant depression. *Biological Psychiatry*, *65*(4), 267–275. DOI: 10.1016/j.biopsych.2008.08.029 PMID: 18842257

Maynard, F. M.Jr, Bracken, M. B., Creasey, G., Ditunno, J. F.Jr, & Donovan, W. H.. (1997). International Standards for Neurological and Functional Classification of Spinal Cord Injury. American Spinal Injury Association. *Spinal Cord*, *35*(5), 266–274. DOI: 10.1038/sj.sc.3100432 PMID: 9160449

Nicolas-Alonso, L. F., & Gomez-Gil, J. (2012). Brain-Computer Interfaces, a Review. *Sensors (Basel)*, *12*(2), 1211–1279. DOI: 10.3390/s120201211 PMID: 22438708

Pahwa, R., Factor, S. A., Lyons, K. E., Ondo, W. G., & Gronseth, G.. (2006). Practice Parameter: treatment of Parkinson's disease with motor fluctuations and dyskinesia (an evidence-based review): report of the Quality Standards Subcommittee of the American Academy of Neurology. *Neurology*, *66*, 983–995. DOI: 10.1212/01.wnl.0000215250.82576.87 PMID: 16606909

Paquette, V., Beauregard, M., & Beaulieu-Prévost, D. (2009). Effect of a psychoneurotherapy on brain electromagnetic tomography in individuals with major depressive disorder. *Psychiatry Research*, *174*(3), 231–239. DOI: 10.1016/j.pscychresns.2009.06.002 PMID: 19914046

Pfurtscheller, G., Muller-Putz, G. R., Scherer, R., & Neuper, C. (2008). Rehabilitation with brain-computer interface systems. *Computer*, *41s*(10), 58–65. DOI: 10.1109/MC.2008.432

Plum, F., & Posner, J. B. (1966). *The diagnosis of stupor and coma*. F.A. Davis.

Rashid, M., & Sulaiman, N., PP Abdul Majeed, A., Musa, R. M., Ab. Nasir, A. F., Bari, B. S., & Khatun, S. (. (2020). Current status, challenges, and possible solutions of EEG-based brain-computer interface: A comprehensive review. *Frontiers in Neurorobotics*, *14*, 25. DOI: 10.3389/fnbot.2020.00025 PMID: 32581758

Santhanam, G., Ryu, S. I., Yu, B. M., Afshar, A., & Shenoy, K. V. (2006). A high-performance brain-computer interface. *Nature*, *442*(7099), 195–198. DOI: 10.1038/nature04968 PMID: 16838020

Scott-Admin. (2024, April 8). *Consortium to develop a fully implantable brain-computer interface to enable communication for people with paralysis*. Wyss Center. https://wysscenter.ch/updates/consortium-to-develop-fully-implantable-brain-computer-interface-to-enable-communication-for-people-with-paralysis/#

Signal preprocessing techniques | Brain-Computer Interfaces Class Notes | Fiveable.(n.d.).https://library.fiveable.me/brain-computer-interfaces/unit-6/signal-preprocessin-techniques/study-guide/04fl2GruJ9mOLNuf

Stanford University. (n.d.-b). *Autism Glass Project*. https://autismglass.stanford.edu/

Sun, F. T., Morrell, M. J., & Wharen, R. E.Jr. (2008). Responsive cortical stimulation for the treatment of epilepsy. *Neurotherapeutics; the Journal of the American Society for Experimental NeuroTherapeutics*, *5*(1), 68–74. DOI: 10.1016/j.nurt.2007.10.069 PMID: 18164485

Yike Sun, Xiaogang Chen (2024). Signal processing and the future of non-invasive BCI systems.

Sun, Y., Chen, X., Liu, B., Liang, L., Wang, Y., Gao, S., & Gao, X. (2022). Multivariate genome-wide association study of depression, cognition, and memory phenotypes and validation analysis identify 12 cross-ethnic variants. *Translational Psychiatry*, *12*(1), 52. DOI: 10.1038/s41398-022-02074-x PMID: 35115488

Sundquist, K., Frank, G., & Sundquist, J. (2004). Urbanisation and incidence of psychosis and depression: A follow-up study of 4.4 million women and men in Sweden. *The British Journal of Psychiatry*, *184*(4), 293–298. DOI: 10.1192/bjp.184.4.293 PMID: 15056572

UC Davis Health-Developed Technology Translates Brain Signals into Speech with 97% Accuracy | AHA. (n.d.-b). American Hospital Association. https://www.aha.org/role-hospital-uc-davis-health-developed-technology-translates-brain-signals-speech-97-accuracy#:~:text=Researchers%20implanted%20sensors%20in%20Harrell's,and%20society%2C%E2%80%9D%20said%20Harrell

Umair, A., Ashfaq, U., & Khan, M. G. (2017). Recent trends, applications, and challenges of brain-computer interfacing (BCI). *International Journal of Intelligent Systems and Applications*, *9*(2), 58–65. DOI: 10.5815/ijisa.2017.02.08

Van Damme, S., Mumford, L., Johnson, A., & Chau, T. (2024). Case report: Novel use of clinical brain-computer interfaces in recreation programming for an autistic adolescent with co-occurring attention deficit hyperactivity disorder. *Frontiers in Human Neuroscience*, *18*, 1434792. Advance online publication. DOI: 10.3389/fnhum.2024.1434792 PMID: 39296916

Vlek, R. J. (2012). Ethical issues in brain-computer interface research, development, and dissemination. *Journal of Neural Engineering*, *9*(3). PMID: 22592066

Vlek, R. J., Steines, D., Szibbo, D., Kübler, A., Schneider, M. J., Haselager, P., & Nijboer, F. (2012). Ethical issues in brain-computer interface research, development, and dissemination. *Journal of Neurologic Physical Therapy; JNPT*, *36*(2), 94–99. DOI: 10.1097/NPT.0b013e31825064cc PMID: 22592066

Wen, D., Fan, Y., Hsu, S., Xu, J., Zhou, Y., Tao, J., Lan, X., & Li, F. (2020). Combining brain-computer interface and virtual reality for rehabilitation in neurological diseases: A narrative review. *Annals of Physical and Rehabilitation Medicine*, *64*(1), 101404. DOI: 10.1016/j.rehab.2020.03.015 PMID: 32561504

Wiz, & Wiz. (2025, March 3). Controlling Devices with Your Mind: The Game-Changing Impact of Brain-Computer Interfaces. *DigitrendZ*. https://digitrendz.blog/tech-news/8168/controlling-devices-with-your-mind-the-game-changing-impact-of-brain-computer-interfaces

Wolpaw, J. R., Birbaumer, N., Heetderks, W. J., ... (2000) Brain-computer interface technology: a review of the first international meeting. EEE Trans Rehabil Eng 8(2): 164–73 DOI: 10.1109/TRE.2000.847807

Zhang, H., Jiao, L., Yang, S., Li, H., Jiang, X., Feng, J., & Wei, B. (2024). Brain–computer interfaces: The innovative key to unlocking neurological conditions. *International Journal of Surgery*, *110*(9), 5745–5762.

Chapter 13
AI as a Mirror of Society Historical Lessons and Sociological Impacts

Anshu Sharma
https://orcid.org/0000-0002-0474-829X
RIMT University, India

Gurtek Singh
https://orcid.org/0009-0008-4207-176X
Akal University, India

Suneet Kaur
https://orcid.org/0009-0004-4260-9639
RIMT University, India

ABSTRACT

The present chapter delves into the dual role of artificial intelligence (AI) in reflecting and modifying society institutions, with a special emphasis on its applications in mental health and education. This chapter will analyze how AI mimics ideals, power dynamics, and biases of society while actively altering these areas, using a historical and sociological lens. By examining important technological breakthroughs from the Industrial Revolution to the AI age, we will analyze the lessons learned from previous sociotechnical systems and their implications for modern AI tools. The chapter will also critically examine the ethical and sociological concerns offered by AI, such as bias, equity, and cultural competence, and provide recommendations for developing more inclusive and socially responsible AI technology.

DOI: 10.4018/979-8-3373-5072-1.ch013

INTRODUCTION

Artificial Intelligence (AI) has become a transformative force in modern society, reshaping industries and redefining human experiences across various domains. Among its most profound applications, AI has begun to influence the deeply human fields of mental health and education, offering tools that promise personalization, accessibility, and efficiency. However, AI systems do not operate in a vacuum, they are deeply embedded in the historical and sociological aspects that shape their design, deployment, and impact. As such, AI serves as a mirror, reflecting the values, biases, and inequalities of the societies that create and use these technologies. The idea of technology as a mirror of society is not new. Historical analyses reveal how tools, from the printing press to the internet, have both mirrored and shaped societal norms, hierarchies, and inequalities (McLuhan, 1964; Latour, 1992). AI continues this tradition but with unprecedented speed and scope. For example, AI-driven mental health diagnostics reflect the datasets on which they are trained, which may carry biases rooted in the historical underrepresentation of marginalized communities (Obermeyer et al., 2019). Similarly, AI-powered educational tools often replicate and amplify existing disparities in access to quality education, echoing long-standing issues of inequality in educational systems (Eubanks, 2018). This chapter explores the dual role of AI as both a reflection of societal structures and an agent of transformation in mental health and education. It delves into the historical roots of sociotechnical systems, examining how past technological advancements inform current AI developments. It also considers the sociological impacts of AI, particularly its potential to reinforce or disrupt existing norms and power dynamics.

Historical Context of AI and Sociotechnical Systems

The development of artificial intelligence (AI) cannot be understood in isolation. It is a product of centuries-long sociotechnical evolution, reflecting the drive to solve complex problems, enhance efficiency, and improve the quality of life of humanity. AI builds upon a historical foundation marked by transformative technological revolutions, including the Industrial Revolution, the computational advancements of the 20th century, and the rapid digitization of the 21st century. Each phase in this progression reveals lessons about the dynamic interplay between technology and society, emphasizing the critical need to consider ethical and equitable implications.

Evolution of Sociotechnical Systems

Sociotechnical systems represent the interdependence between society and technology, shaping how individuals and communities interact with innovations. The Industrial Revolution (late 18th to early 19th century) was a pivotal moment in history when mechanization fundamentally altered social structures. Factories powered by steam engines became the cornerstone of production, replacing traditional handcrafting techniques. This transformation prioritized efficiency and productivity over individual artistry, laying the foundation for modern industrialization (Smith, 1776). The Industrial Revolution reshaped labor systems by introducing specialized roles, leading to a division of labor that emphasized repetition and efficiency. Educational institutions mirrored this shift, adopting regimented structures to prepare students for factory work. Scholars like Tyack (1974) note that schools of this era were often described as "factory models" with strict schedules, uniformity, and centralized authority dominating pedagogical practices. The 20th century marked another significant leap in sociotechnical evolution with the emergence of computing technologies. During World War II, early computational machines, such as the ENIAC, were designed for military applications like ballistic calculations. These machines were later adapted for academic research, business operations, and healthcare (Ceruzzi, 2003). Early examples of computational applications in education include Sidney Pressey's "teaching machine" in the 1920s. This device aimed to automate basic instructional tasks, highlighting the potential for technology to enhance learning efficiency (Watters, 2014). Similarly, the intersection of technology and mental health gained prominence in the mid-20th century with computational psychiatry. Researchers began leveraging computer models to simulate neural activity, diagnose psychological disorders, and predict outcomes (Friston et al., 2014). These innovations laid the groundwork for modern AI applications in diagnosing and treating mental health conditions, despite concerns about the potential depersonalization of care.

Lessons from Historical Integrations of Technology

The historical trajectory of sociotechnical systems reveals recurring themes of both promise and peril. Mechanized educational tools, for instance, were initially lauded for their potential to democratize learning. However, access to such innovations was often limited to elite institutions, reinforcing existing inequalities (Watters, 2014). Pressey's teaching machine exemplifies this paradox: while it aimed to make education more accessible, its widespread adoption was hindered by high costs and institutional resistance. Early computational psychiatry in mental health raised similar concerns. Critics argued that these technologies prioritized quantifiable symptoms over holistic approaches to mental well-being. Rose (1996) contended that this reductionist focus neglected the social and cultural dimensions of mental health, limiting the effectiveness of these tools in diverse populations. These historical lessons underscore the dual nature of technological advancements. While they offer transformative possibilities, they also risk perpetuating systemic biases if not developed and deployed with equity in mind. Technological evolution does not occur in a vacuum as it reflects the values, priorities, and power dynamics of the societies that create it. The Industrial Revolution prioritized economic efficiency, often at the expense of labor rights and environmental sustainability. Similarly, 20th-century advancements in computing prioritized military and industrial applications, with limited consideration for their broader societal implications. Recognizing these patterns is essential to guiding the development of AI in ways that challenge inequities rather than reinforce them.

AI in Historical Perspective

AI is a continuation of humanity's longstanding effort to delegate complex tasks to machines. Unlike previous technological advancements, AI systems possess the capacity to learn, adapt, and make decisions, often without direct human intervention. This capability makes AI both transformative and unpredictable, amplifying its potential for societal impact. In mental health, AI-powered tools like chatbots, diagnostic algorithms, and virtual therapists are redefining care delivery. These innovations build upon the legacy of computational psychiatry but operate with greater precision and accessibility. For instance, AI-based applications can analyze speech patterns, facial expressions, and social media activity to identify early signs of mental health issues, enabling timely interventions (Topol, 2019). Despite these advancements, AI systems inherit biases from their training data, which often reflect historical and cultural inequities. Obermeyer et al. (2019) highlight how predictive algorithms in healthcare can perpetuate racial and socioeconomic disparities, underscoring the need for transparent and inclusive AI development. In education, AI-driven platforms are revolutionizing learning environments. Adaptive learning systems personalize instruction based on individual student performance, while predictive analytics tools help educators identify at-risk students and tailor interventions accordingly. These innovations echo the aspirations of early mechanized teaching tools but operate on a much larger scale. Selwyn (2019) cautions that while AI holds promise for enhancing educational outcomes, it also risks exacerbating inequalities by favouring students and institutions with access to advanced technologies.

Ethical and Equity Considerations in AI Development

The history of AI and sociotechnical systems is a testament to the ingenuity and resilience of humanity. From the mechanized tools of the Industrial Revolution to the sophisticated algorithms of today, each technological leap has reshaped society in profound ways. However, this history also reveals the potential for technology to perpetuate inequities and reinforce existing power structures. Historical patterns in sociotechnical evolution reveal that technology alone cannot solve complex societal problems. Its impact depends on the social, cultural, and economic contexts in which it operates. As AI continues to evolve, it is crucial to address ethical and equity concerns proactively. This includes ensuring that AI systems are designed to reflect diverse perspectives, challenge systemic biases, and promote inclusivity. For example, AI algorithms used in hiring processes have been criticized for replicating gender and racial biases present in historical data (Binns, 2018).

AI AS A SOCIOTECHNICAL MIRROR

AI, as a sociotechnical mirror, is both a reflection and a shaper of societal values and norms. Its design and implementation are deeply entwined with existing power dynamics and cultural biases, yet it holds transformative potential to challenge and reimagine these structures. By critically examining how AI reflects and influences society, we can work towards creating systems that foster equity, inclusivity, and cultural sensitivity in mental health and education. Artificial Intelligence (AI) is not a neutral tool; It is inherently shaped by the societal contexts in which it is developed and deployed. As a sociotechnical system, AI reflects the values, biases, and power dynamics of the societies that create and use it. This mirroring effect makes AI both a product and a perpetuator of societal patterns, capable of reinforcing existing inequalities or challenging them.

Reflection of Societal Values and Biases

AI systems are developed based on data that inherently carries traces of societal norms, prejudices, and historical inequalities. The process of designing and implementing AI is thus deeply influenced by the cultural, political, and economic conditions of its creators. This influence manifests in several ways:-

Bias in Diagnostic Tools

AI-driven diagnostic systems in mental health care are trained on datasets that may underrepresent or misrepresent certain populations. For example, a study by Obermeyer et al. (2019) revealed that an algorithm used to manage healthcare for millions of patients in the United States exhibited racial bias. Black patients were systematically assigned lower risk scores than equally sick white patients, reflecting systemic disparities in access to care and health outcomes. Similarly, AI tools for mental health diagnostics may fail to account for cultural variations in symptom expression, leading to misdiagnoses or neglect of marginalized groups (Bentley et al., 2022).

Disparities in Access to AI-Driven Education Platforms

AI-powered educational tools, such as adaptive learning systems and predictive analytics, hold great promise for personalizing education. However, these technologies often privilege well-resourced schools and communities with access to the necessary infrastructure, leaving underserved populations behind. For instance, rural and low-income schools frequently lack the broadband connectivity or hardware required to implement AI-driven platforms, perpetuating the digital divide (Selwyn, 2019). Furthermore, the content and algorithms of these tools may reflect the biases of their predominantly Western developers, marginalizing non-Western pedagogical approaches and cultural contexts (Smith & Kumar, 2020).

Feedback Loops Between Society and AI

AI not only mirrors societal patterns but also participates in feedback loops that can either reinforce or challenge them.

Reinforcement of Societal Patterns

When AI systems are deployed without addressing underlying societal inequities, they can amplify these inequalities. For example, predictive policing algorithms, which rely on historical crime data, often direct more resources to already over-policed communities, disproportionately targeting minority populations (O'Neil, 2016). In education, AI-driven grading systems have been criticized for penalizing non-native speakers or students from various linguistic backgrounds due to biases in training data (Williamson, 2020).

Challenging Societal Norms

Despite these risks, AI also has the potential to disrupt entrenched societal patterns. For instance, AI tools designed for mental health can provide anonymous and stigma-free access to care, particularly in cultures where discussing mental health is taboo. Chatbots like Woebot and AI-powered platforms like WYSA are helping to democratize mental health resources by making them accessible to individuals who might otherwise avoid traditional therapy due to cultural or economic barriers (Fitzpatrick et al., 2017). In education, AI systems that focus on identifying at-risk students and providing personalized support can help mitigate systemic disadvantages. For example, early intervention tools powered by AI have been used to improve retention rates among first-generation college students, demonstrating how technology can foster equity when implemented thoughtfully (Herzog, 2018).

SOCIOLOGICAL IMPACTS ON MENTAL HEALTH AND EDUCATION

The sociological impacts of AI on mental health and education are multifaceted, offering both opportunities for greater accessibility and risks of deepening existing inequalities. While AI has the potential to address systemic challenges in these fields, its effectiveness depends on how well it incorporates cultural competence, diversity, and a human-centric approach. Thoughtful design and implementation are essential to harness the transformative potential of AI while mitigating its sociological risks. The integration of AI into mental health care and education has generated transformative possibilities while simultaneously introducing new challenges. Sociologically, the impact of AI is shaped by its ability to mediate human relationships, address systemic inequities, and reinforce or disrupt existing social structures. This section explores the dual role of AI as both an enabler and a disruptor in these domains.

Mental Health

AI as a Tool for Accessibility

AI-driven technologies have significantly expanded access to mental health care, particularly for individuals in underserved or remote areas. Chatbots like Wysa and Woebot provide conversational interfaces that mimic therapeutic interactions, offering immediate support for mild to moderate mental health issues (Fitzpatrick et al., 2017). Teletherapy platforms enhanced with AI capabilities enable personalized interventions, including mood tracking and tailored coping strategies (Topol, 2019).

Diagnostic systems powered by machine learning, such as predictive models for depression or anxiety, enable early detection and intervention. These tools can analyze diverse data sources, including social media activity and wearable device metrics, to identify behavioral patterns indicative of mental health challenges (Bentley et al., 2022). Such innovations hold the potential to democratize mental health care, making it more accessible and scalable.

Challenges of Cultural Competence and Bias

Despite these advancements, AI tools in mental health often struggle with cultural competence. Algorithms are typically trained on datasets that overrepresent populations from Western, industrialized nations, resulting in tools that may fail to account for cultural differences in the expression of mental health symptoms (Harris et al., 2020). For example, an AI system trained on Western diagnostic criteria might misinterpret culturally specific behaviors or fail to recognize symptoms prevalent in non-Western communities. Bias in data and design also extends to the stigmatization of certain groups. Studies have shown that minority populations are often underrepresented in datasets, leading to misdiagnoses or inequitable treatment recommendations. Addressing these challenges requires incorporating diverse datasets and involving cross-cultural experts in AI development to ensure inclusivity and relevance across populations (Obermeyer et al., 2019).

Education

Personalization vs. Standardization

Artificial intelligence (AI) has emerged as a transformative force in education, redefining how learning is delivered, assessed, and experienced. One of its most notable impacts is the ability to create highly personalized learning environments. Adaptive learning systems have revolutionized traditional teaching paradigms by tailoring educational content to individual needs. However, the widespread adoption of these technologies also brings significant challenges, particularly regarding the risks of reinforcing standardization and bias.

Adaptive Learning and Personalized Education

AI-powered adaptive learning platforms, such as Khan Academy and Coursera, analyze vast amounts of data to customize educational experiences. These systems leverage machine learning algorithms to assess student performance, identify strengths and weaknesses, and deliver targeted recommendations (Selwyn, 2019).

For example, a student struggling with algebra may receive additional exercises or alternative explanations tailored to their learning style, while an advanced learner may be presented with more challenging content. This level of personalization allows students to progress at their own pace, fostering a deeper understanding of the material. It also provides teachers with actionable insights, enabling them to address individual needs more effectively. For learners with disabilities or those in underserved communities, AI-driven tools offer unprecedented access to educational resources, bridging gaps in equity and inclusion.

Risks of Standardization

Despite these benefits, the reliance on AI systems also risks perpetuating standardization in education. Many algorithms operate on predefined metrics of success, such as test scores or completion rates, which may not align with the diverse learning styles, cultural contexts, or non-traditional pathways of all students (Eubanks, 2018). For instance, predictive analytics tools often assess student potential based on historical data, which may inadvertently reinforce existing disparities. Students from historically marginalized groups, whose performance may have been affected by systemic inequities, could be unfairly labeled as low achievers. This creates a feedback loop where algorithmic biases perpetuate inequalities, further disadvantaging those who do not conform to dominant norms. Additionally, the emphasis on standardized outcomes may stifle creativity and critical thinking. While adaptive systems excel at delivering content aligned with specific objectives, they often struggle to accommodate open-ended exploration or interdisciplinary approaches. This tension highlights the need for a balanced approach that leverages the capabilities of AI without undermining the diversity and richness of human learning.

Addressing Bias and Enhancing Inclusivity

To mitigate these risks, educational institutions and developers must prioritize transparency, inclusivity, and equity in AI design. Incorporating diverse datasets that reflect a wide range of cultural, socioeconomic, and educational backgrounds is essential. Furthermore, involving educators, students, and community stakeholders in the development process can ensure that AI tools align with the values and needs of diverse populations. Ethical frameworks, such as those proposed by Floridi et al. (2018), can guide the responsible integration of AI in education. By prioritizing fairness, accountability, and inclusivity, stakeholders can harness the potential of AI while minimizing its unintended consequences.

The Changing Teacher-Student Relationship in an AI-Mediated Classroom

The integration of AI into classrooms has redefined the traditional roles of teachers and students, creating a dynamic interplay between humans and machines. While AI tools offer powerful capabilities for automating administrative tasks and enhancing instructional efficiency, they also raise fundamental questions about the nature of teaching, learning, and human connection.

Teachers as Facilitators and Overseers

In AI-mediated classrooms, teachers increasingly serve dual roles: facilitators of human interaction and overseers of AI-driven systems. On the one hand, AI tools can handle routine tasks such as grading, attendance tracking, and curriculum management, freeing teachers to focus on higher-order responsibilities. For example, detailed analytics generated by AI systems can provide insights into student progress, enabling educators to identify learning gaps and intervene proactively (Williamson, 2020). On the other hand, the reliance on AI may lead to reduced interpersonal engagement between teachers and students. Traditional classroom dynamics, characterized by empathy, intuition, and personal connection, are difficult to replicate in AI-driven environments. This shift raises concerns about the potential loss of critical elements that contribute to holistic education, such as emotional support, mentorship, and moral guidance.

Enhancing the Human Aspects of Education

When used thoughtfully, AI can complement rather than replace human interaction in education. By automating routine tasks, AI allows teachers to devote more time to fostering creativity, critical thinking, and collaborative skills. For example, educators can use AI-generated insights to design interactive group activities, encourage peer-to-peer learning, and cultivate a culture of curiosity and innovation. Moreover, AI can support differentiated instruction by enabling teachers to address the unique needs of diverse learners. For instance, language translation tools powered by AI can assist non-native speakers in overcoming language barriers, while speech recognition software can aid students with hearing impairments. These applications underscore the potential of AI to enhance inclusivity and equity in education.

Balancing AI Integration

Achieving a harmonious balance between technology and human interaction requires careful integration of AI systems into the educational process. Teachers must be empowered to navigate the complexities of AI tools, ensuring that technology enhances rather than detracts from the learning experience. Professional development programs can equip educators with the skills and knowledge needed to leverage AI effectively, fostering a collaborative relationship between humans and machines. Additionally, educational policies should prioritize the ethical use of AI, emphasizing principles such as transparency, accountability, and student agency. By placing human values at the center of AI integration, stakeholders can create a learning environment that respects and nurtures the individuality of each student.

The Broader Implications of AI in Education

The incorporation of AI into education extends beyond individual classrooms, shaping broader societal, ethical, and economic landscapes. As AI continues to evolve, its implications for education must be considered in the context of lifelong learning, workforce development, and global equity.

Lifelong Learning and Workforce Development

AI-driven education systems have the potential to transform lifelong learning and workforce development. Personalized learning platforms can adapt to the needs of adult learners, providing targeted training and upskilling opportunities. For example, AI tools can identify skill gaps in the workforce and deliver customized training programs to address emerging industry demands (Selwyn, 2019). Furthermore, AI can support micro-credentialing and competency-based education, enabling learners to demonstrate specific skills and knowledge through digital badges and certificates. This shift aligns with the growing demand for flexible, modular learning pathways that accommodate diverse career trajectories.

Global Equity and Access

AI holds promise for addressing global disparities in education by expanding access to quality learning resources. In low-income regions, AI-powered tools can deliver cost-effective, scalable solutions, such as virtual tutors, open educational resources, and remote learning platforms. For example, AI chatbots can provide interactive language instruction, while machine translation tools can make educational content accessible to non-native speakers. However, achieving global equity requires addressing the digital divide, which continues to limit access to technology and connectivity in marginalized communities. Investments in infrastructure, digital literacy, and inclusive design are essential to ensure that AI benefits all learners, regardless of their geographic or socioeconomic background.

ETHICAL CONSIDERATIONS AND CHALLENGES

Bias, access, and accountability are among the most pressing ethical challenges in the application of AI to mental health and education. Addressing these issues requires a multidisciplinary approach that combines technical innovation with sociological and ethical insights. By prioritizing fairness, inclusivity, and transparency, we can harness AI's potential while minimizing its risks and ensuring its benefits are equitably distributed. The integration of artificial intelligence (AI) into mental health care and education presents numerous ethical challenges. As these technologies increasingly influence sensitive aspects of human life, such as mental well-being and learning, they raise critical questions about fairness, access, accountability, and decision-making. This section examines three key ethical considerations: bias in algorithms, access and equity, and agency and accountability.

Bias in Algorithms

AI systems are only as objective as the data they are trained on. Bias in algorithms arises when training datasets reflect existing societal prejudices, resulting in discriminatory outcomes.

Mental Health Diagnostics

AI tools used in mental health care often rely on datasets that underrepresent certain populations, leading to skewed diagnostic outcomes. For example, algorithms trained on data from Western, urban populations may fail to accurately detect or treat mental health conditions in non-Western or rural communities. This bias can exacerbate disparities in mental health care, particularly for marginalized groups already facing systemic barriers to diagnosis and treatment (Bentley et al., 2022).

Educational Platforms

In education, bias in AI systems can manifest in predictive analytics tools that assess student performance or potential. Such tools may disproportionately penalize students from underrepresented or disadvantaged backgrounds, as their training data often reflect historical inequities in education. For instance, students from low-income schools may be inaccurately labeled as "high-risk," perpetuating cycles of disadvantage rather than addressing them (Eubanks, 2018). Mitigating algorithmic bias requires intentional efforts to diversify training datasets, audit AI systems for fairness, and involve stakeholders from diverse backgrounds in the design and implementation processes (Noble, 2018).

Access and Equity

The "digital divide" remains a significant barrier to equitable AI adoption in mental health and education. The "digital divide" is the gap between people who have access to modern technology (like the internet, computers, and smartphones) and those who do not. This can be due to factors like income, education, location, or infrastructure. It creates inequality in opportunities for learning, jobs, and communication.

Mental Health

AI-powered mental health tools like chatbots and teletherapy platforms promise increased accessibility but often require reliable internet access and digital literacy. Marginalized communities, including those in rural areas and low-income households, frequently lack these resources, leaving them excluded from the benefits of AI-driven care (Harris et al., 2020).

Education

In education, disparities in access to AI technologies amplify existing inequities. Schools in affluent areas are more likely to adopt advanced AI tools, while underfunded schools struggle with basic infrastructure. This uneven distribution exacerbates the achievement gap, as students in well-resourced environments gain access to personalized learning opportunities, while others are left behind (Selwyn, 2019). Addressing these disparities requires systemic efforts to bridge the digital divide, including investments in infrastructure, affordable technology, and inclusive policies that prioritize underserved communities.

Agency and Accountability

The delegation of decision-making authority to artificial intelligence (AI) systems has brought about significant ethical dilemmas, particularly in areas like mental health and education. These challenges center on the complex interplay of agency-how much control is ceded to machines-and accountability-who is responsible for the outcomes of AI-driven decisions. Addressing these issues is crucial to fostering trust, fairness, and transparency in the integration of AI technologies into societal structures.

Decision-Making in Mental Health

AI systems in mental health diagnostics and treatment recommendations often function as "black boxes," making decisions that are not easily interpretable by users or practitioners. This opacity raises significant concerns regarding patient agency, as individuals may struggle to understand or challenge the conclusions drawn by these systems. For example, if an AI diagnostic tool misidentifies a psychological condition, the resulting inappropriate treatment could have profound consequences for the well-being of the patient (Topol, 2019). One primary concern is the potential for AI to undermine patient autonomy. Mental health care is deeply personal and requires a level of empathy and individualized understanding that machines struggle to replicate. AI systems, trained on generalized datasets, may fail to account for the unique cultural, social, and personal contexts that shape the mental health of an individual. As a result, patients may feel disempowered when faced with decisions made by a machine, particularly if those decisions are presented as definitive or non-negotiable (Haque & Khan, 2021). Transparency is another critical issue. For patients to trust AI systems, they need to understand how these systems arrive at their conclusions. However, many advanced AI models, such as deep neural networks, operate in ways that are difficult even for experts to fully explain. This "black-box" nature creates barriers to informed consent, a cornerstone of ethical medical practice (Doshi-Velez & Kim, 2017). Patients have the right to know how their data is being used, what factors contribute to AI-driven decisions, and what alternatives exist. Furthermore, accountability becomes a significant concern in cases of misdiagnosis or harm caused by AI recommendations. If an AI system suggests a treatment that leads to adverse effects, determining responsibility can be challenging. Should the blame fall on the developers who designed the algorithm, the healthcare providers who implemented it, or the organizations that failed to establish adequate oversight? Without clear accountability frameworks, patients may be left without recourse, undermining trust in both AI and the healthcare system as a whole.

Accountability in Education

In the education sector, AI-mediated decision-making has become increasingly prevalent, influencing areas such as grading, admissions, and personalized learning. While these technologies offer the promise of efficiency and objectivity, they also raise pressing ethical questions about accountability and fairness. One area of concern is algorithmic grading. AI systems designed to assess student performance often rely on predefined rubrics and historical data to evaluate assignments or exams. While this approach can reduce the workload for educators, it is not immune to bias or error. For instance, an algorithm trained on historical grading data may inadvertently perpetuate existing disparities, such as penalizing non-native speakers for linguistic differences or favoring students from well-resourced schools (Selwyn, 2019).

When Students Receive Unfair Grades Due to Algorithmic Errors, the Question Arises: Who is Accountable?

Admissions processes driven by AI face similar challenges. Many universities and colleges have begun using algorithms to streamline the review of applications, particularly for large applicant pools. However, these systems often operate on opaque criteria, making it difficult for rejected applicants to understand why they were not admitted. Bias in training data-such as an overrepresentation of affluent or majority demographic groups- can lead to discriminatory outcomes, further entrenching educational inequalities (Williamson, 2020). Accountability becomes particularly critical in cases where AI systems disadvantage students or make erroneous decisions. Educational institutions deploying these technologies must establish clear protocols for addressing grievances and ensuring fairness. Without such mechanisms, AI risks eroding public trust in the education system and exacerbating existing inequities.

Ethical Guidelines and Oversight Mechanisms

To address these challenges, it is essential to establish robust ethical guidelines and accountability mechanisms for AI systems. These measures should be designed to ensure transparency, fairness, and human oversight at every stage of AI development and deployment.

Transparency and Explainability

AI systems must be designed to provide clear explanations of their decision-making processes. This involves creating models that prioritize interpretability, enabling users to understand how specific inputs lead to particular outcomes. For example, instead of presenting a diagnostic conclusion as a binary result, AI systems could offer a breakdown of contributing factors and associated probabilities (Ribeiro et al., 2016).In education, transparency could involve providing students and educators with detailed insights into how grades or admissions decisions were determined. This not only fosters trust but also allows stakeholders to identify and address potential biases or errors in the system.

Human Oversight and Review

Human oversight is critical to ensuring that AI systems remain accountable and aligned with ethical standards. In mental health, this could involve requiring that all AI-generated diagnoses or treatment recommendations be reviewed by a qualified healthcare professional before being presented to patients. Similarly, Educators should have the power to override AI decisions when they conflict with professional judgment.

Ethical Training for Developers and Users

Developers and users of AI systems must receive comprehensive ethical training to understand the potential risks and responsibilities associated with these technologies. For developers, this includes learning how to identify and mitigate bias in training data, as well as designing systems that prioritize fairness and inclusivity. For users, such as educators and healthcare providers, training should focus on understanding the limitations of AI and recognizing when human intervention is necessary.

Accountability Frameworks

Establishing clear accountability frameworks is essential for addressing instances of harm or unfairness caused by AI systems. These frameworks should delineate the responsibilities of developers, deployers, and users, ensuring that all parties are held accountable for their actions. For example, developers could be required to conduct regular audits of their algorithms to assess their impact on different demographic groups, while institutions deploying AI systems could establish grievance mechanisms for affected individuals (Floridi et al., 2018).

Balancing Innovation with Responsibility

The integration of AI into mental health and education presents significant opportunities for innovation but also raises complex ethical dilemmas regarding agency and accountability. To navigate these challenges, stakeholders must work collaboratively to establish ethical guidelines, transparency measures, and accountability mechanisms that prioritize fairness and inclusivity. This requires not only technical expertise but also a commitment to the broader social values that underpin trust and equity. As we continue to integrate AI into critical societal domains, we must balance innovation with responsibility.

Mental Health

AI as a Tool for Accessibility

The advent of AI-driven technologies has transformed the landscape of mental health care, significantly enhancing its accessibility and scalability. This is particularly crucial for individuals in underserved or remote areas, where traditional mental health services are often scarce or inaccessible. AI-powered tools like chatbots and teletherapy platforms offer innovative solutions to bridge this gap, democratizing mental health care in unprecedented ways.

AI Chatbots and Conversational Interfaces

AI chatbots such as Wysa and Woebot serve as virtual mental health assistants, providing conversational interfaces that mimic therapeutic interactions. These chatbots use natural language processing (NLP) to engage users in dialogue, offering real-time support for mild to moderate mental health issues such as stress, anxiety, and depression (Fitzpatrick et al., 2017). Unlike traditional therapy, chatbots are available 24/7, enabling users to seek help whenever needed, without the barriers of stigma or cost. The scalability of these tools makes them particularly valuable in resource-constrained settings. For example, during the COVID-19 pandemic, many individuals turned to AI chatbots for mental health support, given the limited availability of in-person services. Studies have shown that these tools can effectively deliver cognitive-behavioral therapy (CBT) techniques, helping users develop coping strategies and improve emotional resilience (Topol, 2019).

AI in Teletherapy Platforms

Teletherapy platforms enhanced with AI capabilities are revolutionizing how mental health services are delivered. These platforms leverage machine learning algorithms to personalize interventions based on individual needs. Features such as mood tracking, predictive analytics, and tailored coping strategies enable therapists to offer more targeted and effective care (Bentley et al., 2022). For instance, AI can analyze data from wearable devices, such as heart rate variability and sleep patterns, to identify early warning signs of mental health issues. This allows for proactive interventions, reducing the risk of escalation and improving overall outcomes. Additionally, teletherapy platforms equipped with AI can match users with therapists based on compatibility metrics, enhancing the therapeutic alliance and treatment efficacy.

Predictive Models for Early Detection

AI-driven diagnostic systems are at the forefront of early detection and intervention in mental health care. These systems use predictive models to analyze diverse data sources, including social media activity, electronic health records, and wearable device metrics, to identify behavioral patterns indicative of mental health challenges (Bentley et al., 2022). For example, algorithms trained to recognize linguistic markers of depression or anxiety in social media posts can flag at-risk individuals for further evaluation. Similarly, wearable devices that monitor physiological indicators, such as heart rate and activity levels, can provide real-time feedback on mental health status.

Challenges of Cultural Competence and Bias

While AI technologies have made significant strides in expanding access to mental health care, they are not without limitations. One of the most pressing challenges is the lack of cultural competence in AI systems, which often stems from biases in training datasets and algorithm design.

Underrepresentation in Datasets

AI algorithms are typically trained on datasets that overrepresent populations from Western, industrialized nations. This results in tools that are optimized for cultural norms and diagnostic criteria prevalent in these regions, often at the expense of global diversity (Harris et al., 2020). For instance, Western diagnostic frameworks for mental health prioritize emotional and psychological symptoms, whereas many non-Western cultures emphasize physical manifestations of distress, such as fatigue or somatic pain. A lack of representation can lead to significant misdiagnoses or the failure to recognize culturally specific symptoms. For example, an AI system trained exclusively on Western data might misinterpret stoicism in certain Asian cultures as a lack of emotional distress, overlooking underlying mental health conditions. Similarly, behaviors considered normative in some cultures, such as communal grieving or spiritual practices, might be incorrectly flagged as pathological by algorithms lacking cultural sensitivity (Obermeyer et al., 2019).

Stigmatization and Bias

Bias in data and design also extends to the stigmatization of certain groups. Minority populations, including racial and ethnic minorities, LGBTQ+ individuals, and people from low-income backgrounds, are often underrepresented in mental health datasets. This underrepresentation exacerbates inequities, as AI systems may fail to account for the unique needs and experiences of these groups (Noble, 2018). For example, studies have shown that Black and Hispanic individuals are more likely to be misdiagnosed with schizophrenia or other severe mental health conditions compared to white individuals.

This disparity arises from both systemic biases in healthcare and algorithmic bias in AI tools trained on skewed datasets. Similarly, LGBTQ+ individuals may face challenges in accessing AI-driven mental health tools that do not recognize or affirm their identities, further marginalizing these communities.

Addressing Cultural Competence

To address these challenges, developers must prioritize the inclusion of diverse datasets that reflect the full spectrum of human experiences. This includes incorporating data from underrepresented populations, as well as engaging cross-cultural experts in the design and validation of AI systems. For example, community-based participatory research (CBPR) can be used to involve marginalized groups in the development process, ensuring that AI tools are inclusive and culturally relevant (Harris et al., 2020). Additionally, integrating explainable AI (XAI) techniques can help mitigate bias by making algorithmic decisions more transparent and interpretable. This allows stakeholders to identify and address potential sources of bias, fostering greater trust and accountability in AI systems (Floridi et al., 2018).

Ethical and Sociological Implications

The integration of AI into mental health care raises broader ethical and sociological questions, particularly regarding equity, agency, and accountability. While AI has the potential to transform mental health care, its implementation must be guided by principles of fairness, inclusivity, and respect for human dignity.

Equity and Access

Ensuring equitable access to AI-driven mental health tools is a critical challenge. The digital divide remains a significant barrier, with marginalized communities often lacking the infrastructure, digital literacy, and resources needed to benefit from these technologies. Addressing this gap requires targeted investments in digital inclusion, as well as the development of low-cost, user-friendly tools that can reach underserved populations (Topol, 2019).

Agency and Accountability

The delegation of decision-making to AI systems raises questions about agency and accountability. For example, if an AI-driven diagnostic tool produces a misdiagnosis, who is responsible—the developer, the healthcare provider, or the end user? Establishing clear accountability frameworks is essential to ensure that ethical principles are upheld in the design and deployment of AI systems (Floridi et al., 2018).

THE WAY FORWARD

The way forward for AI in mental health and education lies in designing technologies that are culturally sensitive, accessible, and aligned with the values of fairness and inclusivity. Interdisciplinary collaboration and thoughtful policy frameworks will be crucial in guiding the development and deployment of AI systems that serve the public good. By prioritizing equity, transparency, and accountability, we can ensure that AI contributes to a more just and inclusive society. As AI technologies continue to shape the future of mental health and education, it is imperative that we actively design and implement systems that promote equity, cultural sensitivity, and ethical use. The challenges and opportunities presented by AI in these domains require thoughtful and collaborative approaches, drawing on insights from multiple disciplines and sectors. This section explores how AI can be leveraged for social good, the importance of interdisciplinary collaboration, and policy recommendations to ensure the ethical deployment of AI in mental health and education.

Leveraging AI for Social Good

AI has immense potential to drive positive change, particularly in the realms of mental health and education, where access to resources is often limited. However, to realize the potential of AI for social good, we must ensure that these technologies are designed with equity, cultural sensitivity, and inclusivity at the forefront.

Equitable and Culturally Sensitive AI Systems

To create equitable AI systems, it is crucial to prioritize diversity in both the development process and the datasets used to train algorithms. This includes ensuring that mental health diagnostic tools and educational platforms are designed to recognize and respect cultural differences in symptom expression, learning styles, and social norms. AI systems in mental health should be capable of addressing diverse needs, whether it's through multilingual interfaces or culturally specific therapeutic approaches (Bentley et al., 2022). In education, adaptive learning platforms should reflect the varied educational backgrounds and experiences of students from different socio-economic, racial, and cultural groups (Eubanks, 2018). Furthermore, AI systems must be designed with a commitment to accessibility. This includes ensuring that tools for mental health support, such as teletherapy platforms and chatbots, are available to those with limited internet access, especially in rural and underserved communities (Harris et al., 2020). Similarly, in education, policymakers and developers must ensure that AI-driven tools are universally accessible, with particular attention paid to bridging the digital divide.

Community Engagement and Feedback

AI systems can also benefit from ongoing community engagement to ensure that they are relevant and effective for the populations they serve. This involves incorporating feedback from individuals who will directly use AI-powered mental health tools and educational platforms. Participatory design models, where end users are actively involved in the creation and evaluation of AI systems, can help ensure that these technologies align with the needs and values of different communities (Williamson, 2020).

Interdisciplinary Collaboration

The complexity of AI and its impact on society necessitates collaboration across various fields of expertise. Sociologists, historians, technologists, and educators must work together to develop and deploy AI systems that are responsible and beneficial.

Sociological and Historical Insights

Sociologists and historians can provide valuable insights into the social and cultural implications of AI in mental health and education. By analyzing historical trends and societal power dynamics, these scholars can help identify potential risks of AI reinforcing existing inequalities. For instance, the study of past technological interventions in education or healthcare can inform the ethical deployment of AI, preventing the replication of past injustices (Noble, 2018). Sociologists can also contribute by examining how AI systems impact different social groups and identifying any unintended consequences, such as deepening disparities in access or outcomes. They can also advocate for the inclusion of diverse voices in the design and governance of AI technologies to ensure that they reflect the values of all communities.

Collaboration with Technologists and Educators

Technologists, including AI engineers and data scientists, must collaborate with sociologists and educators to ensure that AI systems are not only technically sound but also socially responsible. Educators, in particular, have the practical expertise to evaluate how AI technologies impact teaching and learning. Their input can help ensure that AI tools support human connection, creativity, and critical thinking, rather than undermining these essential aspects of education. Furthermore, interdisciplinary teams can collectively advocate for the inclusion of ethics in AI training curricula for technologists, so that developers are equipped to consider the broader social implications of their work from the outset (Topol, 2019).

Policy Recommendations

Effective policy frameworks are essential for addressing the ethical and social challenges of AI in mental health and education. These policies should be designed to ensure the equitable and responsible use of AI while promoting transparency and accountability.

Regulation of AI in Mental Health and Education

Governments should establish clear regulations to ensure that AI tools in mental health and education adhere to strict ethical guidelines. For example, guidelines should mandate the use of diverse and representative datasets to mitigate bias in AI systems. Additionally, regulatory bodies should enforce transparency requirements, including clear explanations of how AI systems make decisions, especially in high-stakes areas like mental health diagnosis and academic evaluation (Obermeyer et al., 2019).

Addressing the Digital Divide

Policies must focus on reducing the digital divide by investing in broadband infrastructure and affordable access to technology in underserved areas. This will help ensure that AI-powered tools are accessible to marginalized communities, including those in rural or low-income areas. Governments could also incentivize the development of low-cost, high-impact AI solutions that prioritize accessibility and inclusivity (Selwyn, 2019).

Ethical Standards and Accountability Mechanisms

Governments and international organizations should also develop ethical standards for AI in mental health and education. These standards should address key concerns such as privacy, data security, and algorithmic fairness. Additionally, policies should include mechanisms for holding developers and institutions accountable when AI systems result in harm or discrimination. This could include the establishment of independent review boards or oversight committees to evaluate the ethical implications of AI systems before they are widely deployed (Williamson, 2020).

Education and Training

Finally, policymakers should support education and training programs for both AI developers and the public to foster a deeper understanding of the ethical and societal implications of AI. By ensuring that technologists are trained in social responsibility and that users are informed about how AI systems work, we can promote a more informed and equitable use of technology.

Reiterating the Thesis

The role of AI in mental health and education is multifaceted, with the technology reflecting existing societal structures and biases while also offering the potential to reshape them. As discussed, AI systems often mirror societal inequalities, such as racial and gender biases, that are embedded in training datasets, leading to skewed outcomes. These biases can perpetuate disparities in access to mental health care and educational opportunities, reinforcing social divides rather than bridging them. At the same time, AI offers transformative possibilities. In mental health, AI-powered diagnostic tools and teletherapy platforms can provide greater access to care, particularly for underserved populations. In education, AI can personalize learning, adapt to individual needs, and improve educational outcomes. Yet, these innovations are not guaranteed to benefit all equally. The potential of technology to address systemic inequities or exacerbate them depends on how it is developed and deployed. As such, AI serves both as a reflection of the societal conditions from which it arises and as a force capable of altering those conditions, for better or worse.

Call to Action: Shaping AI for an Inclusive Future

Artificial intelligence (AI) has emerged as a transformative force, with its applications influencing a wide range of societal domains, including mental health and education. While its potential for innovation and improvement is undeniable, AI also reflects existing societal structures and can inadvertently perpetuate or exacerbate inequalities. Consequently, we must approach AI development and deployment with a steadfast commitment to equity, inclusivity, and ethical responsibility. This call to action extends to all stakeholders—policymakers, developers, educators, and society at large—urging collective action to guide AI toward serving the greater good.

Designing AI with Fairness at Its Core

To achieve equitable outcomes, fairness must be embedded into the foundational principles of AI design. This entails more than merely eliminating bias; it requires creating systems that actively challenge and dismantle entrenched inequities. Bias in AI often originates from the data used to train these systems. Historical and systemic disparities, when embedded in training datasets, can lead to algorithms that replicate and reinforce discrimination (Obermeyer et al., 2019). For instance, AI-driven hiring tools have been criticized for favoring candidates from privileged backgrounds, as their training data disproportionately reflect past hiring practices (Binns, 2018). In mental health, AI systems can inadvertently perpetuate disparities in care accessibility. AI diagnostic tools trained on datasets predominantly drawn from Western populations may fail to account for cultural and ethnic variations in symptom expression. Such limitations risk marginalizing underrepresented communities and reinforcing healthcare disparities (Haque & Khan, 2021). Addressing these challenges requires intentional efforts to diversify datasets and incorporate cultural competence into AI systems.

In education, the implementation of AI-driven adaptive learning tools has shown promise for personalizing instruction. However, these tools often privilege students in well-resourced schools with robust technological infrastructure, leaving those in underfunded districts at a disadvantage (Selwyn, 2019). By designing AI systems with equity as a guiding principle, developers can prioritize accessibility and inclusivity, ensuring that all students benefit from these innovations regardless of their socioeconomic background.

Embedding Ethics into AI Development

The development and deployment of artificial intelligence (AI) have introduced transformative possibilities across industries, from healthcare to education and beyond. However, the rapid evolution of AI technologies also raises profound ethical challenges that require careful consideration. Embedding ethics into AI development is essential to ensure that these technologies align with societal values, prioritize human well-being, and mitigate potential harm. Ethical AI development involves integrating principles such as transparency, accountability, inclusivity, and privacy into every stage of the AI lifecycle- from design and training to implementation and monitoring.

The Role of Transparency in Ethical AI

Transparency is a cornerstone of ethical AI development, ensuring that stakeholders have a clear understanding of how AI systems function. Transparent AI systems are those whose decision-making processes, underlying algorithms, and limitations are comprehensible to users, developers, and regulators alike.

Explainability and Interpretability

Explainability and interpretability are key aspects of transparency. Explainability refers to the ability of an AI system to provide clear and understandable reasons for its decisions or actions. Interpretability, on the other hand, concerns the degree to which humans can understand the internal workings of an AI model (Floridi et al., 2018). Both are essential for fostering trust and accountability, particularly in high-stakes domains such as healthcare, finance, and criminal justice. For example, in predictive models used for medical diagnoses, patients and clinicians must understand the rationale behind a diagnosis or treatment recommendation. Similarly, in credit scoring algorithms, consumers should have access to explanations for their creditworthiness assessments. By providing such insights, transparent AI systems empower users to make informed decisions and hold developers accountable for errors or biases.

Challenges in Achieving Transparency

Despite its importance, achieving transparency in AI is challenging, particularly with complex machine learning models such as deep neural networks. These models often function as "black boxes," making it difficult to discern how specific decisions are reached. To address this, researchers are exploring techniques such as model simplification, visualization tools, and post hoc explanations. Moreover, transparency must extend beyond technical explainability to include organizational transparency. This involves disclosing the data sources, design choices, and objectives underlying AI systems. Organizational transparency fosters public trust and ensures that AI systems align with societal values.

Accountability Mechanisms for Ethical AI

Accountability is critical to ethical AI development, ensuring that developers and deployers are held responsible for the outcomes of their systems. Without robust accountability mechanisms, there is a risk of harm to individuals and communities, particularly those disproportionately affected by biased or flawed AI systems.

Audits and Impact Assessments

Regular audits of AI systems are a vital accountability measure. These audits assess the performance and impact of AI technologies across different demographic groups, identifying potential biases or inequities. For instance, audits of facial recognition systems have revealed significant disparities in accuracy rates across race and gender, prompting calls for improved dataset diversity and algorithmic fairness (Buolamwini & Gebru, 2018). Impact assessments, such as ethical impact assessments (EIAs) or algorithmic impact assessments (AIAs), provide a structured framework for evaluating the societal implications of AI systems. These assessments consider factors such as fairness, privacy, accessibility, and sustainability, guiding developers in mitigating potential harm.

Legal and Regulatory Frameworks

Legal and regulatory frameworks also play a crucial role in ensuring accountability. Governments and international organizations are increasingly recognizing the need for AI-specific regulations that address issues such as data protection, algorithmic bias, and automated decision-making. For example, the European Union's proposed AI Act aims to establish a comprehensive legal framework for trustworthy AI, including requirements for risk assessments, transparency, and human oversight (European Commission, 2021).

Inclusivity and Accessibility in AI Design

Ethical AI development must prioritize inclusivity and accessibility, ensuring that AI systems serve diverse populations equitably. This involves designing technologies that accommodate users with varying abilities, backgrounds, and levels of technological literacy.

Addressing Bias in AI Systems

Bias in AI systems is a significant barrier to inclusivity. Bias can arise from various sources, including unrepresentative training data, biased labeling practices, and flawed algorithmic assumptions. These biases often result in discriminatory outcomes, disproportionately impacting marginalized communities. For example, language models trained predominantly on Western datasets may fail to recognize dialects or cultural expressions from non-Western contexts. Similarly, recruitment algorithms trained on historical hiring data may reinforce gender or racial disparities in employment opportunities. Addressing these issues requires diverse and representative datasets, as well as rigorous bias detection and mitigation techniques during model training and evaluation.

Designing for Accessibility

Accessibility in AI design involves creating systems that are usable by individuals with disabilities or limited technological expertise. This includes incorporating features such as screen readers, voice recognition, and simplified interfaces. For instance, AI-powered language translation tools can facilitate communication for non-native speakers, while speech-to-text software can benefit individuals with hearing impairments. Designing for accessibility also extends to ensuring affordability and connectivity. In low-income regions, access to AI technologies may be limited by cost or infrastructure constraints. Ethical AI development must address these disparities by creating scalable, cost-effective solutions that expand access to underserved communities.

Privacy and Security in AI Development

Privacy and security are fundamental ethical considerations in AI development, particularly in domains where sensitive data is collected and analyzed. Ensuring robust data protection measures is essential to safeguarding individual rights and preventing misuse.

Safeguarding Data Privacy

AI systems often rely on vast amounts of personal data to train models and generate insights. In sectors such as healthcare, finance, and social media, this data may include sensitive information about individuals' health, financial status, or personal behavior. To protect privacy, developers must adhere to stringent data protection standards, such as anonymization, encryption, and secure storage practices. For example, in mental health applications, AI tools must safeguard patient confidentiality by ensuring that sensitive health data cannot be accessed or exploited by unauthorized parties. Compliance with legal frameworks such as the General Data Protection Regulation (GDPR) is essential to maintaining ethical standards and preventing data breaches.

Balancing Privacy and Utility

Balancing privacy with utility is a key challenge in AI development. While protecting user data is paramount, overly restrictive privacy measures may limit the functionality and effectiveness of AI systems. For instance, anonymizing healthcare data can reduce the granularity of insights, potentially hindering the development of predictive models for disease diagnosis or treatment. To address this trade-off, researchers are exploring privacy-preserving techniques such as differential privacy, federated learning, and homomorphic encryption. These methods enable AI systems to analyze data while preserving individual anonymity, striking a balance between privacy and utility.

Ethical AI in Mental Health

The deployment of AI in mental health care highlights the intersection of ethical considerations such as privacy, accountability, and inclusivity. AI tools in this domain have the potential to revolutionize mental health care by enabling early detection, personalized interventions, and scalable support. However, their ethical deployment requires careful attention to patient rights and well-being.

Safeguarding Privacy and Confidentiality

In mental health applications, safeguarding patient privacy is paramount. AI tools that collect sensitive health data, such as mood-tracking apps or chatbots, must adhere to stringent data protection standards to prevent misuse or unauthorized access. Developers should implement robust encryption protocols and secure storage practices to ensure that patient data remains confidential.

Complementing Human Care

Ethical AI deployment in mental health also involves ensuring that AI tools complement, rather than replace, human healthcare providers. While AI chatbots can provide immediate support for mild to moderate mental health issues, they should not be viewed as substitutes for professional care. For instance, tools like Wysa and Woebot can offer initial guidance and coping strategies, but complex cases should be referred to qualified therapists (Topol, 2019). By integrating AI tools into a broader framework of human-centered care, mental health services can enhance accessibility, scalability, and personalization without compromising empathy or compassion.

Interdisciplinary Collaboration for Inclusive AI

The development of AI systems cannot be the sole responsibility of technologists. Interdisciplinary collaboration is essential to ensure that AI serves the broader good of society. Sociologists, historians, educators, psychologists, and other experts bring valuable perspectives that can inform the design and deployment of AI systems. By working together, these stakeholders can identify potential risks and unintended consequences, fostering a more holistic approach to AI development. For instance, sociologists can help developers understand how AI systems may interact with existing social structures, highlighting potential areas of bias or inequality. Historians can provide insights into the long-term impacts of technological advancements, drawing lessons from past innovations to inform current practices. Educators can offer guidance on how AI systems can be tailored to meet the diverse needs of students, while psychologists can ensure that mental health applications prioritize user well-being and ethical care delivery. This collaborative approach is particularly crucial in addressing the digital divide, which remains a significant barrier to equitable AI deployment. The digital divide refers to the gap between those who have access to modern technology and those who do not, often due to socioeconomic disparities. Interdisciplinary teams can work together to develop strategies for bridging this divide, such as implementing affordable and scalable AI solutions for underserved communities.

Advocating for Robust Policy Frameworks

Governments and international bodies play a critical role in shaping the ethical and equitable use of AI through policy and regulation. Robust policy frameworks are needed to establish clear standards for AI development, deployment, and evaluation. These frameworks should prioritize transparency, accountability, and inclusivity, ensuring that AI systems align with societal values and ethical principles. Transparency requirements should include mandating that AI developers disclose information about their algorithms, including the data used for training and the decision-making processes. This allows regulators, researchers, and the public to scrutinize AI systems and hold developers accountable for their impacts (Whittlestone et al., 2019). Accountability mechanisms should also include legal and financial repercussions for organizations that deploy harmful or biased AI systems. These mechanisms incentivize ethical behavior and ensure that AI developers remain committed to creating systems that benefit all users. Inclusivity should be a cornerstone of AI policy, with regulations requiring that AI systems are designed to serve diverse populations. Governments should also invest in initiatives to expand access to AI technologies, such as providing funding for schools in underprivileged areas to adopt AI-driven educational tools or supporting healthcare providers in implementing AI diagnostic systems.

Shaping Trajectory of AI Through Collective Action

As AI continues to evolve, its trajectory will be determined by the collective actions of stakeholders across society. Policymakers must enact and enforce regulations that prioritize ethical and equitable AI deployment. Developers must commit to designing systems that reflect diverse values and experiences, actively challenging inequities. Educators and mental health professionals must advocate for AI systems that enhance, rather than replace, human-centered practices. Moreover, the general public has a role to play in shaping the future of AI. By staying informed about AI developments and engaging in discussions about their societal implications, individuals can contribute to a broader dialogue about the ethical use of these technologies. Public awareness campaigns, community forums, and educational initiatives can empower citizens to participate in decision-making processes and hold stakeholders accountable for their actions.

CONCLUSION

Artificial intelligence holds immense potential to transform mental health and education, offering innovative solutions to longstanding challenges. However, its impact will depend on how it is developed, deployed, and governed. To ensure AI serves as a tool for social good, we must embed fairness, ethics, and inclusivity into its design, foster interdisciplinary collaboration, and advocate for strong policy frameworks. Concrete actions are necessary to achieve this vision. Policymakers should mandate ethical AI audits to ensure transparency and accountability. Developers must prioritize bias detection and mitigation in AI models. Educational institutions should integrate AI ethics into curricula to equip future leaders with the knowledge to create responsible technology. By committing to these measures, we can shape a future where AI reflects the best of society, promoting justice, inclusivity, and human well-being.

REFERENCES

Bentley, G. R., Holliday, E., & Fourie, E. (2022). Addressing cultural bias in AI for mental health care. *Journal of Medical Ethics*, *48*(6), 455–462. DOI: 10.1136/medethics-2021-107764

Binns, R. (2018). Fairness in machine learning: Lessons from political philosophy. *Proceedings of the 2018 Conference on Fairness, Accountability, and Transparency*, 149–159. DOI: 10.1145/3287560.3287598

Cave, S., Dihal, K., & Coughlan, K. (2020). *AI: A critical introduction*. Sage Publications.

Ceruzzi, P. E. (2003). *A history of modern computing* (2nd ed.). MIT Press.

Cukier, W., & Mayer-Schönberger, V. (2019). *The new digital age: Reshaping the future of people, nations, and business*. John Murray.

Dastin, J. (2018). Amazon's AI recruiting tool shows bias against women. *Reuters*. https://www.reuters.com/article/us-amazon-com-jobs-automation-insight-idUSKCN1MK08G

Eubanks, V. (2018). *Automating inequality: How high-tech tools profile, police, and punish the poor*. St. Martin's Press.

Fitzpatrick, K. K., Darcy, A., & Vierhile, M. (2017). Delivering cognitive behavior therapy to young adults with symptoms of depression and anxiety using a fully automated conversational agent (Woebot): A randomized controlled trial. *JMIR Mental Health*, *4*(2), e19. DOI: 10.2196/mental.7785 PMID: 28588005

Floridi, L., Cowls, J., Beltrametti, M., Chatila, R., Chazerand, P., Dignum, V., Luetge, C., Madelin, R., Pagallo, U., Rossi, F., Schafer, B., Valcke, P., & Vayena, E. (2018). AI4People—An ethical framework for a good AI society: Opportunities, risks, principles, and recommendations. *Minds and Machines*, *28*(4), 689–707. DOI: 10.1007/s11023-018-9482-5 PMID: 30930541

Friston, K. J., Stephan, K. E., Montague, R., & Dolan, R. J. (2014). Computational psychiatry: The brain as a phantastic organ. *The Lancet. Psychiatry*, *1*(2), 148–158. DOI: 10.1016/S2215-0366(14)70275-5 PMID: 26360579

Haque, A., & Khan, S. M. (2021). Artificial intelligence and global health: Opportunities and challenges. *Annual Review of Public Health*, *42*, 51–67. DOI: 10.1146/annurev-publhealth-090419-102511

Harris, J., Khan, A., & Cooper, M. (2020). Cultural barriers in mental health AI: Challenges and strategies. *Journal of Cross-Cultural Psychology, 51*(7), 529–541. DOI: 10.1177/0022022120942201

Herzog, S. (2018). Predicting student retention and academic success in higher education. *New Directions for Institutional Research, 2018*(179), 51–64. DOI: 10.1002/ir.20275

Latour, B. (1992). Where are the missing masses? The sociology of a few mundane artifacts. In Bijker, W. E., & Law, J. (Eds.), *Shaping technology/building society: Studies in sociotechnical change* (pp. 225–258). MIT Press.

McLuhan, M. (1964). *Understanding media: The extensions of man.* McGraw-Hill.

Noble, S. U. (2018). *Algorithms of oppression: How search engines reinforce racism.* NYU Press. DOI: 10.18574/nyu/9781479833641.001.0001

O'Neil, C. (2016). *Weapons of math destruction: How big data increases inequality and threatens democracy.* Crown Publishing.

Obermeyer, Z., Powers, B., Vogeli, C., & Mullainathan, S. (2019). Dissecting racial bias in an algorithm used to manage the health of populations. *Science, 366*(6464), 447–453. DOI: 10.1126/science.aax2342 PMID: 31649194

Rose, N. (1996). *Inventing our selves: Psychology, power, and personhood.* Cambridge University Press. DOI: 10.1017/CBO9780511752179

Selwyn, N. (2019). Should robots replace teachers? AI and education: Exploring the implications of AI for schools and teachers. *Learning, Media and Technology, 44*(2), 144–159. DOI: 10.1080/17439884.2019.1601106

Smith, A., & Kumar, P. (2020). Cultural bias in AI-driven education systems: A global perspective. *International Journal of Educational Technology, 7*(4), 309–325. DOI: 10.1080/17439884.2020.1631235

Susskind, R., & Susskind, D. (2015). *The future of the professions: How technology will transform the work of human experts.* Oxford University Press. DOI: 10.1093/oso/9780198713395.001.0001

Topol, E. J. (2019). *Deep medicine: How artificial intelligence can make healthcare human again.* Basic Books.

Tyack, D. (1974). *The one best system: A history of American urban education.* Harvard University Press.

Watters, A. (2014). *The history of the future of education.*

Whittlestone, J., Nyrup, R., Alexandrova, A., & Dihal, K. (2019). The role and limits of principles in AI ethics: Towards a focus on tensions. *Proceedings of the AAAI/ACM Conference on AI, Ethics, and Society*, 195–200. DOI: 10.1145/3306618.3314289

Williamson, B. (2020). Who owns educational data? Datafication and the governance of education. *Learning, Media and Technology*, *45*(3), 218–231. DOI: 10.1080/17439884.2020.1667824

Chapter 14
Artificial Intelligence in Mental Healthcare: Opportunities, Risks, and Regulations

Ashfaq Jafar
https://orcid.org/0009-0007-0867-1617
National Institute of Technology, Kurukshetra, India

Shabnam Shabnam
https://orcid.org/0000-0002-0239-6518
National Institute of Technology, Kurukshetra, India

Azizuddin Khan
Indian Institute of Technology, Bombay, India

ABSTRACT

The domain of mental healthcare has been transforming rapidly against the backdrop of a global pandemic. The scale of mental health crisis that exists in the world is very high with highly prevalent mental health conditions in all countries. In this scenario, incorporating AI systems into mental healthcare marks a significant milestone in addressing the global mental health crisis. This chapter discusses AI's potential in mental healthcare, the extent of AI's capability in supporting mental health, popular AI platforms and their applications, and the risks and regulations grounded in ethical principles. The chapter emphasizes the necessity of adhering to ethical standards in mental health practices while utilizing AI to elevate the mental health field to provide accessible, cost-effective, and readily expandable services. Establishing strong rules, ensuring transparency, validating AI models, and continuously investing in research and development are all necessary to fulfill this potential.

DOI: 10.4018/979-8-3373-5072-1.ch014

INTRODUCTION

"Our future is a race between the growing power of our technology and the wisdom with which we use it. Let's make sure that wisdom wins" (Hawking, 2018, p. 196).

The eminent Nobel Laureate's observation reminds us of technology's immense capacity to transfigure the world and our lives. In the evolution of the human race, we have witnessed the emergence of various technologies in different forms. The ultimate aim of all technologies has been to manipulate the human environment by applying scientific knowledge to practical aims. With all the groundbreaking technologies coming up, humankind is responsible for using our wisdom while utilizing those advanced methods in different contexts.

Following the industrial revolutions powered by steam (1784) and electricity (1870), the information age, guided by the emergence of digital technology since 1969, has now given way to the age of Artificial Intelligence (AI), creating a significant impact since 2011. The rapid advancements in AI technology have been demonstrating substantial changes in various facets of life. People utilize AI-enabled platforms for completing daily tasks in a fast manner, from drafting an official mail to illustrating a graphical picture or preparing an academic presentation. People tend to perceive it as an efficient and effective strategy to complete tasks easily. Fields such as education, finance, marketing, creative production, healthcare, etc., vehemently take advantage of AI technologies to automate tasks, enhance efficiency, and obtain valuable insights for improving outcomes.

Integrating AI into the domain of mental healthcare marks a significant milestone in the evolution of mental health interventions, especially when considering the current situation in which the mental health paradigm is transforming rapidly, creating immense demand against the backdrop of a global pandemic. This chapter attempts to explore one of the remedies that can be efficiently incorporated into mental healthcare to reduce the gap between the demand and supply – integrating artificial intelligence into mental healthcare; its current trends, future paths, the challenges bound with it, and the regulations that need to be taken grounded from an ethical viewpoint.

ARTIFICIAL INTELLIGENCE (AI)

For a long time, human beings have had a curious idea about machines having intelligence. The classic adventure novel "Gulliver's Travels" satirically presents an engine that can be utilized to generate new sentences, books, or ideas for scholars without investing much intellectual effort (Swift, 2003). Swift's satire anticipates the concept of algorithmic text generation, which he articulated in the year 1726. Currently, AI models have been successful in producing ideas in different forms based on the data trained and the algorithms incorporated. Thus, modern AI is doing more than what Swift's fictional engine is supposed to do. From a psychological point of view, intelligence can be defined as the ability to understand complex ideas, adapt effectively to the environment, learn from experience, engage in various forms of reasoning, and overcome obstacles with careful thought. When it comes to intelligence, which is 'artificial', it is something man-made and related to technology.

In 1955, Stanford Professor John McCarthy coined the phrase artificial intelligence (AI) and defined it as "the science and engineering of making intelligent machines". It is "the technology that enables computers and machines to simulate human learning, problem-solving, decision-making, comprehension, creativity, and autonomy" (Ibm, 2024). AI's basis is algorithms that will facilitate computer programs to conduct quick analysis and transmission of data into valid conclusions. Artificial intelligence is a broad term that denotes technologies performing complex tasks that mimic human intelligence to an extent. Machine Learning (ML) is a branch of AI that is an approach or learning mechanism to achieve the capacity of Artificial Intelligence. ML teaches computers to learn and improve from experience. It encompasses various applications such as Natural Language Processing, pattern recognition, signal processing, and expert systems. ML is categorized into two types, namely supervised and unsupervised learning, based on the method of learning data (Cohen, 2021). The Organization for Economic Co-Operation and Development (OECD) Council on Artificial Intelligence defines AI as "a machine-based system that can, for a given set of human-defined objectives, make predictions, recommendations, or decisions influencing real or virtual environments" (OECD, 2021). To date, modern AI technologies have proved to have immense capacities in different forms and for different functions. Artificial intelligence manifests phenomenal capacities, such as analyzing complex datasets, patterns, relationships, etc. (Bajwa et al., 2021). The emergence of generative AI has further magnified the impact across different domains worldwide, transforming the interactions among individuals and societies (Montag et al., 2023). Generative AI can be described as the method of creating seemingly novel and purposeful content and ideas in the form of text, image, video, and music from the training data, employing adequate computational techniques (Feuerriegel et al., 2023). Adobe Firefly, Dall-E, Midjourney, Chat GPT, Gemini, Claude, Jasper, Runway, etc. are some of the well-received platforms that employ generative AI. These platforms have been transforming the way we communicate and build interactions in a multitude of areas. Interestingly, generative AI chatbots have been used for mental health interventions as well (Siddals et al., 2024).

MENTAL HEALTH CRISIS

The scale of the mental health crisis that exists in the world is very high, with highly prevalent mental health conditions in all countries. The World Health Organization (2022) estimates that one in eight persons worldwide suffers from a mental illness, evaluating that 970 million people in the world are living with a mental disorder. Suicide continues to be a top cause of mortality worldwide, and mental illnesses are the primary source of years spent disabled. Mental health disorders have huge economic repercussions; productivity losses greatly outweigh the direct expenses of care. Additionally, there are significant gaps in governance, resources, services, information, and mental health technologies across all global mental health systems. Low health literacy, widespread stigma, and restricted access to high-quality treatments are some of the barriers that prevent people from getting treatment for mental health issues (World Health Organization, 2022). The undisputed statistics show that mental health needs across the globe are high, but responses are insufficient and inadequate. Thus, dedicating resources to mental health would be instrumental in achieving a better life and future for all.

The traditional strategy of mental health interventions is unable to meet the growing demand (Wainberg et al., 2017), with barriers including the prevalent stigma and inadequate resources intensifying the crisis (Olawade et al., 2024). Accessible, cost-effective, and readily expandable mental health services are deeply valued, considering the prevalence of undertreated and under-resourced mental health issues. Additionally, the discrepancy between the supply and demand for therapies in the field of mental health emphasizes how urgently sophisticated and creative solutions are needed. Here, the approach of integrating AI into mental healthcare instills a sense of hope.

AI'S POTENTIAL IN MENTAL HEALTHCARE

The field of mental health significantly takes advantage of psychological science. As a discipline involved in mental health and well-being, psychology possesses four main goals: describe, explain, predict, change, or control human behavior. These goals are achieved through making accurate observations of behavior, resulting in constructive changes in people's lives. These goals help psychologists understand and influence human behavior. Considering the necessity of understanding complex human behaviors and emotions in mental health, AI is instrumental in imparting insights and solutions that were not attainable to that extent with conventional methods (Nilsen et al., 2022).

The history of incorporating AI for mental health intervention can be descended to the middle of the twentieth century. Joseph Weizenbaum, in the late 1960s, created a chatbot called ELIZA. It was a “computer program for the study of natural language communication between man and machine” (Weizenbaum, 1966). ELIZA was characterized by its ability to mimic a Rogerian psychotherapist who encourages people to examine their thoughts, emotions, and feelings by reflecting their statements to them (*Founding Fathers of Artificial Intelligence*, 2023). In fact, ELIZA was not able to provide insightful responses. Rather, it encouraged users to continue the conversation using keyword recognition and some basic rules for producing replies. Still, people got the feeling that, even though they are interacting with a machine, it genuinely understands our feelings and emotions. This phenomenon can be called the Eliza effect (Academy, n.d.), where people attributed human-like understanding to ELIZA. Despite its rudimentary nature, ELIZA’s impact has been significant and is considered one of the first attempts of its kind. This effort successfully paved the way for many such initiatives to give mental health assistance using technology (Basil, 2022).

In the latter half of the 20th century, computerized cognitive-behavioral therapy (CBT) programs have become popular (Blackwell & Heidenreich, 2021). Likewise, many advanced programs supported by the latest technology have emerged to provide expert solutions for common mental health concerns, based on research evidence. The initial attempts were a little less sophisticated than the AI-powered interventions of today. However, it represented a shift toward using technology to improve the accessibility of mental healthcare. The use of AI in mental healthcare increased exponentially as processing capacity increased. Numerous facets of mental healthcare have been impacted by the development of AI in the twenty-first century, including teletherapy advancements, personalized treatment plans, virtual therapists, early detection of mental health issues, and ongoing monitoring (Minerva & Giubilini, 2023). These modern AI technologies have the potential to elevate the field of mental healthcare by enhancing its efficacy, accessibility, and data-drivenness.

Geoffrey Hinton, a pioneer in AI and the 2024 Nobel laureate, highlighted that digital intelligence is capable of learning far more than the average human. He emphasized that, despite having fewer connections, AI has a better learning algorithm than the human brain (Bennett & Cuevas, 2024). Thus, the impressive capability of AI systems can well be utilized in healthcare, specifically in the domain of mental health, where it's crucial to comprehend complex human behavior and emotions. Microsoft Chief Executive Officer Satya Nadella noted that artificial intelligence (AI) is arguably the most revolutionary technology of the modern era, and its most essential use is in healthcare (Microsoft, 2019). AI technologies have the potential to completely transform the mental healthcare industry by offering methods and suggestions that traditional approaches were unable to provide. It will create tangible benefits by potentially enlarging the availability of mental health services, optimizing treatment outcomes, and reducing stigma (Minerva & Giubilini, 2023).

In short, Artificial Intelligence is guiding a transformative advancement in healthcare, including mental healthcare. Mishra et al. (2022) asserted that AI would promisingly transform the area of healthcare. It is already observable that AI is rapidly evolving and taking position as an effective strategy to complete several tasks in healthcare settings, which were accustomed to believing as a human privilege. There are several reasons for considering AI as a potential paradigm-shifter in mental healthcare. The major reason is the ability of AI to efficiently handle extensive datasets and assist in analyzing intricate relationships and patterns (Bajwa et al., 2021). AI appears to be better than humans at diagnosing some diseases due to its immense capacity to deal with intricate data and recognize patterns (Loh, 2018). Presently, AI has been demonstrated beneficial in diagnosing different psychological disorders using methods that are unattainable for human psychologists. AI accesses patient data from various sources, including wearable technology or personal health record systems, social media posts, internet searches, etc. It can combine and analyze that data easily to identify the patterns, helping in the diagnosis (Walsh et al., 2017).

Considering the barriers of conventional mental health interventions, such as social stigma, lack of self-awareness, etc., AI has a beneficial role in overcoming these barriers. On many occasions, people don't reach out for help from professionals even when they are having a psychological illness. It is because of their lack of awareness about the changes in their mental health status (Gilleen et al. 2010). For example, some of the common symptoms of mental illnesses, such as depression, can be attributed to a sedentary lifestyle, reduced sleep, food patterns, etc. Hence, people experiencing those symptoms will not go for medical advice; rather, they tend to try self-medication. It might be useful for eradicating physical symptoms temporarily, but the actual cause may remain untreated. In contexts like these, AI-enabled tools might be useful for better understanding the individual's mental health status and seeking professional help if needed. Moreover, AI-based systems can facilitate real-time monitoring by transferring information from the patient to experienced professionals (Diaz-Asper et al., 2024). There are AI-enabled applications that can track different aspects of individual behavior and advise the user for medical help, then mental health professionals can assess whether the help is needed or not. Here, there are chances of drawbacks, including the probability of false positives, unnecessarily burdening health systems. In the last few years, health monitoring systems, including mobile applications, have surged in popularity (Vegesna et al., 2016). Research evidence shows a possible relationship between smartphone interaction data and brain structure and function (Huckins et al., 2019).

Another important obstacle in promoting mental health is the stigma associated with mental illness. Stigma is defined by the World Health Organization (WHO) as "a mark of shame, disgrace, or disapproval that results in an individual being rejected, discriminated against, and excluded from participating in a number of different areas of society" (World Health Organization, 2001). Many people who deserve mental health services decide not to pursue them or stop the intervention before completing it. One of the major reasons for making such decisions is the stigma (Corrigan, 2004). The stigma is characterized by reluctance to take mental health services even when they are very much aware of their illness, and they can afford the services they want (Corrigan & Watson, 2002). The problem here is so obvious that people don't want to reveal their illness to someone, especially when it is a mental illness. This issue can be resolved by interacting with an AI-enabled system without any requirement to disclose it to another human being. It would be more comfortable to seek help from an AI than a human psychologist in the case of extreme stigma. If a person is highly apprehensive about being stigmatized for his or her mental illness, the two possible alternatives could be availing support with AI or not availing the cure at all. Generally, in healthcare, people with stigmatized health issues increasingly depend on AI over human healthcare providers (An & Boman, 2022). AI-driven interventions possess the capacity to handle the stigma associated with mental illness by employing tools like chatbots, social media analysis, natural language processing systems, etc. (Loies, 2024), making the development of AI in mental healthcare meaningful and rewarding.

In conditions involving the preference for avoiding human-to-human interaction, AI could be more beneficial than a traditional method. Researchers observed that veterans are more susceptible to sharing their thoughts about their condition in the case of post-traumatic stress disorder (PTSD) when they are interacting with virtual interviewers. These virtual interviewers were found to be far better than humans at gathering data that is relevant in the medical context (Fiske et al., 2019). Generally, in psychological science, human-to-human connection plays an essential role in enhancing well-being, but in situations where it is not preferred, AI can be a practical choice. Additionally, in the circumstance of a global shortage of mental health workers, many practitioners believe AI is a practical solution for the shortage of professionals in the field (Doraiswamy et al., 2020). Moreover, there are some shortcomings in traditional mental health practices. There is evidence of limitations in diagnosis, treatment, and behavioral prediction due to the complexity of conditions. There are findings related to the misgivings in the effectiveness of antidepressants (Almohammed et al., 2022), shortcomings in determining treatment based on genetic characteristics (Tansey et al., 2013), limitations in effectively predicting suicides (Franklin et al., 2017), etc. These shortcomings are obvious when humans deal with complex patterns, creating obstacles in mental healthcare. However, AI proposes strategies to solve the challenge. AI algorithms have already succeeded in accurately predicting suicide attempts using extensive datasets (Walsh et al., 2017). AI can also determine the type of antidepressant to be prescribed based on genetic characteristics and predict appropriate therapy (Drysdale et al., 2016). Thus, by effectively identifying the challenges faced by practitioners in mental healthcare, we can determine how to use AI for greater benefits efficiently. The potential of AI for elevating healthcare, including mental healthcare, is evident if it is used responsibly.

AI IN MENTAL HEALTHCARE: CURRENT TOOLS AND THEIR APPLICATIONS

Currently, modern AI systems have been used for early detection, diagnosis, treatment, therapy, monitoring, and follow-up in mental health interventions. Some chatbots provide support for interventions in anxiety, stress, depression, and other varieties of psychological conditions. The extent of involvement of AI systems in the current mental healthcare system is discussed below.

AI in Early Detection and Diagnosis

Early detection refers to identifying and recognizing the signs and symptoms of psychological disorders before they occur. The early detection approach directs individuals at risk phases who are very close to illness, or individuals who have just reached the stage of disorder but have not developed chronic (Lee et al., 2019). Meticulous attempts have been made in mental healthcare to achieve the best outputs in the process. The advent of AI has marked the emergence of a promising tool in the early detection of mental health disorders (D'Alfonso, 2020). How does AI identify individuals at risk for severe mental health conditions? What are the strategies and methods involved? What is the extent of its efficiency? These questions are relevant and originate from curiosity.

As mental health disorders are characterized by complex factors related to the individual, socioeconomic, and clinical aspects, detecting their signs is supposed to be done with the right strategy. Dealing with language is one way. As the popular phrase suggests, language is the window to the human mind. Prominent author and historian Yuval Noah Harari argued that language is the operating system of human beings (Harari, 2023), which is why AI research and efforts have been focused on tackling that system as well. AI-driven tools have succeeded in analyzing the language content in different forms to detect the signs of mental health disorders. Another way can be analyzing electronic health records to detect changes that can be a sign of a mental health condition. Thus, mainly there are two prominent methods in this regard: 1) by analyzing speech, text, and facial expressions, and 2) by analyzing electronic health records.

Analyzing Speech, Text, and Facial Expressions

AI-enabled systems have proven effective in analyzing speech, text, and facial expressions. The language data significant for prediction is being obtained through different technologies to an increasing extent. These systems will also facilitate empathetic conversation for self-management of anxiety and depression (Diaz-Asper et al., 2024). Natural Language Processing techniques can be tailored to obtain significant findings from spoken or written words (Zhang et al., 2022). Another important technique for analyzing language data is sentiment analysis, a subfield of natural language processing. The objective of sentiment analysis is to evaluate the language part generally in the form of text in the digital environment to understand the underlying emotion in a particular situation (Benrouba & Boudour, 2023). Sentiment analysis is characterized by dealing with a large quantity of text to decide whether that expression denotes a positive, negative, or neutral sentiment (Birjali et al., 2021). Sentiment analysis is executed using ML techniques. In this method, the input text and a large list of emotion types would be submitted to the ML pipeline to determine the underlying sentiment. The process generally involves some systematic steps, including preprocessing input data, feature extraction for formulating proper text, feature selection, and sentiment classification. The latest methods of sentiment analysis have implications in several domains such as marketing, politics, sociology, finance, health, etc. For instance, in the field of mental healthcare, sentiment analysis can recognize delicate variations in a person's emotional condition by scrutinizing personal journals, social media posts, or digital conversation records (Uban et al., 2021), which might be instrumental during the early detection of mental illness.

Language can also be articulated in spoken form, involving voice. Voice plays a pivotal role in signaling mental health conditions in advance. Evidence suggests that the human voice may change because of diseases. With the help of technology and AI, we can conduct voice collection and analysis to detect early signs of stress and depression (Tokuno, 2017). A human voice is a versatile way of communication that can produce various sounds. There can be variations in tone, pitch, and rhythm, sometimes as potential signals of psychological disorders. Voice analysis can efficiently identify these variations with the help of AI (Flanagan et al., 2021). Interestingly, ML algorithms can recognize vocal properties that screen persons with psychological disorders (Villongco & Khan, 2020).

Additionally, modern AI technology has the potential to capture and analyze slight changes in involuntary facial expressions that may facilitate the understanding of underlying mental health conditions (Zhao & Li, 2019). Micro-expressions are often nearly impossible to detect with human eyes, making them difficult to analyze (Ekman, 2002). Therefore, AI systems accompanied by computerized vision and machine learning algorithms address this limitation by employing automatic micro-expression analysis.

The ongoing trend in this area involves developing AI systems to make better perceptions of subtle, significant changes in mental health conditions, with high precision. As AI systems continue to advance, they possess the immense capacity to detect the early signs of psychological disorders, contributing to timely intervention and cure.

Analyzing Electronic Health Records

AI systems have been proven to have the potential to analyze data from electronic health records (EHRs), facilitating early diagnosis of psychological problems (Davenport & Kalakota, 2019). ML algorithms have shown an incredible capacity to scrutinize the information obtained from digital records. ML algorithms have been trained to quickly go through large records, including patient histories, details of the diagnostic tests administered, and comprehensive clinical notes to pinpoint specific tendencies and features indicating a psychological disorder (Iyortsuun et al., 2023). Moreover, AI systems can be supportive in organizing and updating a patient's medical data by adding relevant insights from electronic health record systems. This approach will strengthen the effort to maintain a complete health profile of a person, enabling better care while considering the unique characteristic patterns of that individual (Yu et al., 2023). These practices will aid in promoting early detection of mental health disorders, positioning AI as a promising strategy in mental healthcare.

AI in Treatment

Treatments in the domain of mental healthcare can include psychotherapy, medication, lifestyle changes, complementary and alternative medicine, support groups, etc. Generally, a mental health professional will assess the symptoms and discuss the treatment options with the person. An ideal treatment can be carried out by following a biopsychosocial intervention approach, considering the importance of the biological, social, and psychological aspects of the illness. George Engel proposed this model of mental health in 1977 (Engel, 1977). In this regard, three main types of interventions will be worked together: psychotherapy, psychopharmacology, and psychiatric social work. In this context, how AI can be beneficial in elevating the current practices must be discussed. In the treatment of mental healthcare, AI's role is mainly centered on employing virtual therapists and chatbots, personalizing treatment plans, assisting practitioners in various tasks, and monitoring and follow-up.

AI for Personalized Treatment

Understanding individual patients and customizing interventions for each individual has been an important challenge in psychological treatment (Cohen et al., 2021). Optimizing therapy by considering various individual factors can create a better outcome. Traditionally, it has been done with expert clinical assessments, thus, it might have limitations while depending on intuitive judgment. Modern methods grounded in advanced technology have proved effective in developing individualized treatments. Machine learning algorithms can examine large amounts of data to determine the unique attributes of an individual and his or her needs based on the identified features (Mohsin et al., 2023). Individual characteristics include genetic predispositions, medical conditions, personality traits, cognitive abilities, behavioral patterns, socio-economic status, etc. Identifying these characteristics will contribute to the development of personalized treatment plans. Researchers have efficiently established AI algorithms to determine the possible antidepressant outcomes based on a patient's genetic predisposition (Lin et al., 2018). Traditionally, treatment methods followed a single strategy for almost every patient based on the symptoms and the therapist's judgment, without giving much emphasis to the subtle individual differences that may not be obtained with conventional tools. Now, AI systems can facilitate the process of building treatment strategies corresponding to the unique characteristics of individuals (Gual-Montolio et al., 2022). In short, AI-enabled personalization of psychological treatment will enhance efficacy by enabling data-driven decision-making.

AI for Monitoring and Follow-Up

AI systems have been showing groundbreaking applications in the monitoring and follow-up of psychological treatment. AI-based wearable devices transfer data from the client to the therapist, potentially facilitating real-time monitoring (Diaz-Asper et al., 2024). The last few years have shown an increased interest in utilizing AI-driven monitoring systems in psychological science. For instance, Aura Ring is a wearable health monitoring system that observes heart rate variability, sleep patterns, and other biomarkers. The major advantage of wearable devices is their ability to continuously monitor nuanced changes in behavior, contributing to the early detection of mental health conditions. Further, it is quite important to note that these AI-based health monitoring systems have some risk elements concerning the privacy and safety of the individual.

AI for Therapist Assistance

Another application of AI that many of the practicing psychotherapists have been trying and promoting is its potential to be used as an assistance tool in therapy. By its incredible and exceptional capacity to analyze vast data and provide data-driven insights, it can assist therapists in making accurate therapeutic decisions (Alowais et al., 2023). 'Cerebral' is an AI-based online platform that assists mental health practitioners in their professional tasks (Cerebral Inc., n.d.). Additionally, when the client is not responding to the therapeutic technique provided, AI can suggest another possible course of action by analyzing the medical profile to assist the therapist in deciding an alternative. In that way, AI is equipped to help mental health practitioners with a multitude of tasks, including work administration, client monitoring, clinical documentation, and data analysis (Bohr & Memarzadeh, 2020).

Virtual Therapists and Chatbots

AI-based virtual therapists and chatbots have revolutionized the provision of accessible and cost-effective mental health support (Mehta, 2024). They are also a trendsetter these days. The major highlight of these systems is the ability to provide services despite geographical boundaries, time restrictions, or other limitations based on social and cultural aspects. For instance, Chat GPT and other chatbots based on its technology can deliver consequential outcomes to support mental healthcare (Pandya et al., 2024). A chatbot named 'Replika' is used by more than two million people, using a marketing caption, "the AI companion who cares: always here to listen and talk, always on your side" (*Replika*, n.d.). The important thing is that people want someone to listen to and support their mental health. Here, chatbots efficiently take the position by giving support in a human-like, text-based conversation to their physical space at any time. The major advantages of chatbots include anonymity and reduced stigma, specialist referral, the potential for scalability, support for data-driven insights, improved accessibility, continuity of care, and long-term support (Denecke et al., 2021).

Even though chatbots provide an accessible platform for mental health support with several advantages, there are some concerns regarding how these interactions will continue to evolve because of the "black box" characteristics of algorithms (De Freitas et al., 2023). We cannot predict what the response would be from a chatbot. The impact of these technologies on the interaction with people from vulnerable populations is also a concern. Extreme cases of chatbots giving destructive advice could even result in death (Walker, 2023).

POPULAR AI TOOLS IN MENTAL HEALTHCARE

AI-enabled platforms have become trending in mental healthcare because of their accessibility, affordability, and the potential to provide scalable services. Below are some widely used mental health care tools:

1. **BetterHelp:** BetterHelp is an AI-powered online therapy platform that connects clients with the appropriate therapist based on the individual's requirements. AI facilitates the best match between client and therapist. It offers different therapies from around 32000 qualified therapists (BetterHelp, n.d.). It has been reported that the platform significantly helps reduce the symptoms of depression (Marcelle et al., 2018).
2. **Talkspace:** Talkspace is another AI-driven online platform that matches clients with clinicians based on their needs and offers remote counseling and therapy (Talkspace, n.d.).
3. **Woebot:** Woebot is a popular chatbot that provides CBT-based therapy for depression and anxiety (Woebot Health, 2024). The Woebot AI chatbot has been reported to have helped reduce depression symptoms in individuals, making it an influential method in treating and preventing depression (Qi, 2024).
4. **Wysa:** Wysa is a platform for chatbot-based therapy with over five million users. It gives support for different mental health conditions such as depression, anxiety, stress, and disorders related to sleep (*WYSA - Everyday Mental Health*, n.d.). Users reported it as an effective tool for supporting mental well-being (Legaspi et al., 2022).
5. **Calm:** Calm is an app that offers meditation and relaxation techniques through guided practice. It is characterized by providing bed stories and relaxation music for better sleep, mindfulness, and meditation programs, breathing exercises, etc. (*Calm*, n.d.). Users confirmed the app's effectiveness in improving sleep using the meditation components provided (Huberty et al., 2021).
6. **Moodfit:** Moodfit is an AI-enabled app that monitors and analyzes users' moods and emotions. It offers personalized reports to identify the best strategy to manage emotions (*MoodFit*, n.d.)
7. **Happify:** Happify is an app that helps to build skills for lasting happiness by utilizing the latest innovations in positive psychology, CBT, and mindfulness. It also features an AI coach named 'Anna'. Happify is an activity-based, game-oriented platform (*Happify: Science-Based Activities and Games*, n.d.).
8. **Headspace:** Headspace is an AI-enabled app that offers personalized meditation practices for users. It provides guided meditation, AI guidance, sleep resources, and expert-led programs supporting mental health (*Meditation and Sleep Made*

Simple - Headspace, n.d.). It has been reported that using Headspace resulted in beneficial changes in mental health among youngsters (Pierce et al., 2024).

9. **DBT Coach:** DBT Coach is an AI-based emotional health app that provides tools and resources exclusively for practicing dialectical behavior therapy (DBT). DBT focuses on helping people to accept the reality of life and to adapt to change by healthily managing emotions and behavior. DBT involves substituting inappropriate behaviors with effective skills, including mindfulness, interpersonal effectiveness, emotional regulation, and distress tolerance (Linehan & Wilks, 2015).
10. **CBT Companion:** CBT Companion is an AI-driven app that helps users learn about cognitive behavioral therapy (CBT). It is a comprehensive behavioral health platform that facilitates the understanding of CBT principles to support better interaction with the therapist (*CBT Companion - a Comprehensive App for Cognitive Behavioral Therapy*, n.d.).
11. **MindShift CBT:** MindShift CBT is an app that provides CBT practices for anxiety and OCD by providing features including healthy habits training, coping cards, thought journals, belief experiments, etc. It uses interactive cognitive tools for quick relief from anxiety symptoms (*Anxiety Canada*, 2024).
12. **PTSD Coach:** It is a popular personalized mobile app developed by the US Department of Veterans Affairs, which is being used in more than 100 countries. It helps to understand and manage the symptoms of PTSD by providing scientific information about the disorder and its treatment, mechanisms for observing symptoms, quick links for expert support, etc. (*VA.gov | Veterans Affairs*, n.d.). PTSD is an anxiety disorder that occurs as a result of experiencing a traumatic incident (Hamblen, 2009).
13. **SuperBetter:** SuperBetter is an app that uses gamified mechanisms to promote youngsters' mental health. It offers challenges and rewards to enhance self-resilience and motivation (*SuperBetter: Empower Youth Mental Health*, n.d.).
14. **Kintsugi:** Kintsugi is a smart mental health platform that offers voice analysis to provide real-time emotional feedback, mainly to assist therapists (*Kintsugi*, n.d.).
15. **IBM's Watson Health:** IBM Watson Health is a smart healthcare platform that uses artificial intelligence to analyze patient data, suggest diagnoses, make treatment recommendations, etc. It offers AI-powered chatbots for patient-friendly support (*Chatbot for Healthcare - IBM Watsonx Assistant*, n.d.).
16. **Cerebral:** Cerebral is a smart mental health platform designed to support therapists in developing personalized treatment plans for psychological disorders. It also provides several mental health tests for free related to anxiety, depression, ADHD, etc., and facilitates communities of LGBTQIA+ and military veterans (Cerebral Inc., n.d.).

RISKS AND REGULATIONS

"Without these conversations with the chatbot, my husband would still be there". In 2023, a young Belgian man committed suicide after interacting with a chatbot, highlighting the risks of AI in vulnerable populations, especially when it is being implemented in the mental health domain. The above quotation is attributed to the man's widow, according to the reports (Walker, 2023). Recently, a mother in Florida filed a lawsuit against a chatbot for her 14-year-old son's suicide. The mother accused a California-based startup, alleging that the chatbot presented itself as a licensed therapist, encouraged suicidal ideations, and engaged in sexualized conversations, which would be considered serious abuse if it were from a human (Jazeera, 2024). These reports highlight AI's life-threatening risks when presented with human-like interactions. Even in the context of the possible extreme risk of AI with its rapid growth, the ongoing research on safety measures is severely deficient, with an estimated 1-3 percent of publications only (Bengio et al., 2024).

Artificial intelligence is altering the area of well-being and changing the mental healthcare sector. However, this shift raises concerns about ethical issues and regulatory challenges even as it creates possibilities for access, affordability, early diagnosis and action, and customization of treatment programs (Naik et al., 2022). Psychology and healthcare professions have a strong tradition and expectation of adherence to ethical principles. Exploring how AI interacts in the field of mental health is important, where complex human behaviors and emotions are involved. It is essential to ensure the responsible and constructive implementation of these technologies. It has been reported that more people depend upon generative AI chatbots like OpenAI's ChatGPT for mental health support despite knowing its uncertain risks (Gilbert, 2024). The major risks include offering inefficient or dangerous responses, exploiting vulnerable populations, producing biased responses due to possible biases in training data, therapeutic misconceptions, etc. (Khawaja & Bélisle-Pipon, 2023). Additionally, it is even more important to note that the framework of generative AI models hints at its limitations in promising the validity and contextual sensitivity of information, often resulting in inappropriate responses from users (De Freitas et al., 2023).

Yuval Noah Harari argued that it is needed to regulate artificial intelligence carefully, as we have regulated mechanisms to protect humans from nuclear weapons since 1945 (Harari, 2023). He also suggested governments make it mandatory to disclose that it is AI if someone is having an interaction or conversation with an AI-enabled system. Thus, experts raise alarming concerns about the need for intelligible policy frameworks to develop AI systems. Hence, when it comes to mental healthcare, it is even more important as it is a more sensitive area with confidential data involved. Thus, it is imperative to analyze the possible risks of AI and the regulations required while integrating it into the mental health field. Two notable documents of International AI guidelines are *'Ethics and Governance of Artificial Intelligence for Health: WHO Guidance'*, published by the World Health Organization (*WHO Guidance*, 2021), and *'Ethics Guidelines for Trustworthy AI'* (AI HLEG, 2019), published by the European Union. These documents overlap in some significant directions, which emphasizes the emerging international consensus for developing ethical AI systems.

Disadvantages of AI in the Mental Health Field

Scientific research and publications have emphasized the disadvantages of using AI in mental healthcare. Some of them are the following:

- Many AI models are trained on limited or non-diverse datasets, leading to biased or non-generalizable results (Chen et al., 2024; Kourou et al., 2023; Maekawa et al., 2024).
- Most AI tools rely on subjective self-reported data, which results in inaccuracies or biases (Jaroszewski et al., 2019; Kourou et al., 2023).
- In some situations, balancing sensitivity and specificity can be challenging. To achieve a positive outcome in one area, AI models sacrifice or compromise another (Adler et al., 2022; Cook et al., 2016).
- AI models may perform well on training data but fail to generalize to new populations (Bailey et al., 2018; Scodari et al., 2023).
- Data from smartphones or wearables must be securely stored to protect confidentiality to address ethical and privacy concerns (Busk et al., 2020).
- Ensuring transparency and patient autonomy is critical but often inadequately addressed (Nicole Nadine Lonfeldt et al., 2023; Tsui et al., 2021).
- "Black-box" models prevent interpretability, making it difficult to trust or refine their predictions (Choo et al., 2024; Jha et al., 2021).
- High costs and technical complexities create obstacles in implementation, especially in low-income countries or low-resource settings (Kleinau et al., 2024).
- AI chatbots may misunderstand users, provide irrelevant responses, or fail to engage patients effectively (Fulmer et al., 2018; Klos et al., 2021).
- Models trained on specific populations may not work for others, creating bias or inequities, further exacerbating the disparity in the field (Maekawa et al., 2024; Chen et al., 2023).

These disadvantages highlight the need for improved data quality, transparency, and ethical safeguards in the use of AI in the mental health field.

Bias in AI Models

One of the major challenges of using Artificial Intelligence in mental healthcare is the possible bias in its models. Like any other technology, AI requires human input in the training phase, and humans are not free from bias or errors. AI systems often reflect the biases in the training data, resulting in inaccurate suggestions for diagnosing and treating psychological disorders. Researchers and policymakers have expressed apprehensions about the gender and racial bias of different AI-based technologies, especially as AI gains momentum in healthcare (Parikh et al., 2019). Biases can result in serious consequences, especially when they contribute to discrimination or injustice. Biased models have the potential to intensify and deteriorate existing prejudices, often resulting in systemic injustice and inequality. For instance, there is evidence of sex and gender differences in chronic diseases, including mental health conditions (Kuehner, 2017). Thus, gender or sex biases must be eliminated from AI models as it is designed for interventions in mental health. It is imperative to detect possible biases in data and algorithms to promote data-driven decision-making with fairness. Different types of bias can occur in the case of AI from sources such as algorithm, cognitive, exclusion, confirmation, measurement, out-group homogeneity, prejudice, recall, selection, etc. (Holdsworth, 2023). Fairness is fundamental in improving mental health with AI. Biases in training data or algorithms lead to discriminatory care and treatment, increased discrepancies in the diagnosis of psychological disorders, inequalities in accessing mental health support, and errors in treatment outcomes, altogether perpetuating health disparities (Agarwal et al., 2023). For instance, if AI algorithms are mainly trained on data from a specific demographic group, they may not represent individuals from other demographic categories. Depending on different cultural components, psychological disorders and their outcomes might differ for people from various cultures (Bhugra, 2006). So, the representation of every category of people must be ensured to avoid misdiagnosis and inappropriate treatment recommendations. The biases in AI algorithms can exacerbate the condition of individuals with mental illness if they are underrepresented in the training phase (Nazer et al., 2023).

One mitigation strategy to avoid bias is diversifying the training data as much as possible by incorporating contributors from various categories, including practitioners from disempowered and underprivileged groups. This will contribute to making AI systems ethical and efficient for promoting mental health. It is crucial to make sure AI-based therapies are equitable for people from all walks of life who need mental health support. Additionally, it is even more essential to recognize that addressing the possibility of bias in every stage of the AI life cycle is paramount in this regard (Chen et al., 2023). It is also important to train and encourage AI chatbots to use gender-just terminologies which are essential while interacting with people who are the victims of gender-based discrimination or violence (Wang et al., 2023).

In clinical settings, generalizing the task applied for clinical prediction and building different models based on different contexts can be implemented for making unbiased clinical decisions (Shameer et al., 2018). Additionally, algorithmic stewardship programs must be carried out frequently to monitor and evaluate algorithms (Eaneff et al., 2020). Moreover, Reddy et al. (2020) stressed the necessity of setting up a data governance panel comprised of clinical experts, lawmakers, and AI researchers to review the datasets and algorithms to ensure their representative nature and efficiency.

Ultimately, the aim of fully avoiding biases is to ensure inclusivity. The WHO and the EU guidelines for ethical AI have listed inclusiveness, equity, diversity, nondiscrimination, and fairness as the key objectives. The concept of inclusivity suggests that AI systems utilized in mental healthcare should be "intentionally designed to promote the broadest possible and equitable utilization and access, irrespective of factors such as age, gender, income, ability, or other distinguishing characteristics" (Mennella et al., 2024).

Privacy and Security

As far as the discipline of psychology is concerned, maintaining the confidentiality of patient data is indispensable and part of ethical obligations. American Psychological Association (APA) instructed clearly that "psychologists have a primary obligation and take reasonable precautions to protect confidential information obtained through or stored in any medium, recognizing that the extent and limits of confidentiality may be regulated by law or established by institutional rules or professional or scientific relationship." (*Ethical Principles of Psychologists and Code of Conduct*, 2017). Considering this ethical code of conduct related to data privacy, how we can protect the privacy and security of individuals while interacting with AI systems is a matter of concern. Individuals frequently use AI-based systems for mental health support, often letting the AI handle sensitive information without understanding the potential for data breaches. Confidential data can be intercepted if the communication channels are not secured with appropriate encryption (Goodman, 2024). Mobile apps generally face increased data privacy threats (Parker et al., 2019). Users report such experiences resulting in the inhibition of usage of such apps in healthcare (VonHoltz et al., 2015). Hence, AI-based mental health support platforms must follow appropriate guidelines to safeguard sensitive information such as treatment records, behavioral data, or patient histories from unlawful access or breaches. In the context of neural data analytics involving brain-computer interfaces aimed to provide neuroscience interventions, which are significant in mental healthcare, privacy concerns such as mind reading, mental privacy, and threats related to BCI governance must be addressed (Drew, 2019). Additionally, it is even more important to define data ownership and receive consent from the clients (Bukowski et al., 2020). The beneficiaries of health services often emphasize patient autonomy and informed consent as the prime concerns from an ethical viewpoint (Wangmo et al., 2019). Ultimately, individuals must have the authority over the data being shared and the right to know how the data will be utilized for AI-driven interactions (Olawade et al., 2024). Developers need to provide clear disclaimers to the users regarding the system's constraints and encourage them to seek expert help if necessary (Imran et al., 2023).

Maintaining the Human Element

Experts often emphasize the need for human involvement while developing and managing AI systems. They call it ideal technology (Diaz-Asper et al., 2024). The same can be attributed to the limitation that restricts the pace of growth of AI technology when we are stressing human agency in all the phases of development. Yet, most importantly, in the attempt to integrate AI into the domain of mental healthcare, a sufficient amount of human involvement is needed, which is lacking. Preserving the human element is important when AI takes control of the tasks in mental healthcare, which human experts did before. Maintaining the human element refers to protecting the capacity of human beings to control, to an extent, when the decision-making is allocated to AI. For a psychologist, human agency is significantly related to professional autonomy. If decision-making in psychological practice solely depends on AI systems instead of human expert judgment, it will result in the loss of autonomy in the professional context (Zicari et al., 2021). Maintaining the human element in therapy while utilizing AI as a tool is a crucial ethical consideration. AI should enhance rather than replace the therapeutic alliance between patients and therapists (Siala & Wang, 2022). Psychotherapy is generally considered as talk therapy, it is the art of asking questions, empathetically listening, and responding. Here, spontaneous decision-making and a human element are said to be crucial. EU guidelines (AI HLEG 2019) mandate the protection of the human role in the decision-making process. Likewise, the WHO guidance also underscores that human autonomy should not be overshadowed by the extension of machine autonomy (*WHO Guidance*, 2021).

EU guidelines suggest three possible mechanisms to achieve human oversight on AI systems. These are framed as "human-on-the-loop" (human involvement in the design phases and monitoring while it operates), "human-in-the-loop" (humans have complete control over the system and they can sanction or reject any decisions), and "human-in-command" (humans supervise the overall AI system activity and determine when and how to use AI, thus giving more autonomy to humans) (AI HLEG, 2019). The practicability of human involvement in the current areas of AI in psychological science varies based on the intended use of the platform. Diaz-Asper et al (2024) opined that in the case of AI tools that only collect, process, and transmit data, continuous human involvement is not necessary, as the intervention of AI is not directly impacting. But in the case of AI tools discovering high-risk conditions, or managing people with severe psychological issues, a small error would have larger consequences, where human verification is always needed. Most importantly, the human expert must be aware of an AI system's decision-making capacity and limitations. This is to avoid blind trust in AI-made predictions purposefully. This potential problem is called "automation bias" (Goddard et al., 2012), and WHO guidance considers it a threat to human agency. Additionally, an "ethical by design" approach (Leidner & Plachouras, 2017) can be followed to promote ethical practice, ensuring the system has been designed through ethically bound processes.

Transparency and Explainability

Ensuring transparency and explainability of AI systems is crucial to promoting the development of ethical and responsible AI. The system of AI must be understandable for users, developers, policymakers, regulators, and security engineers. The extent of transparency should be documented and shared for scrutiny before designing and implementing the system. Additionally, the document's language explaining the system must be within the comprehension capacity of the intended audience (Mennella et al., 2024). Transparency and intelligibility are frequently debated and discussed challenges of AI (Chandler et al., 2020). The WHO guidance (*WHO Guidance,* 2021) stresses revealing key information about AI systems, datasets, processing strategies, and algorithms. This is intended to give an idea about the merits and demerits of the system, not only to the developers but also to the users of these technologies. The explanation is multifaceted, emphasizing user-centered explainable AI where three categories of recipients or the target audience join: AI researchers and developers, domain experts, and common users (Ribera & Lapedriza, 2019). Regarding the discipline of psychology and mental health, the APA ethics code (American Psychological Association, 2017) mandates psychologists to ensure the explainability of assessment results to the individuals involved. The WHO guidance on AI further directs that AI systems should be "explainable to the extent possible and according to the capacity of those to whom the explanation is directed" (*WHO Guidance,* 2021). However, for most AI tools, the "black box" nature of algorithms restricts transparency and explainability. The black box refers to the nature of AI systems to hide their internal logic from the users (Guidotti et al., 2018). The level of explainability may vary depending on the AI model type.

The ideal strategy to promote explainability is to provide the user with information about the training data, including the data size and ethnic composition, performance, validation, etc. (Gebru et al., 2021). Further, it is important to note that, in mental healthcare, the credibility and trustworthiness of clinical decisions rely on the ability of the psychotherapist to explain the rationale behind choosing a specific AI-driven treatment approach as an effective remedy for a client. Hence, interpretability is the key to building trust in mental healthcare.

Accountability and Responsibility

Accountability and responsibility can be ensured by effectively implementing 'human assurance,' in which clients and health practitioners can supervise the system both in the antecedent and subsequent phases of designing the algorithm. The main objective is to validate the algorithm's effectiveness and ethical accountability to be appropriate for administration in healthcare (Mennella et al., 2024). Accountability for AI system development, clinical data utilization, and evaluation are necessary prerequisite for maintaining a responsible AI system (Norgeot et al., 2020).

Human-Centric AI

In the attempt to integrate AI into mental healthcare, AI systems must meet certain criteria of care to be efficient. There are criticisms of the rapid growth of AI in healthcare, leading to treating humans as commodities rather than individuals (Quinn et al., 2021). For instance, the United Kingdom is witnessing a significant shift in the delivery of mental health services from human experts to AI-driven systems due to their accessibility and cost-effectiveness, without really giving the option to choose (Cotton, 2021). The possible consequence of this would be the distraction of interpersonal processes of psychotherapy. Agarwal et al. (2020) proposed a 'value-centered' approach focusing on the core facets of value: preferences, precision, and process to mitigate this challenge. Bringing humanness by developing human-centric AI that enhances human abilities and well-being rather than replacing human roles is paramount, especially in the mental health field. Humanness is simply the quality of being human. This is characterized by attributes such as empathy, human-like experience, recognition, etc. These elements must be attached to AI systems to satisfy the conditions of care systems (Dalton-Brown, 2020). Despite the awareness that they are interacting with a machine, individuals tend to feel comfortable engaging in empathetic conversation beyond functional purposes with AI systems when they possess some human characteristics (Fosch-Villaronga & Albo-Canals, 2019). One possible pitfall is the chance of deceiving older patients by making them perceive the systems as real humans (Yew, 2020). For instance, in the case of people with neurodegenerative disorders, such as dementia, they may fail to distinguish whether they are interacting with a technology system or a human (Wangmo et al., 2019).

Trustworthy AI

Developing trustworthy AI is of the greatest importance in the mental health domain. EU guidelines (AI HLEG, 2019) stress this dimension. An AI system needs to respect all the relevant laws and regulations and maintain a strong nature from a technical and social standpoint, along with adhering to ethical principles. AI HLEG (2019) proposed seven requirements for trustworthy AI, which are "human agency and oversight (fundamental rights, human agency, and human oversight), technical robustness and safety (resilience to attack and security, fall back plan and general safety, accuracy, reliability, and reproducibility), privacy and data governance (respect for privacy, quality and integrity of data, and access to data), transparency (traceability, explainability, and communication), diversity, non-discrimination, and fairness (avoidance of unfair bias, accessibility and universal design, and stakeholder participation), societal and environmental well-being (sustainability and environmental friendliness, social impact, society, and democracy), and accountability (auditability, minimization and reporting of negative impact, trade-offs, and redress)".

Artificial Wisdom

Technically, the word intelligence does not denote the technological requirements of an evolving society (Siala & Wang, 2022). Especially in mental health, the word wisdom aligns well with the continuing experiences of individuals and society. Even though both terms are related to learning and understanding, there is a difference. Intelligence is "the ability to think logically, to conceptualize and abstract from reality. Wisdom is the ability to grasp human nature, which is paradoxical, contradictory, and subject to continual change" (Clayton, 1983). Therefore, the future demand for AI technology is Artificial Wisdom as suggested by Jeste et al. (2020). The development of Artificial Wisdom necessitates interdisciplinary collaborations (Littmann et al., 2020) and emphasizes understanding and empathy (Wangmo et al., 2019) to promote mutual decision-making in highly uncertain scenarios. It will enhance collaborations among psychologists and other mental health practitioners, as well as experts from AI technology, computer science, neuroscience, and ethics, resulting in better outcomes and promoting greater welfare for humanity (Jeste et al., 2020). The ideal goal of Artificial Wisdom is to mimic human wisdom and morals to handle complex situations with human-like decision-making capabilities. It will elevate the domain of mental healthcare as well.

At present, attempts to establish definite ethical guidelines for AI systems are at the foundational stages. In the professions of psychology and medicine, there is a well-established convention of strictly following ethical standards, both in research and practice. Thus, it is highly expected that clear ethical regulations must be followed while AI is incorporated into mental healthcare. Some AI experts have different opinions regarding the definition of ethics and skepticism about the enforcement of responsibility, making them pessimistic about the ethical design principles of AI (Rainie et al, 2021). They are confused about which framework should be followed, who is responsible, and how AI can be effectively regulated because of its hidden nature. It is hoped that the apprehensions will be resolved immediately in the context of heated debates and discussions on the dangers of AI.

CONCLUSION

Artificial Intelligence can transfigure the health sector, especially mental health. The global mental health crisis can be effectively addressed using AI sensibly. Currently, modern AI systems have been used for early detection, diagnosis, treatment, therapy, monitoring, follow-up, and professional assistance in mental health interventions. Virtual therapists, chatbots, and health record systems are gaining popularity these days. It is understood that AI-driven technology has the potential to cater to personalized, precise, predictive, and accessible solutions, which are instrumental in reducing the disparity between the demand and supply of mental health services. In the disciplines of psychology and medicine, there is a strong tradition of following clear and definite ethical practices; the same standards need to be ensured when AI is being incorporated into mental healthcare. Experts and pioneers in the area are raising alarming concerns about the need for intelligible policy frameworks to develop AI systems. When it comes to mental healthcare, it is even more important as it is a more sensitive area with complex behavior and emotions, and confidential data is involved. At present, ethical guidelines for AI systems are at the foundational stages, with significant attempts made by the WHO and the European Union, along with APA's ethical principles for psychologists. The basic idea is that the benefits of following ethical principles must be greater than the projected benefits without adhering to ethical guidelines. It is important to note that maintaining the human element in mental health interventions while using AI systems is crucial. AI should enhance rather than replace the therapeutic alliance between patients and therapists. Finding the ideal balance between AI-driven methods and human care is paramount.

As mentioned at the beginning of the chapter, human wisdom needs to win in the competition with technology for the greater benefit of humankind.

REFERENCES

Academy, L. I. (n.d.). The story of ELIZA: the AI that fooled the world. *London Intercultural Academy*. Retrieved December 29, 2024, from https://liacademy.co.uk/the-story-of-eliza-the-ai-that-fooled-the-world/

Adler, D. A., Wang, F., Mohr, D. C., & Choudhury, T. (2022). Machine learning for passive mental health symptom prediction: Generalization across different longitudinal mobile sensing studies. *PLoS One*, *17*(4), e0266516. DOI: 10.1371/journal.pone.0266516 PMID: 35476787

Agarwal, R., Bjarnadottir, M., Rhue, L., Dugas, M., Crowley, K., Clark, J., & Gao, G. (2023). Addressing algorithmic bias and the perpetuation of health inequities: An AI bias aware framework. *Health Policy and Technology*, *12*(1), 100702. DOI: 10.1016/j.hlpt.2022.100702

Agarwal, R., Dugas, M., Gao, G., & Kannan, P. K. (2019). Emerging technologies and analytics for a new era of value-centered marketing in healthcare. *Journal of the Academy of Marketing Science*, *48*(1), 9–23. DOI: 10.1007/s11747-019-00692-4

AI, HLEG (2019). *High-Level Expert Group on Artificial Intelligence*. Ethics guidelines for trustworthy AI [Text]. European Commission. Available at: https://ec.europa.eu/digital-single-market/en/news/ethics-guidelines-trustworthy-ai

Almohammed, O. A., Alsalem, A. A., Almangour, A. A., Alotaibi, L. H., Yami, M. S. A., & Lai, L. (2022). Antidepressants and health-related quality of life (HRQoL) for patients with depression: Analysis of the medical expenditure panel survey from the United States. *PLoS One*, *17*(4), e0265928. DOI: 10.1371/journal.pone.0265928 PMID: 35442954

Alowais, S. A., Alghamdi, S. S., Alsuhebany, N., Alqahtani, T., Alshaya, A. I., Almohareb, S. N., Aldairem, A., Alrashed, M., Saleh, K. B., Badreldin, H. A., Yami, M. S. A., Harbi, S. A., & Albekairy, A. M. (2023). Revolutionizing healthcare: The role of artificial intelligence in clinical practice. *BMC Medical Education*, *23*(1), 689. Advance online publication. DOI: 10.1186/s12909-023-04698-z PMID: 37740191

American Psychological Association. (2017). Ethical principles of psychologists and code of conduct (2002, amended effective June 1, 2010, and January 1, 2017). https://www.apa.org/ethics/code

An, L., & Boman, L. (2022). The robot won't judge me: How AI Healthcare Benefits the Stigmatized: An abstract. In *Developments in marketing science: proceedings of the Academy of Marketing Science* (pp. 363–364). https://doi.org/DOI: 10.1007/978-3-030-95346-1_111

Anxiety Canada. (2024, June 25). Anxiety Canada. https://www.anxietycanada.com/resources/mindshift-cbt/

Bailey, N. W., Hoy, K. E., Rogasch, N. C., Thomson, R. H., McQueen, S., Elliot, D., Sullivan, C. M., Fulcher, B. D., Daskalakis, Z. J., & Fitzgerald, P. B. (2018). Responders to rTMS for depression show increased fronto-midline theta and theta connectivity compared to non-responders. *Brain Stimulation*, *11*(1), 190–203. DOI: 10.1016/j.brs.2017.10.015 PMID: 29128490

Bajwa, J., Munir, U., Nori, A., & Williams, B. (2021). Artificial intelligence in healthcare: Transforming the practice of medicine. *Future Healthcare Journal*, *8*(2), e188–e194. DOI: 10.7861/fhj.2021-0095 PMID: 34286183

Basil. (2022, July 7). ELIZA: The chatbot who Revolutionised Human-Machine Interaction [An Introduction]. *Medium*. https://medium.com/nerd-for-tech/eliza-the-chatbot-who-revolutionised-human-machine-interaction-an-introduction-582a7581f91c

Bengio, Y., Hinton, G., Yao, A., Song, D., Abbeel, P., Darrell, T., Harari, Y. N., Zhang, Y., Xue, L., Shalev-Shwartz, S., Hadfield, G., Clune, J., Maharaj, T., Hutter, F., Baydin, A. G., McIlraith, S., Gao, Q., Acharya, A., Krueger, D., & Mindermann, S. (2024). Managing extreme AI risks amid rapid progress. *Science*, *384*(6698), 842–845. DOI: 10.1126/science.adn0117 PMID: 38768279

Bennett, G., & Cuevas, K. (2024, October 8). "Godfather of AI" discusses dangers the developing technologies pose to society. *PBS News*. https://www.pbs.org/newshour/show/godfather-of-ai-discusses-dangers-the-developing-technologies-pose-to-society

Benrouba, F., & Boudour, R. (2023). Emotional sentiment analysis of social media content for mental health safety. *Social Network Analysis and Mining*, *13*(1), 17. Advance online publication. DOI: 10.1007/s13278-022-01000-9

BetterHelp. (n.d.-a). *BetterHelp | Professional therapy with a licensed therapist.* https://www.betterhelp.com/

Bhugra, D. (2006). Severe mental illness across cultures. *Acta Psychiatrica Scandinavica*, *113*(s429), 17–23. DOI: 10.1111/j.1600-0447.2005.00712.x PMID: 16445477

Birjali, M., Kasri, M., & Beni-Hssane, A. (2021). A comprehensive survey on sentiment analysis: Approaches, challenges and trends. *Knowledge-Based Systems*, *226*, 107134. DOI: 10.1016/j.knosys.2021.107134

Blackwell, S. E., & Heidenreich, T. (2021). Cognitive behavior Therapy at the crossroads. *International Journal of Cognitive Therapy*, *14*(1), 1–22. DOI: 10.1007/s41811-021-00104-y PMID: 33584950

Bohr, A., & Memarzadeh, K. (2020). The rise of artificial intelligence in healthcare applications. In *Elsevier eBooks* (pp. 25–60). https://doi.org/DOI: 10.1016/B978-0-12-818438-7.00002-2

Bukowski, M., Farkas, R., Beyan, O., Moll, L., Hahn, H., Kiessling, F., & Schmitz-Rode, T. (2020). Implementation of eHealth and AI integrated diagnostics with multidisciplinary digitized data: Are we ready from an international perspective? *European Radiology*, *30*(10), 5510–5524. DOI: 10.1007/s00330-020-06874-x PMID: 32377810

Busk, J., Faurholt-Jepsen, M., Frost, M., Bardram, J. E., Vedel Kessing, L., & Winther, O. (2020). Forecasting Mood in Bipolar Disorder From Smartphone Self-assessments: Hierarchical Bayesian Approach. *JMIR mHealth and uHealth*, *8*(4), e15028. DOI: 10.2196/15028 PMID: 32234702

Calm. (n.d.). https://www.calm.com/

CBT Companion - A comprehensive app for Cognitive Behavioral Therapy. (n.d.). Resiliens. https://resiliens.com/cbt-companion/

Cerebral Inc. (n.d.). *Online mental health care that caters to you | cerebral | Online therapy | Virtual counseling | Telehealth therapy*. https://cerebral.com/

Chandler, C., Foltz, P. W., & Elvevåg, B. (2019). Using Machine learning in psychiatry: The need to establish a framework that nurtures trustworthiness. *Schizophrenia Bulletin*, sbz105. Advance online publication. DOI: 10.1093/schbul/sbz105 PMID: 31901100

Chatbot for Healthcare - IBM watsonx Assistant. (n.d.). https://www.ibm.com/products/watsonx-assistant/healthcare

Chen, H. H., Hsu, H. T., Lin, P. C., Chen, C.-Y., Hsieh, H. F., & Ko, C. H. (2023). Efficacy of a Smartphone App in Enhancing Medication Adherence and Accuracy in Individuals With Schizophrenia During the COVID-19 Pandemic: Randomized Controlled Trial. *JMIR Mental Health*, *10*, e50806. DOI: 10.2196/50806 PMID: 38096017

Chen, J., Chan, N. Y., Li, C.-T., Chan, J. W. Y., Liu, Y., Li, S. X., Chau, S. W. H., Leung, K. S., Heng, P.-A., Lee, T. M. C., Li, T. M. H., & Wing, Y.-K. (2024). Multimodal digital assessment of depression with actigraphy and app in Hong Kong Chinese. *Translational Psychiatry*, *14*(1), 150. Advance online publication. DOI: 10.1038/s41398-024-02873-4 PMID: 38499546

Chen, Y., Clayton, E. W., Novak, L. L., Anders, S., & Malin, B. (2023). Human-Centered design to address biases in artificial intelligence. *Journal of Medical Internet Research*, *25*, e43251. DOI: 10.2196/43251 PMID: 36961506

Choo, T.-H., Wall, M., Brodsky, B. S., Herzog, S., Mann, J. J., Stanley, B., & Galfalvy, H. (2024). Temporal prediction of suicidal ideation in an ecological momentary assessment study with recurrent neural networks. *Journal of Affective Disorders*, *360*, 268–275. DOI: 10.1016/j.jad.2024.05.093 PMID: 38795778

Clayton, V. (1983). Wisdom and Intelligence: The nature and function of knowledge in the later years. *International Journal of Aging & Human Development*, *15*(4), 315–321. DOI: 10.2190/17TQ-BW3Y-P8J4-TG40 PMID: 7183572

Cohen, S. (2020). The basics of machine learning: strategies and techniques. In *Elsevier eBooks* (pp. 13–40). https://doi.org/DOI: 10.1016/B978-0-323-67538-3.00002-6

Cohen, Z. D., Delgadillo, J., & DeRubeis, R. J. (2021). Personalized treatment approaches. In M. Barkham, W. Lutz, & L. G. Castonguay (Eds.), *Bergin and Garfield's handbook of psychotherapy and behavior change: 50th anniversary edition* (7th ed., pp. 673–703). John Wiley & Sons, Inc.

Cook, B. L., Progovac, A. M., Chen, P., Mullin, B., Hou, S., & Baca-Garcia, E. (2016). Novel Use of Natural Language Processing (NLP) to Predict Suicidal Ideation and Psychiatric Symptoms in a Text-Based Mental Health Intervention in Madrid. *Computational and Mathematical Methods in Medicine*, *2016*, 1–8. DOI: 10.1155/2016/8708434 PMID: 27752278

Corrigan, P. (2004). How stigma interferes with mental health care. *The American Psychologist*, *59*(7), 614–625. DOI: 10.1037/0003-066X.59.7.614 PMID: 15491256

Corrigan, P. W., & Watson, A. C. (2002). Understanding the impact of stigma on people with mental illness. *World Psychiatry; Official Journal of the World Psychiatric Association (WPA)*, *1*(1), 16–20. PMID: 16946807

Cotton, E. (2021, October 1). *Mental health services in England are being 'Uberised' – and that's bad for patients and therapists*. The Conversation. Retrieved January 7, 2025, from https://theconversation.com/mental-health-services-in-england-are-being-uberised-and-thats-bad-for-patients-and-therapists-167065

D'Alfonso, S. (2020). AI in mental health. *Current Opinion in Psychology, 36*, 112–117. DOI: 10.1016/j.copsyc.2020.04.005 PMID: 32604065

Dalton-Brown, S. (2020). The ethics of Medical AI and the Physician-Patient relationship. *Cambridge Quarterly of Healthcare Ethics, 29*(1), 115–121. DOI: 10.1017/S0963180119000847 PMID: 31858938

Davenport, T., & Kalakota, R. (2019). The potential for artificial intelligence in healthcare. *Future Healthcare Journal, 6*(2), 94–98. DOI: 10.7861/futurehosp.6-2-94 PMID: 31363513

De Freitas, J., Uğuralp, A. K., Oğuz-Uğuralp, Z., & Puntoni, S. (2023). Chatbots and mental health: Insights into the safety of generative AI. *Journal of Consumer Psychology, 34*(3), 481–491. DOI: 10.1002/jcpy.1393

Denecke, K., Abd-Alrazaq, A., & Househ, M. (2021). Artificial intelligence for chatbots in mental health: Opportunities and challenges. In *Lecture notes in bioengineering* (pp. 115–128). https://doi.org/DOI: 10.1007/978-3-030-67303-1_10

Diaz-Asper, C., Hauglid, M. K., Chandler, C., Cohen, A. S., Foltz, P. W., & Elvevåg, B. (2024). A framework for language technologies in behavioral research and clinical applications: Ethical challenges, implications, and solutions. *The American Psychologist, 79*(1), 79–91. DOI: 10.1037/amp0001195 PMID: 38236217

Doraiswamy, S., Abraham, A., Mamtani, R., & Cheema, S. (2020). Use of Telehealth during the COVID-19 Pandemic: Scoping review. *Journal of Medical Internet Research, 22*(12), e24087. DOI: 10.2196/24087 PMID: 33147166

Drew, L. (2019). The ethics of brain–computer interfaces. *Nature, 571*(7766), S19–S21. DOI: 10.1038/d41586-019-02214-2 PMID: 31341310

Drysdale, A. T., Grosenick, L., Downar, J., Dunlop, K., Mansouri, F., Meng, Y., Fetcho, R. N., Zebley, B., Oathes, D. J., Etkin, A., Schatzberg, A. F., Sudheimer, K., Keller, J., Mayberg, H. S., Gunning, F. M., Alexopoulos, G. S., Fox, M. D., Pascual-Leone, A., Voss, H. U., & Liston, C. (2016). Resting-state connectivity biomarkers define neurophysiological subtypes of depression. *Nature Medicine, 23*(1), 28–38. DOI: 10.1038/nm.4246 PMID: 27918562

Eaneff, S., Obermeyer, Z., & Butte, A. J. (2020b). The case for algorithmic stewardship for artificial intelligence and machine learning technologies. *Journal of the American Medical Association, 324*(14), 1397. DOI: 10.1001/jama.2020.9371 PMID: 32926087

Ekman, P. (2002). *Microexpression Training Tool (METT)*. University California.

Engel, G. L. (1977). The need for a new medical model: A challenge for biomedicine. *Science, 196*(4286), 129–136. DOI: 10.1126/science.847460 PMID: 847460

Ethical principles of psychologists and code of conduct. (2017). apa.org. Retrieved January 5, 2025, from https://www.apa.org/ethics/code#:~:text=Psychologists%20strive%20to%20benefit%20those,of%20animal%20subjects%20of%20research

Ethics and Governance of Artificial intelligence for Health: WHO guidance. (2021). World Health Organization.

Feuerriegel, S., Hartmann, J., Janiesch, C., & Zschech, P. (2023). Generative AI. *Business & Information Systems Engineering, 66*(1), 111–126. DOI: 10.1007/s12599-023-00834-7

Fiske, A., Henningsen, P., & Buyx, A. (2019). Your robot therapist will see you now: Ethical Implications of Embodied Artificial intelligence in Psychiatry, Psychology, and Psychotherapy. *Journal of Medical Internet Research, 21*(5), e13216. DOI: 10.2196/13216 PMID: 31094356

Flanagan, O., Chan, A., Roop, P., & Sundram, F. (2021). Using acoustic speech patterns from smartphones to investigate mood disorders: Scoping review. *JMIR mHealth and uHealth, 9*(9), e24352. DOI: 10.2196/24352 PMID: 34533465

Fosch-Villaronga, E., & Albo-Canals, J. (2019). "I'll take care of you," said the robot. *Paladyn : Journal of Behavioral Robotics, 10*(1), 77–93. DOI: 10.1515/pjbr-2019-0006

Founding fathers of Artificial Intelligence. (2023, December 28). Quidgest. https://quidgest.com/en/blog-en/ai-founding-fathers/

Franklin, J. C., Ribeiro, J. D., Fox, K. R., Bentley, K. H., Kleiman, E. M., Huang, X., Musacchio, K. M., Jaroszewski, A. C., Chang, B. P., & Nock, M. K. (2017). Risk factors for suicidal thoughts and behaviors: A meta-analysis of 50 years of research. *Psychological Bulletin, 143*(2), 187–232. DOI: 10.1037/bul0000084 PMID: 27841450

Fulmer, R., Joerin, A., Gentile, B., Lakerink, L., & Rauws, M. (2018). Using Psychological Artificial Intelligence (Tess) to Relieve Symptoms of Depression and Anxiety: Randomized Controlled Trial. *JMIR Mental Health, 5*(4), e64. Advance online publication. DOI: 10.2196/mental.9782 PMID: 30545815

Gebru, T., Morgenstern, J., Vecchione, B., Vaughan, J. W., Wallach, H., Daumé, H.III, & Crawford, K. (2021). Datasheets for datasets. *Communications of the ACM, 64*(12), 86–92. DOI: 10.1145/3458723

Gilbert, D. (2024, October 26). *Despite uncertain risks, many turn to AI like ChatGPT for mental health.* washingtonpost.com. Retrieved January 4, 2025, from https://www.washingtonpost.com/business/2024/10/25/ai-therapy-chatgpt-chatbots-mental-health/

Gilleen, J., Greenwood, K., & David, A. S. (2010). Anosognosia in schizophrenia and other neuropsychiatric disorders: similarities and differences. *The study of anosognosia*, 255-290

Goddard, K., Roudsari, A., & Wyatt, J. C. (2011). Automation bias: A systematic review of frequency, effect mediators, and mitigators. *Journal of the American Medical Informatics Association : JAMIA*, *19*(1), 121–127. DOI: 10.1136/amiajnl-2011-000089 PMID: 21685142

Goodman, C. (2024, November 15). *What to know about generative AI chatbots and cybersecurity risks | Balbix.* Balbix. https://www.balbix.com/insights/generative-ai-chatbots-cybersecurity-risks/#:~:text=Eavesdropping%20and%20Interception%3A%20Data%20transmitted,attackers%20from%20intercepting%20sensitive%20information

Gual-Montolio, P., Jaén, I., Martínez-Borba, V., Castilla, D., & Suso-Ribera, C. (2022). Using artificial intelligence to enhance ongoing psychological interventions for emotional problems in Real- or Close to Real-Time: A Systematic review. *International Journal of Environmental Research and Public Health*, *19*(13), 7737. DOI: 10.3390/ijerph19137737 PMID: 35805395

Guidotti, R., Monreale, A., Ruggieri, S., Turini, F., Giannotti, F., & Pedreschi, D. (2018). A survey of methods for explaining black box models. *ACM Computing Surveys*, *51*(5), 1–42. DOI: 10.1145/3236009

Hamblen, J. (2009). What is PTSD. *A Handout From The National Center For PTSD.*

Happify: Science-based activities and games. (n.d.-b). happify.com. https://www.happify.com/

Harari, Y. N. (2023, May 14). *AI and the future of humanity | Yuval Noah Harari at the Frontiers Forum* [Video]. YouTube. https://www.youtube.com/watch?v=LWiM-LuRe6w

Hawking, S. (2018). *Brief answers to the big questions.*

Holdsworth, J. (2023, December 22). AI Bias. *Think.* Retrieved January 5, 2025, from https://www.ibm.com/think/topics/ai-bias

Huberty, J., Puzia, M. E., Larkey, L., Vranceanu, A., & Irwin, M. R. (2021). Can a meditation app help my sleep? A cross-sectional survey of Calm users. *PLoS One*, *16*(10), e0257518. DOI: 10.1371/journal.pone.0257518 PMID: 34679078

Huckins, J. F., daSilva, A. W., Wang, R., Wang, W., Hedlund, E. L., Murphy, E. I., Lopez, R. B., Rogers, C., Holtzheimer, P. E., Kelley, W. M., Heatherton, T. F., Wagner, D. D., Haxby, J. V., & Campbell, A. T. (2019). Fusing mobile phone sensing and brain imaging to assess depression in college students. *Frontiers in Neuroscience*, *13*, 248. Advance online publication. DOI: 10.3389/fnins.2019.00248 PMID: 30949024

Ibm. (2024, December 19). Artificial Intelligence. *Artificial Intelligence*. https://www.ibm.com/topics/artificial-intelligence

Imran, N., Hashmi, A., & Imran, A. (2023). Chat-GPT: Opportunities and Challenges in Child Mental Healthcare. *Pakistan Journal of Medical Sciences*, *39*(4). Advance online publication. DOI: 10.12669/pjms.39.4.8118 PMID: 37492313

Iyortsuun, N. K., Kim, S., Jhon, M., Yang, H., & Pant, S. (2023). A review of machine learning and deep learning approaches on mental health diagnosis. *Health Care*, *11*(3), 285. DOI: 10.3390/healthcare11030285 PMID: 36766860

Jaroszewski, A. C., Morris, R. R., & Nock, M. K. (2019). Randomized controlled trial of an online machine learning-driven risk assessment and intervention platform for increasing the use of crisis services. *Journal of Consulting and Clinical Psychology*, *87*(4), 370–379. DOI: 10.1037/ccp0000389 PMID: 30883164

Jazeera, A. (2024, October 24). US mother says in lawsuit that AI chatbot encouraged son's suicide. *Al Jazeera*. https://www.aljazeera.com/economy/2024/10/24/us-mother-says-in-lawsuit-that-ai-chatbot-encouraged-sons-suicide

Jeste, D. V., Graham, S. A., Nguyen, T. T., Depp, C. A., Lee, E. E., & Kim, H. (2020). Beyond artificial intelligence: Exploring artificial wisdom. *International Psychogeriatrics*, *32*(8), 993–1001. DOI: 10.1017/S1041610220000927 PMID: 32583762

Jha, I. P., Awasthi, R., Kumar, A., Kumar, V., & Sethi, T. (2021). Learning the Mental Health Impact of COVID-19 in the United States With Explainable Artificial Intelligence: Observational Study. *JMIR Mental Health*, *8*(4), e25097. DOI: 10.2196/25097 PMID: 33877051

Khawaja, Z., & Bélisle-Pipon, J. (2023). Your robot therapist is not your therapist: Understanding the role of AI-powered mental health chatbots. *Frontiers in Digital Health*, *5*, 1278186. Advance online publication. DOI: 10.3389/fdgth.2023.1278186 PMID: 38026836

Kleinau, E., Lamba, T., Jaskiewicz, W., Gorentz, K., Hungerbuehler, I., Rahimi, D., Kokota, D., Maliwichi, L., Jamu, E., Zumazuma, A., Negrão, M., Mota, R., Khouri, Y., & Kapps, M. (2024). Effectiveness of a chatbot in improving the mental wellbeing of health workers in Malawi during the COVID-19 pandemic: A randomized, controlled trial. *PLoS One*, *19*(5), e0303370. DOI: 10.1371/journal.pone.0303370 PMID: 38805444

Klos, M. C., Escoredo, M., Joerin, A., Lemos, V. N., Rauws, M., & Bunge, E. L. (2021). Artificial Intelligence Chatbot for Anxiety and Depression in University Students: A Pilot Randomized Controlled Trial (Preprint). *JMIR Formative Research*, *5*(8), e20678. Advance online publication. DOI: 10.2196/20678 PMID: 34092548

Kourou, K., Manikis, G., Mylona, E., Poikonen-Saksela, P., Mazzocco, K., Pat-Horenczyk, R., Sousa, B., Oliveira-Maia, A. J., Mattson, J., Roziner, I., Pettini, G., Kondylakis, H., Marias, K., Nuutinen, M., Karademas, E., Simos, P., & Fotiadis, D. I. (2023). Personalized prediction of one-year mental health deterioration using adaptive learning algorithms: A multicenter breast cancer prospective study. *Scientific Reports*, *13*(1), 7059. Advance online publication. DOI: 10.1038/s41598-023-33281-1 PMID: 37120428

Kuehner, C. (2017). Why is depression more common among women than among men? *The Lancet. Psychiatry*, *4*(2), 146–158. DOI: 10.1016/S2215-0366(16)30263-2 PMID: 27856392

Lee, T. Y., Kim, M., & Kwon, J. S. (2019). Early identification of psychiatric disorders. *Advances in Experimental Medicine and Biology*, *1192*, 341–352. DOI: 10.1007/978-981-32-9721-0_18 PMID: 31705504

Legaspi, C. M.Jr, Pacana, T. R., Loja, K., Sing, C., & Ong, E. (2022). *User Perception of Wysa as a Mental Well-being Support Tool during the COVID-19 Pandemic.*, DOI: 10.1145/3516492.3559064

Lin, E., Kuo, P., Liu, Y., Yu, Y. W., Yang, A. C., & Tsai, S. (2018). A deep learning approach for predicting antidepressant response in major depression using clinical and genetic biomarkers. *Frontiers in Psychiatry*, *9*, 290. Advance online publication. DOI: 10.3389/fpsyt.2018.00290 PMID: 30034349

Linehan, M. M., & Wilks, C. R. (2015). The course and Evolution of Dialectical Behavior Therapy. *American Journal of Psychotherapy*, *69*(2), 97–110. DOI: 10.1176/appi.psychotherapy.2015.69.2.97 PMID: 26160617

Littmann, M., Selig, K., Cohen-Lavi, L., Frank, Y., Hönigschmid, P., Kataka, E., Mösch, A., Qian, K., Ron, A., Schmid, S., Sorbie, A., Szlak, L., Dagan-Wiener, A., Ben-Tal, N., Niv, M. Y., Razansky, D., Schuller, B. W., Ankerst, D., Hertz, T., & Rost, B. (2020). Validity of machine learning in biology and medicine increased through collaborations across fields of expertise. *Nature Machine Intelligence*, *2*(1), 18–24. DOI: 10.1038/s42256-019-0139-8

Loh, E. (2018). Medicine and the rise of the robots: A qualitative review of recent advances of artificial intelligence in health. *BMJ Leader*, *2*(2), 59–63. DOI: 10.1136/leader-2018-000071

Loies, S. E. (2024). Combating mental health stigma with artificial intelligence. In *Advances in psychology, mental health, and behavioral studies (APMHBS) book series* (pp. 75–92). https://doi.org/DOI: 10.4018/979-8-3693-3673-1.ch005

Lønfeldt, N. N., Olesen, K. V., Das, S., Mora-Jensen, A.-R. C., Pagsberg, A. K., & Clemmensen, L. K. H. (2023). Predicting obsessive-compulsive disorder episodes in adolescents using a wearable biosensor—A wrist angel feasibility study. *Frontiers in Psychiatry*, *14*, 1231024. Advance online publication. DOI: 10.3389/fpsyt.2023.1231024 PMID: 37850105

Maekawa, E., Grua, E. M., Nakamura, C. A., Scazufca, M., Araya, R., Peters, T., & van de Ven, P. (2024). Bayesian Networks for Prescreening in Depression: Algorithm Development and Validation. *JMIR Mental Health*, *11*, e52045. DOI: 10.2196/52045 PMID: 38963925

Marcelle, E. T., Nolting, L., Hinshaw, S. P., & Aguilera, A. (2018). Effectiveness of a multimodal digital Psychotherapy platform for Adult Depression: A Naturalistic Feasibility Study. *JMIR mHealth and uHealth*, *7*(1), e10948. DOI: 10.2196/10948 PMID: 30674448

Meditation and sleep made simple - Headspace. (n.d.). Headspace. https://www.headspace.com/

Mehta, P. (2024). Pioneering the future of mental health with AI. In *Advances in medical technologies and clinical practice book series* (pp. 277–304). https://doi.org/DOI: 10.4018/979-8-3693-4422-4.ch014

Mennella, C., Maniscalco, U., De Pietro, G., & Esposito, M. (2024). Ethical and regulatory challenges of AI technologies in healthcare: A narrative review. *Heliyon*, *10*(4), e26297. DOI: 10.1016/j.heliyon.2024.e26297 PMID: 38384518

Microsoft. (2019, October 1). *Satya Nadella announces strategic collaboration with Novartis* [Video]. YouTube. https://www.youtube.com/watch?v=wMfsQE-D2q4

Minerva, F., & Giubilini, A. (2023). Is AI the future of mental healthcare? *Topoi*, *42*(3), 809–817. DOI: 10.1007/s11245-023-09932-3 PMID: 37361723

Mishra, A., Savulescu, J., & Giubilini, A. (2022). The Ethics of Medical AI. In *Oxford University Press eBooks* (pp. 487–507). https://doi.org/DOI: 10.1093/oxfordhb/9780198857815.013.25

Mohsin, S. N., Gapizov, A., Ekhator, C., Ain, N. U., Ahmad, S., Khan, M., Barker, C., Hussain, M., Malineni, J., Ramadhan, A., & Nagaraj, R. H. (2023). The role of artificial intelligence in prediction, risk stratification, and personalized treatment planning for congenital heart diseases. *Cureus*. Advance online publication. DOI: 10.7759/cureus.44374 PMID: 37664359

Montag, C., Ali, R., Al-Thani, D., & Hall, B. J. (2023). On artificial intelligence and global mental health. *Asian Journal of Psychiatry*, *91*, 103855. DOI: 10.1016/j.ajp.2023.103855 PMID: 38113698

MoodFit | Tools & Insights for your Mental health. (n.d.-b). Moodfit. https://www.getmoodfit.com/

Naik, N., Hameed, B. M. Z., Shetty, D. K., Swain, D., Shah, M., Paul, R., Aggarwal, K., Ibrahim, S., Patil, V., Smriti, K., Shetty, S., Rai, B. P., Chlosta, P., & Somani, B. K. (2022b). Legal and ethical consideration in artificial intelligence in healthcare: Who takes responsibility? *Frontiers in Surgery*, *9*, 862322. Advance online publication. DOI: 10.3389/fsurg.2022.862322 PMID: 35360424

Nazer, L. H., Zatarah, R., Waldrip, S., Ke, J. X. C., Moukheiber, M., Khanna, A. K., Hicklen, R. S., Moukheiber, L., Moukheiber, D., Ma, H., & Mathur, P. (2023). Bias in artificial intelligence algorithms and recommendations for mitigation. *PLOS Digital Health*, *2*(6), e0000278. DOI: 10.1371/journal.pdig.0000278 PMID: 37347721

Nilsen, P., Svedberg, P., Nygren, J., Frideros, M., Johansson, J., & Schueller, S. (2022). Accelerating the impact of artificial intelligence in mental healthcare through implementation science. *Implementation Research and Practice*, *3*, 26334895221112033. Advance online publication. DOI: 10.1177/26334895221112033 PMID: 37091110

Norgeot, B., Quer, G., Beaulieu-Jones, B. K., Torkamani, A., Dias, R., Gianfrancesco, M., Arnaout, R., Kohane, I. S., Saria, S., Topol, E., Obermeyer, Z., Yu, B., & Butte, A. J. (2020). Minimum information about clinical artificial intelligence modeling: The MI-CLAIM checklist. *Nature Medicine*, *26*(9), 1320–1324. DOI: 10.1038/s41591-020-1041-y PMID: 32908275

OECD. (2021). *Artificial intelligence & responsible business conduct*. https://mneguidelines.oecd.org/RBC-and-artificial-intelligence.pdf

Olawade, D. B., Wada, O. Z., Odetayo, A., David-Olawade, A. C., Asaolu, F., & Eberhardt, J. (2024). Enhancing mental health with Artificial Intelligence: Current trends and future prospects. *Journal of Medicine, Surgery, and Public Health, 3*, 100099. DOI: 10.1016/j.glmedi.2024.100099

Pandya, A., Lodha, P., & Ganatra, A. (2024). Is ChatGPT ready to change mental healthcare? Challenges and considerations: A reality-check. *Frontiers in Human Dynamics, 5*, 1289255. Advance online publication. DOI: 10.3389/fhumd.2023.1289255

Parikh, R. B., Teeple, S., & Navathe, A. S. (2019). Addressing bias in artificial intelligence in health care. *Journal of the American Medical Association, 322*(24), 2377. DOI: 10.1001/jama.2019.18058 PMID: 31755905

Parker, L., Halter, V., Karliychuk, T., & Grundy, Q. (2019). How private is your mental health app data? An empirical study of mental health app privacy policies and practices. *International Journal of Law and Psychiatry, 64*, 198–204. DOI: 10.1016/j.ijlp.2019.04.002 PMID: 31122630

Pierce, M. E., Mirabito, G., & Verhaeghen, P. (2024). Mind the app: More time spent on headspace leads to beneficial day-to-day changes in mindfulness, depression, anxiety and stress in college students. *Cogent Mental Health, 3*(1), 1–23. DOI: 10.1080/28324765.2024.2400878 PMID: 38550624

Qi, Y. (2024). Pilot Quasi-Experimental Research on the Effectiveness of the Woebot AI Chatbot for Reducing Mild Depression Symptoms among Athletes. *International Journal of Human-Computer Interaction*, •••, 1–8. DOI: 10.1080/10447318.2023.2301256

Quinn, T. P., Senadeera, M., Jacobs, S., Coghlan, S., & Le, V. (2021). Trust and medical AI: The challenges we face and the expertise needed to overcome them. *Journal of the American Medical Informatics Association : JAMIA, 28*(4), 890–894. DOI: 10.1093/jamia/ocaa268 PMID: 33340404

Rainie, L., Anderson, J., & Vogels, A. E. (2021, June 16). *Worries about developments in AI*. Pew Research Center. Retrieved January 8, 2025, from https://www.pewresearch.org/internet/2021/06/16/1-worries-about-developments-in-ai/

Reddy, S., Allan, S., Coghlan, S., & Cooper, P. (2019). A governance model for the application of AI in health care. *Journal of the American Medical Informatics Association : JAMIA, 27*(3), 491–497. DOI: 10.1093/jamia/ocz192 PMID: 31682262

Replika. (n.d.). replika.com. https://replika.com/

Ribera, M., & Lapedriza, A. (2019). Can we do better explanations? A proposal of user-centered explainable AI. *Joint proceedings of the ACM IUI 2019 workshops* (pp. 38–44). https://ceur-ws.org/Vol-2327/IUI19WSExSS2019-12.pdf

Scodari, B. T., Chacko, S., Matsumura, R., & Jacobson, N. C. (2023). Using machine learning to forecast symptom changes among subclinical depression patients receiving stepped care or usual care. *Journal of Affective Disorders*, *340*, 213–220. DOI: 10.1016/j.jad.2023.08.004 PMID: 37541599

Shameer, K., Johnson, K. W., Glicksberg, B. S., Dudley, J. T., & Sengupta, P. P. (2018). Machine learning in cardiovascular medicine: Are we there yet? *Heart (British Cardiac Society)*, *104*(14), 1156–1164. DOI: 10.1136/heartjnl-2017-311198 PMID: 29352006

Siala, H., & Wang, Y. (2022). SHIFTing artificial intelligence to be responsible in healthcare: A systematic review. *Social Science & Medicine*, *296*, 114782. DOI: 10.1016/j.socscimed.2022.114782 PMID: 35152047

Siddals, S., Torous, J., & Coxon, A. (2024). "It happened to be the perfect thing": Experiences of generative AI chatbots for mental health. *Npj Mental Health Research*, *3*(1), 48. Advance online publication. DOI: 10.1038/s44184-024-00097-4 PMID: 39465310

SuperBetter: Empower Youth Mental Health. (n.d.). https://superbetter.com/

Swift, J. (2003). *Gulliver's Travels*. Penguin.

Talkspace. (n.d.-b). *TalkSpace - #1 rated online therapy, 1 million+ users*. Talkspace. https://www.talkspace.com/

Tansey, K. E., Guipponi, M., Hu, X., Domenici, E., Lewis, G., Malafosse, A., Wendland, J. R., Lewis, C. M., McGuffin, P., & Uher, R. (2013). Contribution of common genetic variants to antidepressant response. *Biological Psychiatry*, *73*(7), 679–682. DOI: 10.1016/j.biopsych.2012.10.030 PMID: 23237317

Tokuno, S. (2017). Pathophysiological voice analysis for diagnosis and monitoring of depression. In *Springer eBooks* (pp. 83–95). https://doi.org/DOI: 10.1007/978-981-10-6577-4_6

Tsui, F. R., Shi, L., Ruiz, V., Ryan, N. D., Biernesser, C., Iyengar, S., Walsh, C. G., & Brent, D. A. (2021). Natural language processing and machine learning of electronic health records for prediction of first-time suicide attempts. *JAMIA Open*, *4*(1), ooab011. Advance online publication. DOI: 10.1093/jamiaopen/ooab011 PMID: 33758800

Uban, A., Chulvi, B., & Rosso, P. (2021). An emotion and cognitive based analysis of mental health disorders from social media data. *Future Generation Computer Systems*, *124*, 480–494. DOI: 10.1016/j.future.2021.05.032

VA.gov | Veterans Affairs. (n.d.). https://www.ptsd.va.gov/appvid/mobile/ptsdcoach_app.asp

Vegesna, A., Tran, M., Angelaccio, M., & Arcona, S. (2016). Remote Patient Monitoring via Non-Invasive Digital Technologies: A Systematic review. *Telemedicine Journal and e-Health*, *23*(1), 3–17. DOI: 10.1089/tmj.2016.0051 PMID: 27116181

Villongco, C., & Khan, F. (2020). "Sorry I didn't hear you." The ethics of voice computing and AI in high risk mental health populations. *AJOB Neuroscience*, *11*(2), 105–112. DOI: 10.1080/21507740.2020.1740355 PMID: 32228383

VonHoltz, L. H., Hypolite, K. A., Carr, B. G., Shofer, F. S., Winston, F. K., Hanson, C. W.III, & Merchant, R. M. (2015). Use of mobile apps: A patient-centered approach. *Academic Emergency Medicine*, *22*(6), 765–768. DOI: 10.1111/acem.12675 PMID: 25998446

Wainberg, M. L., Scorza, P., Shultz, J. M., Helpman, L., Mootz, J. J., Johnson, K. A., Neria, Y., Bradford, J. E., Oquendo, M. A., & Arbuckle, M. R. (2017). Challenges and Opportunities in Global Mental Health: A Research-to-Practice Perspective. *Current Psychiatry Reports*, *19*(5), 28. Advance online publication. DOI: 10.1007/s11920-017-0780-z PMID: 28425023

Walker, L. (2023, March 28). Belgian man dies by suicide following exchanges with chatbot. The Brussels Times. https://www.brusselstimes.com/430098/belgian-man-commits-suicide-following-exchanges-with-chatgpt

Walsh, C. G., Ribeiro, J. D., & Franklin, J. C. (2017). Predicting risk of suicide attempts over time through machine learning. *Clinical Psychological Science*, *5*(3), 457–469. DOI: 10.1177/2167702617691560

Wang, X., Sanders, H. M., Liu, Y., Seang, K., Tran, B. X., Atanasov, A. G., Qiu, Y., Tang, S., Car, J., Wang, Y. X., Wong, T. Y., Tham, Y., & Chung, K. C. (2023). ChatGPT: Promise and challenges for deployment in low- and middle-income countries. *The Lancet Regional Health. Western Pacific*, *41*, 100905. DOI: 10.1016/j.lanwpc.2023.100905 PMID: 37731897

Wangmo, T., Lipps, M., Kressig, R. W., & Ienca, M. (2019). Ethical concerns with the use of intelligent assistive technology: Findings from a qualitative study with professional stakeholders. *BMC Medical Ethics*, *20*(1), 98. Advance online publication. DOI: 10.1186/s12910-019-0437-z PMID: 31856798

Weizenbaum, J. (1966). ELIZA—A computer program for the study of natural language communication between man and machine. *Communications of the ACM*, *9*(1), 36–45. DOI: 10.1145/365153.365168

Woebot Health. (2024b, December 4). *Scalable enterprise solution for mental health | Woebot Health*. https://woebothealth.com/

World Health Organization. (2001). [*Mental Health: New Understanding, New Hope*. World Health Organization.]. *World Health Report*, •••, 2001.

WYSA - Everyday Mental Health. (n.d.-b). Wysa - Everyday Mental Health. https://www.wysa.com/

Yew, G. C. K. (2020). Trust in and ethical design of carebots: The case for Ethics of care. *International Journal of Social Robotics*, *13*(4), 629–645. DOI: 10.1007/s12369-020-00653-w PMID: 32837630

Yu, J., Shen, N., Conway, S., Hiebert, M., Lai-Zhao, B., McCann, M., Mehta, R. R., Miranda, M., Putterman, C., Santisteban, J. A., Thomson, N., Young, C., Chiuccariello, L., Hunter, K., & Hill, S. (2023). A holistic approach to integrating patient, family, and lived experience voices in the development of the BrainHealth Databank: A digital learning health system to enable artificial intelligence in the clinic. *Frontiers in Health Services*, *3*, 1198195. Advance online publication. DOI: 10.3389/frhs.2023.1198195 PMID: 37927443

Zhang, T., Schoene, A. M., Ji, S., & Ananiadou, S. (2022). Natural language processing applied to mental illness detection: A narrative review. *NPJ Digital Medicine*, *5*(1), 46. Advance online publication. DOI: 10.1038/s41746-022-00589-7 PMID: 35396451

Zicari, R. V., Brusseau, J., Blomberg, S. N., Christensen, H. C., Coffee, M., Ganapini, M. B., Gerke, S., Gilbert, T. K., Hickman, E., Hildt, E., Holm, S., Kühne, U., Madai, V. I., Osika, W., Spezzatti, A., Schnebel, E., Tithi, J. J., Vetter, D., Westerlund, M., & Kararigas, G. (2021). On assessing trustworthy AI in healthcare. Machine learning as a supportive tool to recognize cardiac arrest in emergency calls. *Frontiers in Human Dynamics*, *3*, 673104. Advance online publication. DOI: 10.3389/fhumd.2021.673104

KEY TERMS AND DEFINITIONS

Artificial Intelligence (AI): Scientific discipline of developing intelligent machines by simulating human intelligence to accomplish tasks that require learning, reasoning, and decision-making.

Automation Bias: Tendency of humans to over-trust automated decision-making systems over their judgment.

Black box algorithm: The Nature of AI models to hide the internal mechanisms used to create an outcome due to the absence of transparency and interpretability.

Brain-Computer Interface (BCI): A system that allows users to control a device using neural signals by acquiring, analyzing, and translating brain data.

Electronic Health Records (EHR): Digital collection of patients' health information obtained through different technologies and transferred to medical practitioners.

Generative AI: A type of AI capable of creating novel content in different forms by learning patterns and structures of training data.

Machine Learning (ML): A subset of AI that equips computer systems to learn from data and improve performance through experience without explicit programming.

Mental Health: The state of well-being encompasses emotional, psychological, and social aspects influencing how people think, feel, and behave.

Natural Language Processing (NLP): Subfield of AI to understand, analyze, generate, and interact with human language both spoken and written form in a meaningful way.

Chapter 15
Leveraging AI and Big Data for Sustainable Mental Health and Education Solutions Through a Green HRM Lens

Sonia Najam Shaikh
https://orcid.org/0009-0004-8358-7077
Jiangsu University, China

Li Zhen
Jiangsu University, China

Jan Muhammad Sohu
Sukkur IBA University, Pakistan

Saeed Abbas Shah
Sukkur IBA University, Pakistan

Hassan Abbas Soomro
Sukkur IBA University, Pakistan

ABSTRACT

This chapter explores the integration of Artificial Intelligence (AI), Big Data, and Green Human Resource Management (GHRM) to address mental health challenges in

DOI: 10.4018/979-8-3373-5072-1.ch015

Pakistan's higher education institutions (HEIs). Mental health issues such as stress, anxiety, and burnout significantly impact students and staff, hindering academic performance and well-being. AI-driven tools offer real-time, personalized mental health support, while Big Data enables institutions to identify risks and implement timely interventions. Green HRM complements these technologies by fostering sustainable practices, such as flexible work policies and eco-friendly campuses, that promote mental wellness and environmental responsibility. By combining these approaches, this chapter presents a holistic framework to improve mental health outcomes while aligning with sustainability goals, addressing challenges unique to Pakistan's HEIs, and offering actionable solutions for fostering resilient, supportive educational environments.

INTRODUCTION

Mental health has become a critical concern in Pakistan's higher education institutions (HEIs), where the pressures of academic success, financial constraints, and inadequate access to mental health resources create significant challenges for students and staff. The Pakistan Mental Health Survey 2020 revealed that over 35% of young people in the country face mental health issues, severely affecting their academic achievements and quality of life. Similarly, staff members in HEIs report high levels of stress and burnout, driven by excessive workloads, inadequate institutional support, and insufficient work-life balance. Addressing these issues is vital for improving individual well-being and creating an environment conducive to academic and professional growth.

New solutions especially AI and Big Data have the potential to give a solution to these problems. Mental health self-treatment applications like chatbots, voice assistants, and digital therapy apps help people contact mental health care instantly. By incorporating smart algorithms, it brings timely interferences, de-stigmatization, and affordable alternatives in a system. For instance, Woebot employs Cognitive Behavioral Therapy (CBT) to assist users in dealing with stress and anxiety (Boucher et al. 2021).

The potential benefits of integrating AI, Big Data, and Green HRM to support sustainable mental health and well-being are clear. However, to fully realize these benefits, there is a pressing need for continued research into the effectiveness of these technologies in different contexts, as well as their ethical implications (Alshuaibi et al. 2024). Moreover, policy makers, educational leaders, and HR professionals must be encouraged to adopt these integrated approaches and ensure that they are implemented with accessibility, equity, and sustainability in mind.

Future research should explore how these technologies can be applied in more underrepresented communities and address the mental health challenges specific to those populations. Additionally, the development of frameworks for integrating AI and Big Data while safeguarding privacy and adhering to ethical standards is essential. Innovative solutions combining sustainability and technology will lead the way for future mental health initiatives, particularly in educational and workplace settings, helping to create more resilient, supportive environments for future generations (Gu et al. 2022).

Big Data supports AI through providing institutions the opportunity to track large datasets, such as attendance records, academic achievements, and engagement rates. Using the risk factors and patterns at HEIs, early mitigation measures could be implemented on the students and staff that require it (Shaikh et al. 2024). Business intelligence and analytics from Big Data helps institutions take preventive measures with regards to mental health issues, creating a culture of early detection and treatment.

However, in Pakistan there is scarcity of mental health resources; people still have conservative mental health attitudes which discourages them from seeking help; therefore, deployment of these technologies should be cost effective and culturally appropriate. AI and Big Data have to be aligned with Green HRM as it gives the framework for tackling these issues more holistically. Green HRM, which identify activity that is friendly to environment and society, holds the potential for a firm to promote well-being at the same time as the firm minimizes damaging effects on the environment (Ali et al. 2023). Consequently, Green HRM in the context of HEIs includes measures such as flexible working arrangements, environmentally friendly campus layouts and designs, wellness promotions focusing on mental health as well as other green promotions.

BACKGROUND: THE ROLE OF AI, BIG DATA, AND SUSTAINABILITY

Artificial Intelligence and Big data have the potential to revolutionize mental health care and education in Pakistan's higher education institutions. For example, AI systems can analyze mood and emotions, monitor students' activities, and recommend actions to mitigate potential mental health issues such as anxiety and stress (Gu et al. 2022).

Big data, however, gathers large datasets from different sources, which may include the students' records, their attendance, and behaviours among other things. Big Data highlights trends and interdependencies that HEIs need to act upon to strengthen and enhance academic and mental health results (Thakkar, Gupta, and

De Sousa 2024). For instance, performance data in an institution may reveal the student who is likely to perform dismally or worse, drop out so institutions make necessary interventions to modify adverse future behavior.

When **AI** and **Big Data** are integrated, they become adaptive tools to address mental health issues. Real-time data can be processed by predictive algorithms to identify situations that may lead to the development of mental health concerns, while sentiment analysis can analyze interactions of students on the social network or other platforms to determine their well-being (Patel, Hung, and Katapally 2025).These technologies enable the HEIs in Pakistan to respond to mental health issues in an appropriate, timely and proactive manner which makes them helping instruments in creation of conducive learning environment.

However, in Pakistan, the scarcity of mental health resources and the prevalent stigma around mental health care continue to pose significant barriers. Therefore, the deployment of AI and Big Data technologies must be both cost-effective and culturally appropriate. Moreover, these technologies should be aligned with Green HRM practices, which promote both well-being and environmental sustainability. Green HRM which focuses on environmentally friendly activities holds the potential for institutions to foster mental well-being while minimizing environmental harm (Ali et al., 2023). In the context of HEIs, Green HRM includes flexible working arrangements, eco-friendly campus designs, wellness programs, and other green initiatives that promote mental health.

ETHICAL AND PRIVACY CONCERNS

While AI and Big Data offer promising solutions for mental health care, their use raises significant ethical concerns, particularly around data privacy and security. The collection and analysis of personal mental health data involve sensitive information that must be handled with the utmost care. In Pakistan's context, where mental health is often stigmatized, ensuring that individuals' data is kept private and secure is paramount. There is also the concern of algorithmic biases that could result in inaccurate or discriminatory outcomes. If AI systems are trained on biased data, they may perpetuate or even exacerbate inequalities in mental health care, particularly for marginalized groups. Therefore, it is crucial that AI and Big Data systems be developed with built-in mechanisms to prevent bias and ensure fairness, transparency, and accountability in how data is used. Ensuring ethical standards are met will help build trust in these technologies and encourage their adoption in sensitive areas like mental health.

MENTAL HEALTH CHALLENGES IN PAKISTAN'S HEIS

Pakistan's HEIs face significant challenges in managing mental health due to the unique sociocultural and institutional pressures within the country. Students also have higher stress rates due to academic competition, financial issues, or lack of appropriate help in groups. Lack of qualified mental health workers, prejudices and the stigma associated with mental health also contributes to the problem. Similarly, faculty and staff experience severe workload pressures, unrealistic expectations and organisational support leaving them highly stressed and burnt out (Javaid, Chen, and Ramzan 2024).

Barriers to Technology Adoption in Pakistan's HEIs

While AI and Big Data present promising solutions for mental health challenges in Pakistan's HEIs, several barriers to their adoption remain. Lack of infrastructure is a major obstacle, as many institutions struggle with limited access to high-speed internet, reliable electricity, and necessary hardware. Additionally, financial constraints prevent many HEIs from investing in the technology and skilled personnel required to implement AI and Big Data solutions effectively. Technological limitations, including outdated software and insufficient technical support, further hinder the integration of these tools into educational and administrative systems. Moreover, resistance from staff due to unfamiliarity with these technologies, fears of job displacement, or reluctance to adopt new methodologies complicates the process of implementing AI-driven mental health solutions. These challenges must be addressed in order to unlock the full potential of AI and Big Data in improving mental health outcomes within HEIs.

AI and Big Data offer new ways to solve these problems successfully. For students, it can track changes in their behavior like lack of participation, frequent absenteeism or withdrawal which might signify stress or anxiety. These patterns can be recognized in advance through predictive analytics so that these learning institutions can provide early detection and interventions including counselling, mentoring or academic adjustment for the particular problem. Likewise, Big Data can they describe institutional policies' influence on mental health, making it easier to assess how teaching models, workload organization, or assessment schedules affect general well-being (Lin and Chen 2024).

Faculty and staff also stand to benefit from AI-powered systems designed to monitor workplace stress. For instance, besides monitoring productivity indicators, an analysis of emails and communication activity can identify the first symptoms of burnout or dissatisfaction. After these signals are identified, institutions can then bring about work arrangements including flexible work schedules, or mindfulness and wellness sessions. All of these steps help not only to decrease the risks of mental health issues but also to increase the level of activation, satisfaction, and effectiveness of institutions and organizations.

Green HRM in Pakistan's HEIs

Green HRM has a central role to address and adopt sustainable mental health practices in Pakistan's HEIs. That is why integration of sustainability into HR polices is an approach of Green HRM that a creates suitable conditions for mental health of students and staff. Measures like incorporating energy conservation in hall designs, having greeneries and less littering do not only make operation environmentally friendly but help reduce stress and increase concentration levels (Ali 2023; Shaikh et al. 2024).

It is also Green HRM practice that allows the best flexibility of work policies where faculty have adequate working and personal life balance, thus minimizing on burnout. Altogether, learning environments that are environmentally friendly such as light, plants, and ergonomically friendly area relieve students of academic stress. Some of the Green HRM practices include mental health workshops, counselling services, and wellness programs which provide solutions to psychological issues and promote a healthy environment (Kamaruddin et al. 2018).

Combining AI, Big Data, and Green HRM

This integration thus provides a systematic approach of addressing issues to do with mental health, within the Pakistani context of HEIs under the influence of AI, Big Data and Green HRM. Big data can be analyzed to ascertain and find out probable mental health issues and give timely intervention through AI software. For instance, AI-powered systems can suggest ways to manage stress, therapy, or curriculum changes with the patterns learned through the Big Data analysis. Green HRM supports these initiatives by creating sustainable, effective environments like offering flexible working hours, greens spaces and wellness programs in collaboration with AI mental health tactics that are sought after (Sabale and Dr.S 2022).

However, Green HRM initiations can also be supported by the help of AI and Big Data in educational organizations to assess the effectiveness of these practices. For instance, big data can analyse the effects that the green designs of campus have on engagement, satisfaction, and health among students (Shahid et al. 2023). These strategies can be enhanced and expanded by AI-powered systems based also on analyses on aspects like where green areas could be allocated more efficiently or where members of the community can receive help to address mental health issues (Sohu et al. 2024). It creates a constant feedback system, which ensures that mental health interventions being implemented are not only efficacious but also feasible that will build a strong resilience to the environment among the institutions.

By integrating these technologies and strategies, HEIs in Pakistan can meet the multifaceted tasks in mental health with an integrated and evidence-based approach. They found that AI and Big Data offer effectiveness and extensiveness in scale, while Green HRM would ensure that those interventions are sustainable and healthy. Collectively, they work to foster conditions that enhance wellbeing, academic achievement, and institutional viability at a global level.

SUSTAINABILITY AND GREEN HRM

Sustainability in organizational practices has expanded to address not just environmental concerns but also employee and student well-being. Sustainability has gone beyond being observed in organizational processes relating to environmental impacts but also the physical and psychological health of employees and students (Renwick, Redman, and Maguire 2013). By incorporating sustainability into people management, Green HRM reflects this paradigm change and encourages people to match the organisational commitment. Some of the Green HRM practices include flexible work schedules access to mental health facilities and work environment being created to reduce burn out while improving satisfaction (Shaikh et al. 2024)

AI and Big data enhance the ability of Green HRM through the generation of insights on well-being. Sentiment analysis or behavioral analysis for stress indicates the need for AI algorithms, while Big Data points to systematic stress that needs to be addressed at a particular level. For instance, AI-based artificial companion apps provide weekly gratitude logs, guided relaxation sessions, and feedback with counselling sessions to help these targets immediately and be adequately mentally treated as students and employees (García-Madurga et al. 2024).

On the academic level, the combined use of AI, Big Data, and Green HRM helps detect stress levels, develop, and launch relevant health promotion programs, and develop environmentally friendly policies (Murugesan et al. 2023). It fosters such circumstances that would enhance the understanding of resilience and satisfaction, fulfilling the purposes of the HEIs in terms of mental health and sustainable objectives. When applied to advancing technology within the HEIs, sound human resource management interventions for mental health support can be embraced alongside themes of innovation, sustainability.

AI-DRIVEN SOLUTIONS FOR MENTAL HEALTH

AI has transformed mental health care, making it more accessible, personalized, and stigma-free. Thus, AI tools such as chatbots, digital therapy platforms, and monitoring systems offer sophisticated approaches to overcome mental well-being issues, including workplaces, schools, and communities (Balcombe 2023). Digital platforms support care even more due the possibility to tailor it on person's specific needs. With the help of artificial intelligence, these systems process user responses to serve up therapeutic content at the time when it is needed, be it a mindfulness exercise or a set of writing prompts. With help of AI monitoring systems, such parameters as sleep, activity and social interaction are analyzed to note deterioration in a patient's state and take corrective measures.

AI is also strongly involved in workplaces as one of the key instruments in advance mental health support. Self-evaluation tools used in workplaces check for signs of stress during communication processes, while wearables track the physical signs of stress such as heart rate and sleep patterns (García et al. 2024). Such observations make it possible to organize workload for employees, encourage the practice of mindfulness, or provide counselling to ensure that the employees do not deteriorate psychologically. Of all the valuable roles that AI plays, the most apparent is its capability of eradicating stigma. In its way, providing both anonymous and private spaces, it makes it possible for an individual to look for help without worrying for them to be stigmatized. They encourage people to seek help with mental disorders as much as they seek help with any physical ailment, improving schools, workplaces, and communities.

Big Data and Mental Health in Educational Institutions

Big Data is revolutionizing education by enabling institutions to support students academically, socially, and emotionally. Big Data helps compound crucial academic records with the assessments of behavior and social relations to design complete and personalized mental health strategies that contribute to the students' well-being. In educational paradigms, educational Big Data monitors student activity within classes, course attendance, interactions, as well as submitted assignments. It enables educators to understand the students who may be in danger of poor performance hence giving them the required attention (Sohu et al. 2025).

Except for academics, Big Data evaluates the patient's emotional and psychological self. Social media posts, surveys and feedback analysis reveals signs of stress, anxiety or/and depression among individuals. For instance, lack of participation or even frequent absenteeism might indicate the onset of mental health problems that call for early treatment (Maples-Keller et al. 2017). Another area of Big Data is the application called predictive analytics which, for example, expounds on students prone to some risk factors with the reference to such data examples as academic achievements, interactions with peers, and health. Any changes of conduct which include late submission, reduced contribution, may be symptoms of emotional problems. Institutions can then react with proper resources like counselling, peer support, and wellness programs.

The opportunities of Big Data also include a differentiated approach, especially when it comes to education. Failure rates could be lowered and stress levels decreased at the individual student level by evaluating the way in which they use the content. In addition, it is important to use assessment data in relation to the mental health programs with a view to improving on the strategies used to implement the programs.

Big Data in Identifying Institutional Patterns

Big Data plays a crucial role in identifying emergent patterns which might impact the students. Tess Truth A conceptual framework that is important for Big Data to ascertain regularly occurring patterns influencing the students' welfare. For instance, it encompasses stressors like difficulty level of the course, how workload is shared and the methods, which are used when teaching. These findings can be used by institutions to modify curricula or develop extra assistance to assist stressed programs (Qasim, Qureshi, and Shaikh 2025). The survey results show that the level of social engagement helps to determine students' belongingness. This implies that student who seldom participate in campus activities or have a weakening peer support normally face more severe mental health issues. These challenges can be dealt with by promoting diversity through some key functions passing through a special mentoring programme, extracurricular club, or SPAR functionality event in institutions.

Big Data also reveals disparities in patients' mental health by gender or race, and/or some students, like international or underrepresented ones. Through inequitable support structures, universities help to eliminate inequalities towards the improvement of health and well-being of all learners as stated by (Renwick et al. 2013).

Integrating Technologies for Holistic Solutions

The integration of AI, Big Data, and Green HRM provides a comprehensive framework for addressing mental health challenges while promoting sustainability. AI provides more accurate outcomes at the particular time; Big Data provides overall patterns and trends and Green HRM constructs conditions that will promote employees' health. It is through these approaches that institutions can approach mental health in a programmatic style and push the sustainability agenda forward (Jin et al.

2023). For instance, AI and Big Data evaluate outcomes of Green HRM policies including flexible working, green areas, and mental health seminars to students and staff. Since they deliver support according to evaluated mental health needs, these technologies guarantee that the plan offered is relevant to the individual, as well. It creates responsive resilience, assertiveness for inclusion and correctness, satisfaction, better, health, and sustainability in the educational and organizational communities.

Green HRM: Integrating Sustainable Mental Health Practices

Green HRM is the environmental friendly HRM framework which incorporate both better environment and improved employee's mental health successfully. This gives a very balanced approach that would help and suffice the individual self and the organizational self as well as the society self. Green HRM combats both sustainability and psychological concerns by incorporating environmental sustainability strategies into human resource management and policies, specifically focusing on mental health assistance (Jackson et al. 2012).

Another Green HRM practice is work options flexibility, which helps employees balance their work-life to ensure they meet the environmental objectives. Teleworking possibilities, flexible schedules, and shortened workweeks are meant to help employees decrease stress and gain more schedule flexibility. At the same time, these practices reduce commuting requirements and cut resource utilization in offices, thus supporting other sustainable development goals (Lee, Chong, and Ojo 2024).

Another factor is creating favourable conditions for work, and a friendly environment and conditions for the surrounding environment. Offices with elements of natural lighting, some indoor greenery and sustainable materials cause calming, positive effect in the mental and social health of workers (Iqbal et al. 2023). Studies have also revealed that when people are taken through nature, or they work close to natural factors, their stress levels decrease and they concentrate well (Lygum et al. 2023).

Mental health programs are organisational components of Green HRM where the employees are offered the appropriate counselling, Mindfulness workshops and the tools for wellbeing. They minimize the culture of concealed illness and help individuals take action in early stages concerning their mental health. Third, digital wellness tools are equally useful as they provide immediate assistance to all stress, anxiety, or other emotional issues that employees might be facing, making mental health a more attainable and customizable solution (Wu et al. 2021).

Green HRM is also agreed on its focus of engagement arising from sustainability. Businesses that champion for environmentally friendly policies and practices including recycling, power conservation and green transportation commute policies encourage employee commitment and corporate culture conformity. Ribeiro et al.

(2022) posited that employees who feel better about social impact of their organisations job are more committed, satisfied and hence, more loyal and productive.

Green HRM and Employee Engagement

Green HRM is a key element that helps organizations enhance employees' commitment through promoting health and green the organization's operations. This way committed employees are productive, satisfied with their work and exhibit positive . Organizations that cultivate a culture of well-being emphasizing flexibility, mental health resources, and eco-conscious practices—empower employees to thrive and contribute meaningfully to organizational goals (Gyensare and Adomako 2023).

Moreover, Green HRM fosters collaboration and communication by encouraging open discussions about wellness programs and green initiatives. This transparency strengthens employee relationships, reduces feelings of isolation, and promotes teamwork. Employees are more likely to feel connected and motivated in workplaces that support both their emotional needs and environmental values. Alignment of organizational and individual values is another driver of engagement (Yang and Li 2023). Employees resonate strongly with workplaces that champion sustainability and prioritize mental health. For example, initiatives such as reducing waste, using renewable energy, or promoting mindfulness exercises in natural settings can foster a sense of pride and deeper commitment to the organization's mission (Monteiro and Joseph 2023).

Big Data in Identifying Institutional Patterns Affecting Well-Being

Big Data serves as a powerful tool for understanding and improving well-being in both workplaces and educational institutions. By analyzing large and complex datasets, organizations can identify patterns, address systemic challenges, and implement evidence-based interventions to support mental health (Dash et al. 2019).

In educational institutions, Big Data helps uncover academic stressors such as demanding course structures or ineffective teaching methods. This information enables administrators to refine curricula and reduce workload pressures, creating a more supportive environment for students (Dumont, Shen, and Deng 2016). Similarly, data on student participation in campus events and extracurricular activities can highlight areas of isolation or disengagement, allowing institutions to promote inclusivity and foster a stronger sense of community (Sweeney et al., 2020). Big Data also plays a critical role in addressing equity in mental health support. By analyzing data across demographics, organizations and institutions can identify disparities in well-being and tailor interventions to meet the needs of specific groups, such as international students or those from underrepresented backgrounds (Samuel and Extension 2024).

Predictive analytics, a core application of Big Data, enables proactive mental health management. By monitoring indicators such as attendance, performance, and behavior, institutions can identify at-risk individuals and provide timely interventions. For example, behavioral changes or declining engagement may signal underlying mental health challenges, prompting personalized support through counselling or mentoring programs.

Synergizing AI, Big Data, and Green HRM

The combination of AI, Big data, and Green HRM form a revolutionary model that offers an integrated solution to mental health issues. AI delivers immediate prescriptive feedback for the behavior of people, Big Data identifies embedded systematic trends, while Green HRM promotes both environment and mindset.

With the help of AI capabilities, employees' engagement and stress levels can be monitored and further suggestions for improvement can be introduced in form of breathing techniques or flexible working hours. Big Data provides information on the performance of Green HRM, given developments that can be implemented to improve strategies and results. For instance, information regarding the effects of green office designs or flexible working hours on the wellbeing of workers assist organisations in enhancing their initiatives (Baig, Shuib, and Yadegaridehkordi 2020). One of the other areas that has been highlighted to features AI and Green HRM include environmentally sensitive mental health practices. Mental health can be improved through outdoor mindfulness sessions or utilization of nature activates for relaxation, all in pursuit of environmental initiatives. These two cases give a cyclical boost where sustainability initiatives improve well-being as well as vice versa.

Challenges And Solutions

Despite its potential, the implementation of Green HRM, AI, and Big Data is not without challenges. Privacy concerns are a significant barrier, particularly when collecting and analyzing sensitive mental health data. Organizations must ensure compliance with data protection regulations and maintain transparency to build trust with employees and students (Sohu et al. 2023).

Resource constraints also pose a challenge, especially for smaller organizations or institutions with limited budgets. Gradual adoption of affordable AI tools, combined with targeted training for staff, can help overcome these barriers. Finally, resistance to change is a common obstacle. Transparent communication about the benefits of these initiatives and active involvement of employees in program design can foster acceptance and engagement.

Green HRM, when integrated with AI and Big Data, offers a comprehensive solution to the intertwined challenges of mental health and sustainability. By leveraging these tools and practices, organizations and institutions can create inclusive, resilient, and eco-conscious environments. This innovative approach enhances individual well-being, aligns with environmental objectives, and fosters a culture of engagement and collaboration. As organizations adopt these integrated strategies, they pave the way for a future where mental health is prioritized alongside sustainability. Through thoughtful implementation and collaboration, Green HRM, AI, and Big Data can help build healthier, more equitable, and sustainable workplaces and educational institutions, benefiting individuals and society as a whole.

AI, Big Data, and Green HRM in Educational Settings

Educational institutions face growing challenges in addressing student mental health amidst rising stress, anxiety, and other psychological issues. Traditional methods of student support are no longer sufficient to meet these challenges. The integration of AI, Big Data, and GHRM offers innovative and comprehensive solutions to revolutionize mental health and well-being in educational environments.

AI and Big Data for Student Well-Being

AI technologies like chatbots and virtual assistants provide real-time mental health support by analyzing student behaviors, emotional states, and engagement patterns through sentiment analysis and interaction tracking (Nuwasiima, Metogbe, and Kadiri 2024). Big Data enhances this process by offering real-time insights from diverse sources, including attendance records, academic performance metrics, and student surveys. By identifying patterns and early warning signs of mental health challenges, Big Data enables educators and mental health professionals to intervene proactively (Monteiro and Joseph 2023). This predictive capability ensures that institutions can provide targeted support to students before issues escalate, creating a safer and more supportive learning environment.

Personalized learning paths further integrate mental health support into academic experiences. By leveraging AI and Big Data, institutions can adjust coursework difficulty, recommend breaks, or suggest wellness activities tailored to a student's emotional state or stress levels (Sohu et al. 2023). This holistic approach ensures students receive both academic and emotional support, empowering them to achieve success while maintaining mental well-being.

Green HRM in Educational Institutions

Green HRM integrates sustainability and mental health practices into educational settings, promoting eco-conscious initiatives that benefit students and staff. Sustainable, eco-friendly campuses—featuring energy-efficient buildings, natural lighting, and green spaces—create calming environments that reduce stress and foster mental well-being (K.M, Aithal, and K R S 2024).

Educational institutions adopting Green HRM focus on policies that balance academic responsibilities with mental health priorities. Flexible scheduling for faculty, wellness programs for students, and initiatives to reduce campus waste are integral to these efforts. Additionally, educators can incorporate Green HRM principles into curricula, fostering a culture of sustainability and mental wellness awareness. This holistic approach empowers students to connect with nature, enhance their focus, and improve their overall emotional health (Ababneh 2021).

Case Studies of Green HRM in Action

To better understand how Green HRM practices positively influence both employee well-being and engagement, here are a few case studies of organizations that have implemented successful Green HRM strategies. Google is another example of an organization that integrates Green HRM principles to support mental health and employee engagement. The company offers a wide range of wellness programs, including on-site fitness centers, mental health workshops, and access to counselling services. Google's workspaces feature green designs with natural lighting, open spaces, and eco-friendly furniture, which promote employee well-being and creativity. These initiatives have contributed to Google's reputation as an employer of choice, with employees citing the company's focus on well-being as a key factor in their job satisfaction (Rapo 2024).

Unilever is committed to integrating sustainability into every aspect of its operations, including its HR practices. The company has launched various mental health initiatives, such as employee assistance programs and mindfulness training, and promotes work-life balance through flexible work hours and remote work options. Unilever's eco-friendly office spaces also contribute to employee well-being by reducing stress and creating a more comfortable work environment. These Green HRM practices have resulted in improved employee engagement and reduced levels of burnout (Haque, Islam, and Soh 2024).

Green HRM offers a holistic approach that integrates sustainability with employee well-being, fostering a work environment that promotes mental health, engagement, and productivity. By adopting sustainable HR practices, such as flexible work arrangements, mental health support programs, and eco-friendly office designs, organizations can improve their employees' mental health, reduce stress, and enhance overall job satisfaction. The case studies of Patagonia, Google, and Unilever illustrate the positive outcomes of Green HRM, showing that organizations that prioritize both environmental responsibility and employee well-being enjoy higher engagement and productivity levels. Green HRM provides a win-win solution for organizations seeking to achieve both environmental sustainability and employee mental health.

Case Study of Successful Integration

There are several case studies of educational institutions successfully integrating AI, Big Data, and Green HRM practices to support student mental health. For instance, Stanford University has integrated AI-powered mental health platforms, like Woebot, alongside their campus-wide mental wellness programs to offer students personalized mental health support. Woebot uses AI to engage with students through conversations, providing coping strategies for stress, anxiety, and depression. Meanwhile, Stanford also encourages sustainability through their Green HRM policies, including a campus initiative focused on mental health awareness and eco-friendly initiatives, such as the development of green spaces and energy-efficient buildings that contribute to the students' well-being (Khan et al. 2024).

These case studies demonstrate that when AI, Big Data, and Green HRM practices are combined, educational institutions can significantly improve their ability to support student mental health while simultaneously promoting environmental sustainability.

FUTURE DIRECTIONS: EMERGING TRENDS AND OPPORTUNITIES

The future of AI and Big Data in mental health is marked by a shift toward more personalized, accurate, and accessible solutions. Deep learning algorithms, which have already shown great promise in fields like image and speech recognition, are increasingly being applied to mental health diagnostics. These algorithms can analyze complex datasets, such as brain scans and voice patterns, to detect early signs of mental health disorders like depression and anxiety with high accuracy (Rebelo et al. 2023). The continued development of these technologies will likely lead to more precise mental health diagnoses and early intervention strategies.

Another emerging trend is real-time mental health monitoring through wearable devices and mobile apps. These tools, powered by AI and Big Data, can track users' physiological and psychological states in real time, providing continuous feedback and intervention. For example, wearables that monitor heart rate, sleep patterns, and activity levels can be integrated with AI tools to offer insights into a person's mental health, alerting them to potential issues before they escalate (Shajari et al. 2023). This could significantly improve outcomes by allowing individuals and healthcare providers to intervene earlier.

Virtual Reality (VR) is also emerging as a promising tool in mental health care. VR has been shown to be effective in treating conditions like PTSD, anxiety, and depression by immersing users in controlled environments where they can confront and manage their symptoms in a safe space (Soomro et al. 2024). As VR technologies become more sophisticated, they may become a central component of digital mental health strategies, offering highly personalized and interactive treatment options.

Opportunities for Green HRM in the Future

The future of Green HRM will be shaped by the growing recognition of the importance of sustainability in both the workplace and educational institutions. As environmental concerns become more pressing, organizations will increasingly adopt Green HRM strategies to reduce their ecological footprint while enhancing employee and student well-being. The link between sustainability and mental health is already well-documented, and Green HRM practices such as flexible working arrangements, eco-friendly office spaces, and promoting environmental responsibility will become even more integral to organizational culture (Gupta and Jangra 2024).

As sustainability becomes a higher priority globally, Green HRM will evolve to include more robust mental health strategies that are tied to environmental outcomes. For instance, AI and Big Data may play a key role in assessing the effectiveness of Green HRM strategies, providing insights into how specific sustainability initiatives, such as reducing carbon emissions or promoting green spaces, affect employee and student mental health (Aftab et al. 2023).

Innovative Solutions for Sustainable Mental Health and Education

Looking forward, the integration of AI, Big Data, and Green HRM will lead to more personalized, accessible, and sustainable mental health solutions. Future research will likely explore how these technologies can be better integrated into existing healthcare and education systems to improve access and outcomes for diverse populations. As AI and Big Data become more sophisticated, their ability to address mental health in underrepresented communities or individuals with chronic conditions will improve, making mental health support more equitable and inclusive.

In education, AI-powered tools will enable more adaptive learning environments that not only promote academic success but also prioritize emotional and psychological development. Schools and universities will continue to innovate by integrating sustainability into both their physical infrastructure and their curriculum, helping students connect with nature and understand the importance of maintaining their mental health while caring for the planet (Kamalov, Santandreu Calonge, and Gurrib 2023).

Shaping the Future of Sustainable Mental Health and Education

This chapter has explored the transformative role that AI, Big Data, and Green HRM can play in fostering sustainable mental health and education solutions. As we have seen, these three forces are increasingly intertwined, creating opportunities for more personalized, accessible, and environmentally responsible strategies to address the growing mental health challenges in educational and workplace settings.

At the core of this integration, AI technologies, such as chatbots, natural language processing, and predictive analytics, offer substantial promise in improving mental health management. (Manole et al. 2024). AI's ability to process large amounts of data and provide tailored, real-time interventions makes it an essential tool in combating mental health issues that have traditionally been difficult to address, especially in institutional settings. By analyzing vast quantities of data and giving responsive, individualized interventions, AI is an indispensable resource in fighting mental disorders, which are especially hard to manage, particularly in facilities. Through AI apps such as Woebot and Wysa or through the use of other technologies like sentiment analysis, burnout detection, AI creates an early intervention method and generates proactive approaches for students and employees (Jiang et al. 2024). Further, the advanced ability of artificial intelligence to power predictive models makes it easier for institutions to detect mental health issues before they become crises, and address the need of timely intervention and individual patient care.

Big Data performs a similarly significant role in contributing to AI, as it serves as the basis for its work. Using metrics from a scale of academic and social performance and health through Big Data tools, institutions can get an invaluable look at the health of their student and employee populations (Ikegwu et al. 2022). In particular, through Big Data's means of monitoring in real-time, it can detect otherwise unnoticed signals of developing mental health problems, including increased stress, potential signs of depression, or the likelihood of burnout. In addition, Big Data can be used to provide a more individualized approach with mental health resources and learning opportunities, whether it be in learning modules, mental health check-in and assistance, and creating programmatic tactics based on previous experiences (Aebi et al. 2021).

In the similar vein, Green HRM has evolved as an effective tool for addressing the concerns of employee, student, and environment at large. Green HRM focuses on integrating sustainable initiatives in organizational systems including work flexibility, environment friendly workplace, and health management systems. These practices lead to lower stress, higher morale and a better work or learning climate (Zihan, Makhbul, and Alam 2024). Environmental sustainability and interpersonal health are now linked with research showing that exposure to green environments and carrying out environmental friendly activates helps reduce anxiety, promote rest and enhance concentration. Green HRM initiatives not only helps in constructing a better form which is effective for the mental health of the employees but also ensures the overall culture of sustainability which is so highly concerned in today's global environment.

The integration of these technologies provides a broader perspective of mental health that provides solutions beyond the conventional medical model of practice placed in individual therapy, social and physical environment, and working organizations. Sustainability can be implemented into mental health programs for employees and students and also into organizational practices and policies that would lead to environmental sustainability of the world (Feijt et al. 2023).

CONCLUSION

Future focus areas include sustainability, mental health, and technology as key drivers that will define the future of well-being within educational and workplace settings. Since technology is always improving AI and Big Data will probably play an even bigger role in mental health interventions as more advanced techniques for the early diagnosis, individual approach and prognosis of patients with mental disorders can be developed. On the other hand, the emphasis on Green HRM will persist to remain relevant as more organisations and educational facility adapt more usually HRM practices that improvement the mental-and-physical health of employees and students.

Such merging of technology and sustainability brings new hope to enhance mental health in the context of the world continuing to be a single village while having technology interconnected with sustainability. Increased awareness of the connection between people's mental health and environmental factors, including natural areas, clean air, and environmentally friendly practices demonstrates the need for integrated approaches that address both mental health and the environment. The more organizational and educational institutions adopt these integrated models, then we are likely to have more individualised, scable, and sustainable system for tackling mental health issues within the targeted population.

Nevertheless, with the AI, Big data, and Green HRM there are opportunities to help the society and improve mental health and well being of people; yet there are lots of challenges. Challenges that relate to problems like the lack of data privacy, employee resistance, and digital gap must be worked out for these technologies to work to the maximum potential. However, it is also important there is increased research conducted so that there is increased understanding in relation to the appropriateness and consequences of the utilization of these technologies and practices.

However, all these have to be done under one important aspect; integration which requires working under one roof. Thus, educational institutions, human resources departments, and mental health workers must contemplate how they can build environments in which learners and employees thrive emotionally and mentally, and organizations are sustainable. This can involve mobile applications for the treatment of mental disorders, Big data for monitoring stress and academic outcomes, and of the advocacy for green HRM practices. Organizations and institutions that adopt this broad approach will be in a better place to address care and mental health and also incorporate sustainability in every operational activities.

Call to Action

From this perspective, the opportunities of AI, Big Data, Green HRM for the establishment of effective practices promoting sustainable mental health and well-being can be numerous. However, for the realisation of these potential benefits, more work is needed to establish how effective these technologies are in those, as well as the ethics of using such technologies. Furthermore, the policy makers, educational leaders and the Human resource professionals must be encouraged to adopt these integrated approaches to provide for access, equity, and sustainability.

Further research should be conducted on how these technologies could be used in other diverse areas and to recruit minorities, understand the existing mental health disorders affecting these groups of people. Further, the concept of implementing AI and Big Data together, and how to do so with an emphasis on privacy and ethical use will emerge as important. Sustainable approaches and technological integration will be novel futures for mental health intervention in specific areas of education and workplace to produce healthier generations.

In sum, it would be pertinent to underscore that a synthesis of the AI, Big Data and Green HRM offers an innovative and promising avenue in the endeavour to finding suitable and sustainable solutions towards the mental health crisis. The intersection of mental health, technology, and sustainability promises a future where both people and the planet can thrive. This vision will require ongoing commitment, research, and collaboration among all stakeholders, but the potential to reshape how we support mental health and well-being in educational and workplace settings is immense.

REFERENCES

Ababneh, O. M. A. (2021). How Do Green HRM Practices Affect Employees' Green Behaviors? The Role of Employee Engagement and Personality Attributes. *Journal of Environmental Planning and Management, 64*(7), 1204–1226. DOI: 10.1080/09640568.2020.1814708

Aebi, N. J., De Ridder, D., Ochoa, C., Petrovic, D., Fadda, M., Elayan, S., Sykora, M., Puhan, M., Naslund, J. A., Mooney, S. J., & Gruebner, O. (2021). Can Big Data Be Used to Monitor the Mental Health Consequences of COVID-19? *International Journal of Public Health, 66*, 633451. DOI: 10.3389/ijph.2021.633451 PMID: 34744586

Aftab, J., Abid, N., Cucari, N., & Savastano, M. (2023). Green Human Resource Management and Environmental Performance: The Role of Green Innovation and Environmental Strategy in a Developing Country. *Business Strategy and the Environment, 32*(4), 1782–1798. DOI: 10.1002/bse.3219

Ali, A. (2023). GREEN HRM IMPACT ON SUSTAINABILITY IN PAKISTANI UNIVERSITIES. *Journal for Business Education and Management, 3*(2), 177–196. DOI: 10.56596/jbem.v3i2.85

Ali, Q. M., Nisar, Q. A., Abidin, R. Z., Qammar, R., & Abbass, K. (2023). Greening the Workforce in Higher Educational Institutions: The Pursuance of Environmental Performance. *Environmental Science and Pollution Research International, 30*(60), 124474–124487. DOI: 10.1007/s11356-022-19888-3 PMID: 35349063

Alshuaibi, M. S. I., Alhebri, A., Khan, S. N., & Sheikh, A. A. (2024). Big Data Analytics, GHRM Practices, and Green Digital Learning Paving the Way towards Green Innovation and Sustainable Firm Performance. *Journal of Open Innovation, 10*(4), 100396. DOI: 10.1016/j.joitmc.2024.100396

Baig, M. I., Shuib, L., & Yadegaridehkordi, E. (2020). Big Data in Education: A State of the Art, Limitations, and Future Research Directions. *International Journal of Educational Technology in Higher Education, 17*(1), 44. DOI: 10.1186/s41239-020-00223-0

Balcombe, L. (2023). AI Chatbots in Digital Mental Health. *Informatics (MDPI), 10*(4), 82. DOI: 10.3390/informatics10040082

Boucher, E. M., Harake, N. R., Ward, H. E., Stoeckl, S. E., Vargas, J., Minkel, J., ... & Zilca, R. (2021). Artificially intelligent chatbots in digital mental health interventions: a review. Expert Review of Medical Devices, 18(sup1), 37-49.

Dash, S., Shakyawar, S. K., Sharma, M., & Kaushik, S. (2019). Big Data in Healthcare: Management, Analysis and Future Prospects. *Journal of Big Data*, *6*(1), 54. DOI: 10.1186/s40537-019-0217-0

Dumont, J., Shen, J., & Deng, X. (2016). Effects of Green HRM Practices on Employee Workplace Green Behavior: The Role of Psychological Green Climate and Employee Green Values: Effect of Green HRM on Employee Workplace Green Behavior. *Human Resource Management*, *56*(4), 613–627. Advance online publication. DOI: 10.1002/hrm.21792

Feijt, M., de Kort, Y., Westerink, J., Bierbooms, J., Bongers, I., & IJsselsteijn, W. (2023). Integrating Technology in Mental Healthcare Practice: A Repeated Cross-Sectional Survey Study on Professionals' Adoption of Digital Mental Health before and during COVID-19. *Frontiers in Psychiatry*, *13*, 1040023. DOI: 10.3389/fpsyt.2022.1040023 PMID: 36874171

García, M., Gil-Lacruz, A.-I., Gil, I., & Gil-Lacruz, M. (2024). The Role of Artificial Intelligence in Improving Workplace Well-Being: A Systematic Review. *Businesses*, *4*(3), 389–410. DOI: 10.3390/businesses4030024

García-Madurga, M.-Á., Gil-Lacruz, A.-I., Saz-Gil, I., & Gil-Lacruz, M. (2024). The Role of Artificial Intelligence in Improving Workplace Well-Being: A Systematic Review. *Businesses*, *4*(3), 389–410. DOI: 10.3390/businesses4030024

Gu, Z., Li, P., Zhang, A., Xu, X., & Gu, F. (2022). The Role of Mental Health and Sustainable Learning Behavior of Students in Education Sector Influences Sustainable Environment. *Frontiers in Psychology*, *13*, 822751. Advance online publication. DOI: 10.3389/fpsyg.2022.822751 PMID: 35211067

Gupta, A., & Jangra, S. (2024). Green Human Resource Management and Work Engagement: Linking HRM Performance Attributions. *Sustainable Futures : An Applied Journal of Technology, Environment and Society*, *7*, 100174. DOI: 10.1016/j.sftr.2024.100174

Gyensare, M., Adomako, S., & Amankwah-Amoah, J. (2023). Green HRM Practices, Employee Well-being, and Sustainable Work Behavior: Examining the Moderating Role of Resource Commitment. *Business Strategy and the Environment*, *33*(4), 3129–3141. Advance online publication. DOI: 10.1002/bse.3642

Haque, M. A., Islam, M. A., & Soh, S. H. (2024). Green HRM Practices and Green Work Engagement: The Roles of Green Knowledge Sharing and Green Group Cohesion. *Global Business and Organizational Excellence*, *44*(1), 16–31. DOI: 10.1002/joe.22266

Ikegwu, A., Nweke, H., Anikwe, C., Alo, U., & Okonkwo, O. (2022). Big Data Analytics for Data-Driven Industry: A Review of Data Sources, Tools, Challenges, Solutions, and Research Directions. *Cluster Computing*, *25*(5), 3343–3387. Advance online publication. DOI: 10.1007/s10586-022-03568-5

Iqbal, S., Akhtar, S., Anwar, F., Kayani, A. J., Sohu, J. M., & Khan, A. S. (2023). Linking Green Innovation Performance and Green Innovative Human Resource Practices in SMEs; a Moderation and Mediation Analysis Using PLS-SEM. *Current Psychology (New Brunswick, N.J.)*, *42*(13), 11250–11267. DOI: 10.1007/s12144-021-02403-1

Jackson, E. M., Rossi, M. E., Hoover, E. R., & Johnson, R. E. (2012). Relationships of Leader Reward Behavior with Employee Behavior Fairness and Morale as Key Mediators. *Leadership and Organization Development Journal*, *33*(7), 646–661. DOI: 10.1108/01437731211265232

Javaid, Z. K., Chen, Z., & Ramzan, M. (2024). Assessing Stress Causing Factors and Language Related Challenges among First Year Students in Higher Institutions in Pakistan. *Acta Psychologica*, *248*, 104356. DOI: 10.1016/j.actpsy.2024.104356 PMID: 38885578

Jiang, M., Zhao, Q., Li, J., Wang, F., He, T., Cheng, X., . . . Fu, G. (2024). A Generic Review of Integrating Artificial Intelligence in Cognitive Behavioral Therapy. arXiv preprint arXiv:2407.19422.

Jin, K. W., Li, Q., Xie, Y., & Xiao, G. (2023). Artificial Intelligence in Mental Healthcare: An Overview and Future Perspectives. *The British Journal of Radiology*, *96*(1150), 20230213. DOI: 10.1259/bjr.20230213 PMID: 37698582

Kamalov, F., Calonge, D. S., & Gurrib, I. (2023). New Era of Artificial Intelligence in Education: Towards a Sustainable Multifaceted Revolution. *Sustainability (Basel)*, *15*(16), 12451. DOI: 10.3390/su151612451

Kamaruddin, N. F., Ahmad, A. A., Omar, K., Mat, N. H. N., Salleh, A. M. M., Fatini Kamaruddin, N., & Ahmad, A. (2018). Green work life balance, green human resource management practices on employee satisfaction. European Proceedings of Social and Behavioural Sciences, 40.

Khan, M., Hussain, A., Kousar, R. & Anitha, S. (2024). "A Study on Leveraging Artificial Intelligence in Educational Institutions: Enhancing Human Resource Management Practices." Pp. 84–90 in *QTanalytics Publication (Books)*.

Lee, S. H., Chin, W. C., & Ojo, A. O. (2024). Influence of Workplace Flexibility on Employee Engagement among Young Generation. *Cogent Business & Management, 11*(1), 2309705. DOI: 10.1080/23311975.2024.2309705

Lin, H., & Chen, Q. (2024). Artificial Intelligence (AI) -Integrated Educational Applications and College Students' Creativity and Academic Emotions: Students and Teachers' Perceptions and Attitudes. *BMC Psychology, 12*(1), 487. DOI: 10.1186/s40359-024-01979-0 PMID: 39285268

Lygum, V. L., Dupret, K., Bentsen, P., Djernis, D., Grangaard, S., Ladegaard, Y., & Troije, C. P. (2023). Greenspace as Workplace: Benefits, Challenges and Essentialities in the Physical Environment. *International Journal of Environmental Research and Public Health, 20*(17), 6689. DOI: 10.3390/ijerph20176689 PMID: 37681829

Mahesh, K. M., Aithal, P. S., & Sharma, K. R. S. (2024). Green HRM and teaching sustainability in higher education institutions: For promoting sustainable education and sustainable development goals. [IJCSBE]. *Education, 8*(1), 261–271.

Manole, A., Cârciumaru, R., Brînza , R., & Manole, F. (2024). Harnessing AI in Anxiety Management: A Chatbot-Based Intervention for Personalized Mental Health Support. *Information (Basel), 15*(12), 768. DOI: 10.3390/info15120768

Maples-Keller, J. L., Bunnell, B. E., Kim, S.-J., & Rothbaum, B. O. (2017). The Use of Virtual Reality Technology in the Treatment of Anxiety and Other Psychiatric Disorders. *Harvard Review of Psychiatry, 25*(3), 103–113. DOI: 10.1097/HRP.0000000000000138 PMID: 28475502

Monteiro, E., & Joseph, J. (2023). A review on the impact of workplace culture on employee mental health and well-being. International Journal of Case Studies in Business [IJCSBE]. *IT and Education, 7*(2), 291–317.

Murugesan, U., Subramanian, P., Srivastava, S., & Dwivedi, A. (2023). A Study of Artificial Intelligence Impacts on Human Resource Digitalization in Industry 4.0. *Decision Analytics Journal, 7*, 100249. DOI: 10.1016/j.dajour.2023.100249

Nuwasiima, M., Metogbe, P., & Kadiri, C. (2024). The Role of Artificial Intelligence (AI) and Machine Learning in Social Work Practice. *World Journal of Advanced Research and Reviews, 24*(1), 080–097. Advance online publication. DOI: 10.30574/wjarr.2024.24.1.2998

Patel, J., Hung, C., & Katapally, T. R. (2025). Evaluating Predictive Artificial Intelligence Approaches Used in Mobile Health Platforms to Forecast Mental Health Symptoms among Youth: A Systematic Review. *Psychiatry Research, 343*, 116277. DOI: 10.1016/j.psychres.2024.116277 PMID: 39616981

Qasim, S., Qureshi, M. A., & Shaikh, S. N. (2025). "Green Management and Sustainability in SMEs: A Pathway to a Greener Economy." Pp. 115–44 in *Examining Green Human Resources Management and Nascent Entrepreneurship*. IGI Global Scientific Publishing.

Rapo, M. (2024). Exploring the Influence of Green HRM Practices on Employee Motivation and Sustainable Performance: A Focus on Organizations in the Service Industry in Tirana. *Economicus, 23*(1), 35–55. DOI: 10.58944/rbxx6764

Rebelo, A. D., Verboom, D. E., Rebelo dos Santos, N., & Willem de Graaf, J. (2023). The Impact of Artificial Intelligence on the Tasks of Mental Healthcare Workers: A Scoping Review. *Computers in Human Behavior: Artificial Humans, 1*(2), 100008. DOI: 10.1016/j.chbah.2023.100008

Renwick, D. W. S., Redman, T., & Maguire, S. (2013). Green Human Resource Management: A Review and Research Agenda*. *International Journal of Management Reviews, 15*(1), 1–14. DOI: 10.1111/j.1468-2370.2011.00328.x

Ribeiro, N., Gomes, D. R., Ortega, E., Gomes, G. P., & Semedo, A. S. (2022). The Impact of Green HRM on Employees' Eco-Friendly Behavior: The Mediator Role of Organizational Identification. *Sustainability (Basel), 14*(5), 2897. DOI: 10.3390/su14052897

Sabale, Anjali, & Dr, Gomathi.S. (2022). Artificial Intelligence Supported Green HRM Practices For Socially Responsible And. *Environmental Sustainability, 58*, 115.

Samuel, K.Kiu Publication Extension. (2024).. . *The Role of Extracurricular Activities in Student Development.*, *5*, 26–30.

Shahid, T. A. S. T. A., Muhammad, K. M. K., Sami-Ullah, S.-U., & Abubakar, K. A. K. (2023). Opening a New Horizon in Green HRM Practices with Big Data Analytics and Its Analogy to Circular Economy Performance an Empirical Evidence. *International Journal of Business & Finance Implications, 4*(1).

Shaikh, S. N., Zhen, L., Sohu, J. M., Soomro, S., Akhtar, S., Kherazi, F. Z., & Najam, S. (2024). How green HRM practices foster green competitive advantage through big data analytics capability and are amplified by managerial environmental concern. *Kybernetes*.

Shajari, S., Kuruvinashetti, K., Komeili, A., & Sundararaj, U. (2023). The Emergence of AI-Based Wearable Sensors for Digital Health Technology: A Review. *Sensors (Basel), 23*(23), 9498. DOI: 10.3390/s23239498 PMID: 38067871

Sohu, J. M., Mirani, M. A., Shaikh, S. N., Memon, U., Bhanbhro, A., & Kherazi, F. Z. (2025). "Integrating Green Human Resource Management and Big Data Analytics Capability for Sustainable Environmental Performance in SMEs." Pp. 145–72 in *Examining Green Human Resources Management and Nascent Entrepreneurship*. IGI Global Scientific Publishing.

Sohu, J. M., Tian, H., Hussain, F., & Akbar, U. S. (2023). Digital Innovation, Digital Transformation, and Digital Platform Capability: Detrimental Impact of Big Data Analytics Capability on Innovation Performance. *International Research Journal of Management and Social Sciences*, *IV*, 265–281.

Sohu, J. M., Tian, H., Junejo, I., Akhtar, S., Ejaz, F., Dunay, A., & Hossain, M. B. (2024). Driving Sustainable Competitiveness: Unveiling the Nexus of Green Intellectual Capital and Environmental Regulations on Greening SME Performance. *Frontiers in Environmental Science*, *12*, 1348994. Advance online publication. DOI: 10.3389/fenvs.2024.1348994

Soomro, S., Fan, M., Sohu, J. M., Soomro, S., & Shaikh, S. N. (2024). AI adoption: A bridge or a barrier? The moderating role of organizational support in the path toward employee well-being. *Kybernetes*.

Thakkar, A., Gupta, A., & De Sousa, A. (2024). Artificial Intelligence in Positive Mental Health: A Narrative Review. *Frontiers in Digital Health*, *6*, 1280235. DOI: 10.3389/fdgth.2024.1280235 PMID: 38562663

Wu, A., Roemer, E. C., Kent, K. B., Ballard, D. W., & Goetzel, R. Z. (2021). Organizational Best Practices Supporting Mental Health in the Workplace. *Journal of Occupational and Environmental Medicine*, *63*(12), e925–e931. DOI: 10.1097/JOM.0000000000002407 PMID: 34840320

Yang, M., & Li, Z. (2023). The Influence of Green Human Resource Management on Employees' Green Innovation Behavior: The Role of Green Organizational Commitment and Knowledge Sharing. *Heliyon*, *9*(11), e22161. DOI: 10.1016/j.heliyon.2023.e22161 PMID: 38034614

Zihan, W., Zafir, K. M. M., & Alam, S. S. (2024). Green Human Resource Management in Practice: Assessing the Impact of Readiness and Corporate Social Responsibility on Organizational Change. *Sustainability (Basel)*, *16*(3), 1153. DOI: 10.3390/su16031153

Chapter 16
The Hidden Cost of AI: How Tools Are Undermining the Mental Agility of Youth

Arun Agrawal
https://orcid.org/0000-0001-7233-6660
Institute of Technology and Management, Gwalior, India

Yogita Deepak Mane
https://orcid.org/0000-0002-7097-2193
Thakur College of Engineering and Technology, India

S. Pavithra
Sri Venkateshwaraa College of Engineering and Technology, Puducherry, India

Vijay Kalmani
https://orcid.org/0000-0003-0738-3211
Rajarambapu Institute of Technology, Shivaji Univerity, Kolhapur, India

Ritika Sharma
Panipat Institute of Engineering and Technology, India

Deepak Gupta
https://orcid.org/0000-0003-3929-1362
Institute of Technology and Management, Gwalior, India

Neeta P. Patil
https://orcid.org/0009-0003-1532-3996
Thakur College of Engineering and Technology, India

Atul Kumar
Dr. D.Y. Patil B-School, India

ABSTRACT

This article focuses on understanding the hidden impacts of Artificial Intelligence (AI) on youth mental development. It explains how AI tools can weaken their mental agility. Although AI promises improvements in efficiency and features but its excessive use in education, entertainment, and daily life is making young people dependent on it. This is weakening their critical thinking, problem-solving abilities, creativity, and memory. The constant use of AI platforms and applications reduces the need to engage deeply in intellectual tasks, shortens attention span, and discourages in-

DOI: 10.4018/979-8-3373-5072-1.ch016

dependent thinking. The article also examines the psychological and social effects of AI such as decreased motivation, resilience, and intellectual curiosity. Through case studies and real-life examples, it illustrates what the long-term impact of AI might be on young minds and what role education and policies can play in reducing these negative effects. Finally, the article emphasizes the need for balanced use of AI so that its benefits can be utilized without hampering mental development.

INTRODUCTION

While the rapid development of Artificial Intelligence (AI) and its integration into every sector of society has brought many significant benefits and created several challenges. AI tools have now become an integral part of education, entertainment, and daily life, changing how we learn, work, and interact with technology (Dandotiya, Gupta, Dandotiya, & Sharma, 2024). Although these advancements have made tasks more efficient and easier but raising concerns about their impact on young people's mental development. The continuous use of AI may have unexpected consequences on how young people think, learn, and develop crucial cognitive skills.

Integration of AI in Education, Entertainment, and Daily Life

Artificial Intelligence (AI) is deeply influencing young people's lives, especially in education, entertainment, and daily routines. AI-powered learning platforms and virtual tutoring systems offer personalized educational experiences, adapting to each learner's needs (Kaswan, Dhatterwal, & Ojha, 2024). While beneficial, these tools risk reducing students' engagement in essential skills like independent problem-solving and self-directed learning—skills crucial for both academic and career success.

In entertainment, AI algorithms power streaming services, social media, and video games by recommending content based on user behavior (Prasad & Makesh, 2024). While this personalization keeps users engaged, it also encourages passive consumption and instant gratification. Over time, this can limit young people's ability to explore new ideas and diminish critical thinking and creativity.

Beyond education and entertainment, AI has become part of everyday life. Virtual assistants like Siri and Alexa, and tools like Google Maps, make tasks more convenient (Mahmoudi, Camboim, & Brovelli, 2023). However, constant reliance on such tools can reduce the use of memory and problem-solving skills.

This growing dependence on AI should prompt careful reflection. While technological progress should be welcomed, it is vital to ensure that AI supports rather than replaces foundational cognitive abilities. A balanced, mindful use of AI is essential for healthy youth development.

AI's Impact on Cognitive Development, Especially in Young People

As AI becomes more integrated into daily life, its impact on the cognitive development of young people is becoming increasingly clear. Cognitive development involves how individuals acquire, organize, and apply knowledge to think, learn, and solve problems—skills crucial during youth.

While AI tools offer convenience and personalization, they may unintentionally hinder mental growth. Tools that provide instant answers reduce the need for critical thinking and problem-solving (Lee, 2025). For instance, using AI to solve a math problem may save time but prevents students from developing persistence and analytical strategies.

AI also externalizes memory. In the past, students memorized facts and recalled them when needed. Today, AI-powered search engines replace this effort, which weakens memory retention and processing skills.

Creativity is similarly affected. Entertainment algorithms recommend content based on past behavior, limiting exposure to new perspectives and reducing opportunities for imaginative thinking (Chandramouli & Margetis, 2024).

Finally, AI-driven platforms are designed to capture attention through notifications, scrolling, and visuals. This can shorten attention spans and reduce the ability to focus on complex tasks.

While AI improves efficiency and access, its overuse may impact how young minds develop essential cognitive skills—raising the need for mindful, balanced usage.

UNDERSTANDING AI TOOLS

Artificial intelligence is a powerful 21st-century technology shaping industries like healthcare and finance (Khalil, 2023). It plays a crucial role in education, entertainment, and daily life. As this technology evolves, it's essential to understand what AI is, its uses, and its potential impact on the lives of young people. This section explores the concept of AI, examines the tools commonly used by young people, and highlights the advantages they bring, especially in terms of accessibility, ease of use, and enhanced learning experiences.

Definition of AI and its Applications

Artificial intelligence, in simple terms, refers to machines, particularly computer systems that imitate human intelligence processes. These processes include learning (the ability to improve performance over time), reasoning (drawing conclusions), problem-solving, perception (recognizing patterns or objects), and natural language processing (understanding and responding to human language). The purpose of AI is to replicate human cognitive abilities, allowing machines to perform tasks that would normally require human intelligence, often with greater efficiency.

AI can be broadly classified into two types: narrow AI (or weak AI) and general AI (or strong AI). Narrow AI refers to systems designed to perform specific tasks such as facial recognition, language translation, or medical diagnosis (Sabry, 2023). These systems are already integrated into various applications, from voice assistants on smart-phones to autonomous vehicles. General AI, on the other hand, refers to AI that can understand, learn, and apply knowledge like humans, although this type of AI has not yet been fully developed.

AI is utilized across various fields. In healthcare, AI assists in diagnosing diseases and suggesting treatment plans. In retail, AI enhances recommendation engines that suggest products consumers may like. In education, AI is incorporated into adaptive learning platforms, personalizing the learning experience for students. In entertainment, AI is used for gaming, recommending content, and even creating interactive media formats. Social media platforms like Instagram, TikTok, and Facebook use AI to curate personalized content for users, based on their past behaviors.

Types of AI Tools Commonly Used by Youth

AI has a significant presence in the daily lives of young people, often through tools that they use for learning, entertainment, and social interaction. Below are some of the most common AI tools that youth engage with:

AI-Powered Learning Assistants

AI-powered learning platforms and virtual assistants are gaining popularity in education. Tools like Duolingo, Khan Academy, and Google Assistant offer personalized learning experiences by adjusting to the user's learning style, pace, and preferences (Yekollu et al., 2024). For example, AI tutors can identify a student's strengths and weaknesses and tailor lessons to provide targeted help. These platforms also allow students to access educational content anytime and anywhere, making learning more flexible and accessible. Additionally, AI tools like Grammarly analyze writing and suggest improvements, helping students enhance their writing skills instantly (Fitria, 2021).

Social Media Algorithms

One of the most impactful uses of AI in the lives of young people is through social media platforms like Instagram, TikTok, and YouTube. These platforms use AI algorithms to analyze users' behaviors and preferences, delivering content that is highly personalized. AI decides which videos, posts, or ads to show based on a user's previous interactions, such as likes, comments, and shares (Lozano-Blasco, Mira-Aladrén, & Gil-Lamata, 2023). This personalization helps keep users engaged, often leading to longer usage times. While this can improve user experience by showing relevant content, it also raises concerns about limiting exposure to different viewpoints and promoting content that may not foster critical thinking or creativity.

Gaming

AI is heavily embedded in the gaming industry, enhancing both game design and player experiences. It is used to create dynamic and responsive environments, where non-player characters (NPCs) can react to player actions in real time. This makes the gaming experience more immersive and interactive. Games like Mine craft, Fortnite, and The Sims use AI to build complex, ever-changing worlds that adapt to player decisions (Champandard, 2003). AI also powers smart in-game assistants, offering tips, hints, or navigation help, which makes games more accessible, especially for younger or new players. Additionally, AI is used to generate procedural content, such as unique game levels or maps, ensuring that game play remains fresh and engaging.

Entertainment and Content Recommendations

AI plays a key role in how young people consume entertainment, especially on streaming platforms like Netflix, Spotify, and YouTube. These platforms use AI algorithms to analyze users' viewing or listening habits and suggest content that matches their preferences. For instance, Netflix recommends movies and TV shows based on past viewing, while YouTube suggests videos based on previous content watched (Chan, Hogaboam, & Cao, 2022). AI helps users easily discover new entertainment tailored to their interests. However, this reliance on AI for content curation also raises concerns about the "filter bubble," where users are shown similar types of content repeatedly, limiting exposure to diverse ideas or new genres.

Benefits of AI: Accessibility, convenience, and learning enhancement.

AI tools offer a wide range of benefits, particularly in terms of accessibility, convenience, and enhancing learning experiences. These benefits are particularly evident for young people, who are growing up in a world where technology plays an integral role in their personal and academic lives.

Accessibility

AI significantly enhances accessibility for individuals with diverse needs. In education, AI-powered tools can be customized to accommodate various learning styles and abilities. For example, students with dyslexia can use text-to-speech software, while those with visual impairments can benefit from voice-activated assistants or screen readers. AI tools like **Google Translate** provide real-time translations, breaking down language barriers and enabling students from different linguistic backgrounds to access educational materials. Similarly, AI-based apps that convert sign language into text or speech make communication more accessible for individuals with hearing impairments (Kumar & Nagar, 2024).

Convenience

AI streamlines everyday tasks, making life more convenient for youth. Virtual assistants, like Siri, Alexa, and Google Assistant, help young people manage their time, set reminders, and search for information instantly. In education, AI tools help students with tasks like scheduling study sessions, tracking progress, and organizing notes. In entertainment, AI curates content, saving users time by recommending shows, movies, or music that match their preferences. Overall, AI provides convenience by handling repetitive or time-consuming tasks, allowing young people to focus on more complex or creative activities.

Learning Enhancement

AI can significantly enhance the learning experience by personalizing educational content. AI-powered tools can adapt lessons to fit the individual needs of students, providing extra support where needed and accelerating learning in areas of strength. This personalized approach ensures that students are challenged at the right level and can progress at their own pace. Moreover, AI tools can help students with real-time feedback, identifying areas for improvement and providing targeted exercises to strengthen skills. Tools like **Quizlet** and **Kahoot!** make learning interactive and fun, while AI-driven platforms like **Coursera** and **Edmodo** offer students access to high-quality courses and educational content from around the world (Renacido & Biray, 2025).

AI tools have become an integral part of youth's daily lives, enhancing their learning, entertainment, and social interactions. While these tools offer many benefits, including accessibility, convenience, and personalized learning experiences, they also raise questions about the long-term effects on cognitive development. Understanding the nature of these AI tools and their applications is crucial for recognizing both their potential and their limitations in shaping the minds of the next generation.

COGNITIVE DEVELOPMENT IN YOUTH

Cognitive development refers to the process by which young people acquire, organize, and use knowledge and skills to think, learn, and solve problems. This process is especially critical during adolescence, a period when the brain undergoes significant changes that shape a young person's ability to reason, understand, and interact with the world. The development of cognitive skills such as problem-solving, creativity, and critical thinking is fundamental to overall mental agility, which is the capacity to think quickly and clearly, adapt to new situations, and handle complex tasks (Byrnes & Bernacki, 2013). In this section, we will explore the cognitive development that occurs during adolescence, the role of problem-solving, creativity, and critical thinking in brain development, and how traditional learning methods support the development of mental agility.

Overview of Mental Agility and Cognitive Development During Adolescence

Adolescence is a crucial stage in cognitive development, typically occurring between the ages of 12 and 18, when significant changes in the brain contribute to the development of advanced cognitive functions. During this period, the brain's prefrontal cortex the area responsible for decision-making, planning, and impulse control undergoes significant maturation. The brain is highly plastic during adolescence, meaning it is flexible and capable of adapting to new experiences and learning opportunities (Steinberg, 2005).

Mental agility, the ability to think, adapt, and solve problems effectively, develops significantly during adolescence. At this stage, the brain enhances its capacity for abstract thinking, future planning, and understanding consequences. Adolescents move from concrete to more complex, abstract reasoning. This cognitive growth is shaped by their environment—education, social interactions, and technology use—all of which influence how they adapt, make decisions, and handle challenges.

The Role of Problem-solving, Creativity, and Critical Thinking in Brain Development

Problem-solving, creativity, and critical thinking are foundational to cognitive development and are key components of mental agility. These skills help young people navigate the world, understand complex issues, and make decisions (Pherson & Pherson, 2020). Here's how each of these skills plays a role in brain development:

Problem-Solving

Problem-solving involves identifying an issue, considering possible solutions, and selecting the most appropriate action. For adolescents, problem-solving skills are critical in both academic and everyday contexts. As the brain matures, adolescents begin to develop more sophisticated problem-solving strategies, moving beyond trial and error to apply logic, analyze situations, and predict outcomes. The ability to solve problems builds mental agility by enhancing the brain's capacity to handle complexity and uncertainty. Engaging in problem-solving activities whether through academic challenges, puzzles, or real-life situations helps strengthen neural connections in the brain, improving overall cognitive function (Greiff et al., 2014).

Creativity

Creativity is the ability to think outside the box and generate novel ideas or solutions. It is essential not only in the arts but also in science, business, and everyday life. During adolescence, the brain undergoes changes that enhance creative thinking, particularly in the areas of innovation and abstraction. Creative activities such as artistic expression, writing, or experimental thinking stimulate neural networks that connect different regions of the brain, fostering new connections and promoting cognitive flexibility. Creativity is a key aspect of mental agility, as it allows individuals to approach problems from multiple angles and come up with unique solutions (van der Zanden, Meijer, & Beghetto, 2020).

Critical Thinking

Critical thinking is the ability to analyze information objectively, evaluate arguments, and make reasoned judgments. It is a skill that involves questioning assumptions, identifying biases, and considering various perspectives before reaching a conclusion. For adolescents, critical thinking is vital because it enables them to navigate the vast amounts of information they encounter in school, media, and social interactions. Developing critical thinking skills strengthens cognitive agility by enhancing the brain's ability to process information, make decisions, and evaluate potential outcomes. Adolescents who practice critical thinking are better equipped to analyze problems, understand different viewpoints, and make informed choices (Facione, 2011).

Together, problem-solving, creativity, and critical thinking contribute to a young person's cognitive development by strengthening the brain's ability to process information, adapt to new situations, and solve complex problems. These skills form the foundation of mental agility, which is crucial for success in both academic and real-life situations.

How Traditional Learning Methods Foster Mental Agility

Traditional learning methods have long been a cornerstone of education, providing structured opportunities for cognitive development and mental agility. These methods, which often emphasize direct instruction, hands-on learning, and interactive problem-solving, help young people develop essential cognitive skills. Here are some ways traditional learning fosters mental agility:

Active Engagement and Hands-On Learning

One of the most effective ways to build mental agility is through active engagement in learning. In traditional classrooms, students are often encouraged to participate in discussions, solve problems in groups, and apply their knowledge to real-world scenarios. Hands-on learning experiences, such as science experiments, field trips, or project-based learning, allow students to engage deeply with the material, encouraging them to think critically, analyze data, and develop solutions to problems. This active engagement strengthens cognitive skills by requiring students to apply what they've learned in practical situations (Al Shloul et al., 2024).

Problem-Based Learning (PBL)

In many traditional educational settings, problem-based learning is used to encourage critical thinking and problem-solving. In PBL, students are presented with complex, real-world problems and are required to work collaboratively to find solutions. This method encourages them to think critically, research solutions, and test hypotheses. By engaging in PBL, students develop mental agility as they learn to navigate challenges, consider multiple viewpoints, and evaluate possible outcomes

(Hmelo-Silver, 2004). The problem-solving nature of PBL helps adolescents practice cognitive flexibility, which is an essential component of mental agility.

Structured Curriculum and Scaffolding

Traditional education often follows a structured curriculum designed to gradually build a student's knowledge and skills. This gradual progression allows students to master foundational concepts before moving on to more complex material. By starting with basic concepts and scaffolding learning experiences, students are given the support they need to tackle more difficult problems over time. This approach helps build mental agility by ensuring that students develop a strong cognitive foundation that they can build upon. Furthermore, this structured learning process encourages the development of perseverance, as students learn to overcome challenges and think critically to solve problems (Reiser, 2023).

Discipline and Focus

Traditional classrooms also encourage the development of discipline and focus—two key elements of mental agility. Students are often required to pay attention to lectures, follow instructions, and complete assignments on time. This structured environment helps students develop the ability to concentrate for extended periods, an important skill for solving complex problems. The ability to focus on tasks, despite distractions, is essential for building mental agility, as it strengthens the brain's capacity to process information and stay on track when faced with challenges (Gardner, 2021).

Traditional learning methods provide invaluable opportunities for young people to develop the cognitive skills needed to enhance mental agility. Problem-solving, creativity, and critical thinking are fostered through active engagement, problem-based learning, and structured curricula, all of which play a crucial role in brain development. These traditional methods are vital for ensuring that young people not only acquire knowledge but also develop the cognitive flexibility and resilience needed to navigate an increasingly complex world.

THE ROLE OF AI IN EVERYDAY LIFE

Artificial Intelligence (AI) has become an integral part of modern life, influencing a wide range of activities from education to entertainment and even decision-making. The tools powered by AI are embedded in daily routines, shaping the way young people learn, interact, and solve problems. As AI tools become more pervasive, it's important to explore how they impact various aspects of life, especially in areas like education, entertainment, and cognitive decision-making. This section will delve into the ubiquity of AI in education, its influence in entertainment and social media, and how it shapes decision-making and problem-solving skills in young people.

The Ubiquity of AI Tools in Education

AI tools have dramatically transformed education by enhancing accessibility, personalization, and engagement. Today, AI is used in various aspects of education, from tutoring platforms to e-learning apps and virtual classrooms. These technologies not only support students' learning but also provide opportunities for independent, tailored education outside of traditional classroom settings.

AI-Powered Tutoring Platforms

AI-driven tutoring platforms like **Khan Academy**, **Duolingo**, and **Socratic** offer personalized learning experiences by adapting to a student's individual progress and learning style. These platforms utilize AI to analyze the learner's strengths and weaknesses, tailoring lessons to meet specific needs. AI tutors are available 24/7, allowing students to access help whenever they need it, making learning more flexible and accessible. This constant availability reduces barriers to education, particularly for students who may not have access to in-person tutoring. These platforms can also identify gaps in knowledge, offering targeted exercises to address those areas, helping students improve at their own pace (Bojadjiev, 2024).

E-Learning Apps

AI is also prevalent in e-learning apps, which have become a staple for many students, particularly during the shift to online education. Apps like **Google Classroom**, **Quizlet**, and **Edmodo** use AI to streamline the management of coursework, assignments, and communication between teachers and students. AI algorithms in these platforms track students' learning patterns, providing feedback and adjusting learning activities based on performance. These features ensure that learning is not one-size-fits-all but is instead customized to maximize each student's potential (Kurni, Mohammed, & Srinivasa, 2023).

Virtual Classrooms

With the rise of remote learning, virtual classrooms have become a central part of the educational experience. Platforms such as **Zoom** and **Microsoft Teams** integrate AI features like automatic transcription, virtual assistants, and real-time language translation, making learning more inclusive and effective. AI can also track students' engagement during virtual lessons, alerting educators to any signs of disengagement or difficulty, which allows for timely intervention. These features contribute to a more personalized learning environment, even in virtual settings, and ensure that students continue to receive the support they need in an increasingly digital world (Swargiary, 2024).

AI's Influence in Entertainment and Social Media

AI has also reshaped the entertainment and social media landscape, influencing everything from gaming to content creation and consumption. Young people, in particular, are heavily influenced by AI-driven experiences in these areas, which have become central to their social lives and leisure activities.

Gaming

The gaming industry has long utilized AI to enhance player experiences, making games more interactive, immersive, and dynamic. AI is used to design adaptive game environments where non-player characters (NPCs) respond intelligently to a player's actions. Games like **Minecraft** and **Fortnite** use AI to create vast, evolving worlds that change based on player decisions, encouraging exploration and creativity. Additionally, AI is employed to create more realistic game physics and smarter AI opponents that mimic human behavior, providing a challenging and engaging experience (Bhambri, 2025). AI-driven gaming also includes personalized content, with games adapting in difficulty based on the player's skill level, ensuring that they remain challenged but not overwhelmed.

Content Curation in Social Media

Social media platforms such as **Instagram**, **TikTok**, and **YouTube** are heavily powered by AI algorithms that curate content to match users' interests and behaviors. These algorithms analyze users' past interactions—what they like, share, and comment on—to predict and recommend posts, videos, and advertisements. This personalized feed keeps users engaged for longer periods and influences the content they consume. While this can enhance user experience by presenting relevant content, it also raises concerns about the filter bubble effect, where users are primarily exposed to content that reinforces their existing beliefs or preferences. For young people, this may limit their exposure to diverse viewpoints and ideas, potentially stunting their critical thinking and cognitive flexibility (Singh & Pathania, 2024).

AI in Content Creation

AI is also involved in content creation, from generating music using platforms like **Amper Music** to creating personalized video recommendations on streaming services like **Netflix** and **Spotify** (Filimowicz, 2023). These platforms use AI to analyze users' preferences and predict what content they might enjoy based on their viewing or listening habits. This makes entertainment more accessible and convenient, but it also shapes the type of content young people are exposed to. AI's role in content creation also means that the lines between human creativity and machine-generated content are becoming increasingly blurred, leading to new forms of media and entertainment that were previously unimagined.

How AI Shapes Decision-Making and Problem-Solving in Young People

AI tools are increasingly influencing how young people make decisions and solve problems, both in their academic work and personal lives. The ability of AI to provide personalized recommendations and automated solutions has a profound effect on the cognitive processes involved in decision-making and problem-solving.

Decision-Making

AI tools play a significant role in shaping the way young people make decisions, particularly when it comes to navigating information and determining next steps. AI-powered recommendation systems, such as those used in social media, streaming platforms, and e-commerce sites, present users with suggestions based on previous behaviors. While these recommendations are convenient and help streamline decision-making, they can also limit the variety of choices young people consider. The constant reliance on AI-driven suggestions may reduce the need for young people to critically assess multiple options or make independent decisions, potentially stifling their decision-making skills.

In education, AI tools also influence how students make decisions about their learning paths. AI-powered apps help students choose which courses to take or what study methods to adopt based on their performance and preferences. While these tools provide guidance, they may unintentionally limit students' ability to explore different learning styles or subjects outside their immediate interests.

Problem-Solving

AI tools play a significant role in assisting young people with problem-solving by offering instant answers and step-by-step guidance, especially in areas like math and coding. These tools help reinforce knowledge and support learning, but they can also limit opportunities for independent thinking. Relying too heavily on AI may reduce the need for students to explore creative or critical solutions on their own, potentially weakening their problem-solving abilities over time.

In gaming and interactive platforms, AI creates engaging challenges that enhance strategic thinking and adaptability. These environments can foster cognitive flexibility, encouraging users to shift strategies and think quickly. However, the immediate feedback and assistance provided by AI may reduce the chance for users to struggle productively and develop solutions independently.

Beyond education and gaming, AI influences entertainment, social media, and decision-making. From personalized content on social platforms to adaptive learning in virtual classrooms, AI is deeply woven into young people's daily lives. While it enhances accessibility and engagement, its pervasive role in guiding decisions and offering solutions raises concerns. Overdependence on AI may hinder the development of essential cognitive skills such as creativity, critical thinking, and independent problem-solving—abilities that are crucial for long-term intellectual growth and adaptability.

HOW AI TOOLS UNDERMINE MENTAL AGILITY

As artificial intelligence (AI) tools continue to grow in prominence, their widespread use is reshaping cognitive processes, particularly in the younger generation. While AI has many benefits, such as accessibility and convenience, it also comes with certain drawbacks that may undermine the mental agility of users. Mental agility—the ability to think quickly, adapt, and solve complex problems—relies on a delicate balance of critical thinking, memory retention, creativity, and problem-solving. AI tools, however, have the potential to erode these cognitive skills by reducing reliance on critical thinking, externalizing memory, shortening attention spans, diminishing creativity, and limiting problem-solving skills. This section explores the specific ways in which AI tools may weaken mental agility.

Reduced Reliance on Critical Thinking: Over-Dependence on AI for Answers

One of the most significant impacts of AI on cognitive development is the growing over-dependence on these tools for answers. AI-powered search engines, virtual assistants, and tutoring platforms provide instant solutions to a wide range of queries, from solving math problems to answering general knowledge questions. While this accessibility has benefits, it also diminishes the need for young people to engage in deep thinking and problem-solving processes (Shah & Asad, 2024).

Critical thinking involves analyzing and evaluating information, forming judgments, and making decisions based on logic and reasoning. In contrast, when AI tools instantly provide answers, users may be less inclined to engage in the analytical processes required to arrive at conclusions on their own. For example, when students use AI-based math solvers or writing assistants, they may simply accept the answers or suggestions without fully understanding the underlying concepts or reasoning processes. Over time, this reduces their ability to assess situations critically, leading to a dependency on AI rather than fostering independent thought (Duenas & Ruiz, 2024).

Additionally, many AI tools, particularly in education, are designed to offer step-by-step guidance, which further diminishes the need for users to think critically about the steps they would take on their own. The mental shortcut provided by AI may feel convenient, but it significantly stunts cognitive growth by failing to engage users in the deeper cognitive processes involved in learning.

The Diminishing Role of Memory: AI's Role in Externalizing Memory and Knowledge

AI can undermine mental agility by affecting memory retention. Traditionally, people engaged deeply with material to remember facts and concepts. Now, AI tools like Siri and Google Assistant store and retrieve information instantly, reducing the need to memorize. While convenient, this reliance weakens the brain's engagement with information, leading to decreased recall and retention. Memory isn't just for storing facts—it supports reasoning, creativity, and problem-solving. Outsourcing memory to AI may hinder the brain's natural processes, resulting in reduced cognitive development. Over time, this can cause cognitive atrophy, where the brain's ability to remember and process information declines due to lack of use. Ultimately, over-dependence on AI tools may diminish critical mental functions and the development of independent thinking and memory skills.

Shortened Attention Spans: AI-Driven Distractions in Media and Social Platforms

The constant flow of AI-curated content on platforms like Instagram, TikTok, and YouTube is contributing to shorter attention spans, especially in young people. AI algorithms track user behavior to deliver an endless stream of personalized content, encouraging frequent shifts in focus and reducing the ability to concentrate on one task for long. This cycle of instant gratification weakens attention span and focus, essential skills for deep thinking and problem-solving. Research links rapid content consumption with diminished cognitive engagement, making it harder for individuals to stay focused on long-form tasks such as studying or reading. For young people, whose cognitive abilities are still developing, this is particularly concerning. Reduced attention span directly impacts mental agility, hindering critical thinking, creativity, and the ability to tackle complex problems effectively.

Decreased Creativity: The Impact of AI-Assisted Content Creation on Creative Thinking

Creativity is a vital component of mental agility, enabling individuals to think innovatively and approach problems from new perspectives. However, AI tools used in content creation—such as ChatGPT for writing or Canva for design—may reduce the need for personal imagination and originality. While these tools streamline the creative process, they can limit users' opportunities to develop their own ideas, skills, and problem-solving abilities. By relying on AI to generate content, individuals may become passive consumers rather than active creators.

This dependence can also lead to homogenized outputs, as AI generates content based on existing data patterns rather than novel thinking. For young people especially, this can hinder the growth of creativity by discouraging experimentation, risk-taking, and learning through trial and error. Over time, such reliance may weaken the very skills needed for original and adaptive thinking.

Lack of Problem-Solving Skills: How AI Tools Solve Problems for the User

AI tools, while highly efficient, can hinder the development of essential problem-solving skills, especially in young people. Platforms like Google Search, Wolfram Alpha, and AI-based calculators offer instant solutions, bypassing the need for critical thinking and reasoning. Students using AI-powered homework apps often receive step-by-step answers, leaving little room for them to engage in their own thought processes or explore different problem-solving strategies.

This immediate access to answers limits cognitive flexibility—the ability to adapt and apply knowledge in various contexts—which is crucial for long-term mental agility. True problem-solving is developed through practice, experimentation, and learning from mistakes. When AI removes these steps, young people miss valuable opportunities to build resilience and adaptability.

Furthermore, over-reliance on AI can reduce persistence in the face of challenges. Problem-solving involves trial and error, hypothesis testing, and strategy revision, all of which are bypassed when solutions are readily provided. This undermines the development of independent thinking and creativity.

While AI offers clear advantages in speed and convenience, it also poses risks to mental agility by weakening critical cognitive processes. To preserve and enhance problem-solving skills, it's important to encourage thoughtful engagement and balance AI use with opportunities for active, independent learning.

THE PSYCHOLOGICAL AND SOCIAL IMPACTS OF AI

As AI tools become increasingly integrated into everyday life, their influence extends beyond cognitive and mental agility. They also have profound psychological and social impacts, particularly on young people. While AI provides convenience, accessibility, and instant gratification, it also contributes to psychological dependency, unhealthy social comparison, and a reduction in resilience. This section explores how AI affects motivation, social interactions, dependency, and emotional well-being, ultimately reshaping the psychological landscape of the younger generation (Shanmugasundaram & Tamilarasu, 2023).

Impact on Motivation: Instant Gratification Through AI-Driven Content

One of the most significant psychological effects of AI is the way it fosters a culture of instant gratification. AI-driven platforms, such as social media, streaming services, and online shopping, continuously deliver content that aligns with users' preferences. These tools use algorithms to predict and provide personalized experiences, making it easy for individuals to obtain what they want with minimal effort.

The constant availability of instant content can have a negative impact on intrinsic motivation. When young people can access entertainment, information, and social validation at the click of a button, it diminishes the need for patience and effort. For example, social media platforms like **Instagram** and **TikTok** offer immediate rewards in the form of likes, comments, and shares, which can quickly become addictive. Similarly, platforms like **Netflix** or **YouTube** provide on-demand entertainment, offering instant access to thousands of hours of content.

This instant gratification discourages long-term goal setting and the persistence required to achieve meaningful accomplishments. When AI tools make it so easy to access rewards without significant effort, young people may struggle to develop the delayed gratification skills necessary for academic achievement, career success, and personal growth. Over time, this can lead to a decrease in motivation to engage in tasks that require sustained effort and patience, as the immediate rewards provided by AI tools become more appealing.

Social Comparison: AI Tools Fostering Unrealistic

AI-driven social media platforms play a significant role in fostering social comparison, especially among young people. Algorithms on apps like Instagram, Facebook, and TikTok are designed to promote content that receives the most likes, shares, and engagement—often highlighting idealized versions of people's lives. These curated posts, filled with filtered images, luxurious lifestyles, and carefully crafted personas, create a distorted view of reality. For young users, repeated exposure to such content can lead to negative self-evaluation, feelings of inadequacy, and diminished self-esteem. Research indicates that the more time individuals spend on social media, the more likely they are to compare themselves negatively to others, increasing the risk of anxiety, depression, and loneliness. AI amplifies this issue by continually reinforcing similar content based on user behavior, trapping individuals in a cycle of comparison and unrealistic expectations. As a result, many young people may begin to perceive their own lives as lacking, even though real life is far more nuanced and complex than what is portrayed online. This ongoing exposure to idealized content can undermine emotional well-being and self-worth, making it crucial to recognize and address the psychological impacts of AI-curated social media experiences.

Dependency: The Psychological Toll of Relying on AI Tools for Intellectual Tasks

Over-reliance on AI tools for intellectual tasks can also have a profound psychological impact. As AI systems increasingly take over tasks such as writing, problem-solving, and research, individuals become less inclined to engage their cognitive faculties in these areas. Tools like **Grammarly**, **Google Search**, or **AI-based writing assistants** enable users to avoid the mental effort required for tasks like composing essays, solving math problems, or conducting research. While these tools can be helpful, they may lead to a growing dependency on AI for tasks that once required critical thinking, creativity, and intellectual engagement.

Psychologically, this dependency can lead to a sense of diminished self-efficacy the belief in one's ability to accomplish tasks independently. When young people rely on AI for intellectual tasks, they may lose confidence in their own abilities and feel inadequate without the assistance of technology. This can create a cycle where individuals become increasingly dependent on AI, which in turn leads to greater difficulty in tackling tasks on their own.

Moreover, this reliance on AI tools can also diminish cognitive resilience, as individuals may struggle to adapt to situations where AI assistance is unavailable. In environments where AI tools are not accessible, young people may feel overwhelmed or incapable of completing tasks, resulting in higher levels of stress, frustration, and anxiety.

Isolation: How AI Can Replace Social Interactions and Reduce Cognitive Development Opportunities

AI tools in communication and entertainment can contribute to social isolation, particularly among young people. While platforms like Facebook, WhatsApp, and Snapchat facilitate virtual connections, they cannot replace in-person interactions, which are essential for developing emotional intelligence, empathy, and social skills (Baruah, 2024). Increased engagement with AI-powered systems and AI-curated content may lead youth to spend less time in face-to-face settings, thereby missing critical opportunities for cognitive and emotional development. For example, instead of participating in group activities, some students may choose solo video gaming experiences, where AI-generated opponents substitute human players. Although entertaining, such experiences lack the depth of real-world social learning. In-person interactions help individuals develop problem-solving abilities in social contexts and adaptability to diverse environments. Furthermore, AI can foster digital echo chambers by continuously reinforcing similar viewpoints, limiting exposure to differing ideas and perspectives. This not only reduces critical thinking but also hampers the development of cognitive flexibility and openness (Baruah, 2024).

The Erosion of Resilience: Avoidance of Challenges Due to AI's Problem-Solving Capabilities

AI tools, designed for quick and efficient problem-solving, can undermine resilience, particularly in young people. Platforms like Google Search, Wolfram Alpha, and AI-based tutoring provide immediate solutions to complex problems, making it easier for users to bypass the challenges of independent problem-solving

(Banerjee, 2024). Resilience is built through overcoming obstacles and learning from adversity, but when AI tools offer instant answers, young people miss out on these valuable learning experiences. For instance, students may rely on AI-powered platforms to complete assignments, skipping over difficult sections that would help develop critical thinking and problem-solving skills.

This avoidance of challenges can have significant psychological consequences. Without the experience of tackling difficulties independently, young people may develop feelings of helplessness when confronted with setbacks. Over time, this can erode emotional resilience, increase stress, and hinder personal growth. The lack of resilience can lead to a diminished ability to cope with failure and reduced motivation to engage in intellectually challenging tasks. As AI continues to shape daily life, it is crucial to address these psychological impacts to ensure that young people can develop the cognitive, emotional, and social skills needed for healthy psychological development in the digital age.

CASE STUDIES AND REAL-WORLD EXAMPLES

The impact of AI tools on cognitive development, mental agility, and social behavior can be better understood through real-world case studies. These examples highlight how AI is shaping the thinking, creativity, and problem-solving skills of young people across different contexts, from education to entertainment and even the workplace.

Case Study 1: Students Using AI-Driven Educational Tools and Their Cognitive Outcomes

In a study conducted at a large urban university, a cohort of students was provided with access to AI-powered educational tools like **AI-based tutoring platforms** and **personalized learning apps**. These tools were designed to assist students in subjects ranging from mathematics to writing. Students using these tools had access to instant solutions, step-by-step explanations, and feedback on their assignments (Aliabadi, 2023).

While initial results showed improvements in test scores, long-term studies revealed significant gaps in students' deeper understanding of the subject matter. Many students relying on AI-driven tools for homework and assignments showed a diminished ability to solve similar problems without the assistance of the AI tools. This trend was especially noticeable in subjects that required critical thinking, such as calculus or logic-based problem solving. Students often became accustomed to receiving instant solutions without engaging with the reasoning behind them. As a result, while their grades improved in the short term, their ability to tackle complex problems independently, and their critical thinking skills, did not develop as robustly as expected.

This case study illustrates that while AI tools provide convenience and short-term academic improvement, they may hinder cognitive skills like problem-solving and independent learning.

Case Study 2: Young People Engaging in AI-Powered Gaming and Social Media Platforms and its Impact on Mental Agility

A prominent example of the impact of AI tools in entertainment and social media is the use of AI-powered gaming and social media platforms among young people. A group of teenagers who regularly played AI-driven video games and spent considerable time on social media platforms like **Instagram** and **TikTok** was studied. AI algorithms on these platforms curate personalized content based on user behavior, promoting an environment of constant novelty and instant gratification. Similarly, in AI-based video games, players often face non-human opponents whose behavior adapts in real-time to the player's actions, creating a highly interactive experience (Van Der Wal, Valkenburg, & van Driel, 2024).

Psychological assessments of the teenagers in this study showed a marked reduction in attention span. On social media, students exhibited lower concentration levels on academic tasks and showed an increased need for instant rewards. In gaming, although players demonstrated quick reflexes and adaptability in response to the AI-driven challenges, they struggled to apply the same level of mental engagement to real-world tasks that required sustained focus, such as studying or problem-solving. The AI-driven experiences, while engaging, also contributed to decreased patience and an over-reliance on external stimuli for stimulation, which in turn impacted their ability to think critically and engage in tasks that required deep focus.

This case study suggests that while AI-powered entertainment and social media may foster quick decision-making and adaptability, they also contribute to diminished cognitive stamina, shortened attention spans, and a reduced capacity for sustained intellectual effort.

Case Study 3: AI in the Workplace and its Effects on Young Professionals' Problem-Solving Skills

A case study conducted by a consulting firm observed young professionals in the tech industry using AI tools, such as chatbots, automated customer service platforms, and analytics tools, to perform daily tasks. These AI systems helped save time and reduce manual labor by automating tasks like answering client queries, generating reports, and analyzing large datasets (De Wever et al., 2023). However, reliance on these tools led to a decline in problem-solving skills. Employees became dependent on AI to identify patterns and analyze data, which diminished their ability to troubleshoot, think creatively, and analyze data without assistance. This dependency became apparent when a team of young professionals struggled to manually analyze data and create a customized report for a client request outside the scope of their AI systems. The lack of hands-on problem-solving experience made the task more difficult. This case underscores how extensive use of AI tools in the workplace can reduce critical thinking and creativity, making young professionals less adaptable in situations where AI is unavailable. It highlights the need to balance AI usage with traditional methods that encourage independent thinking, creativity, and resilience.

THE ROLE OF EDUCATION AND POLICY IN ADDRESSING AI'S IMPACT

As AI tools continue to infiltrate every aspect of life, their effects on cognitive development, mental agility, and emotional well-being are becoming more apparent, especially among the youth. Educational systems and policymakers play a critical role in mitigating the potential negative impacts of AI while maximizing its benefits. By fostering digital literacy, critical thinking, and responsible AI usage, education and policy can help young people navigate the AI-driven world more effectively and develop the cognitive and social skills needed for the future (Chan, 2023).

How Educational Systems are Adapting to AI Tools

Educational systems worldwide are recognizing the significance of AI tools in enhancing the learning experience, but they are also aware of the challenges posed by over-reliance on these technologies. Many schools, colleges, and universities are integrating AI-driven learning platforms, personalized tutoring systems, and virtual classrooms to assist students in their academic journeys. These tools offer personalized learning experiences, helping students progress at their own pace and providing real-time feedback (Cho, 2022).

However, the integration of AI tools into education has raised concerns about their impact on cognitive development. Some institutions are adopting hybrid learning models, where traditional classroom activities are balanced with AI-powered resources. For example, AI-based platforms like **Duolingo** for language learning or **Khan Academy** for mathematics provide personalized learning paths, but educators are still encouraged to monitor student progress and ensure that learners are engaged in critical thinking exercises beyond the scope of AI tools (Mounkoro et al., 2024).

In some cases, educational institutions are introducing courses and curricula aimed at teaching students how to use AI tools responsibly, while also emphasizing the importance of independent problem-solving and creativity. These adaptive teaching methods aim to maintain a balance between leveraging the benefits of AI and fostering essential cognitive skills like analytical thinking, problem-solving, and creativity that AI cannot replicate.

The Importance of Teaching Digital Literacy and Critical Thinking

As AI continues to influence education and communication, digital literacy has become an essential skill. It involves not only using digital tools but also understanding their ethical implications and critically assessing their impact on society (Banerjee, 2024). For young people, digital literacy extends beyond basic device navigation to include evaluating information, detecting misinformation, and making informed decisions. Critical thinking is especially important when using AI tools like Google or ChatGPT, as students must learn to question AI-generated results, understand algorithms, and identify biases (Banerjee, 2024). Educators are increasingly integrating critical thinking and digital literacy into the curriculum, helping students become discerning digital citizens. These programs teach students how to evaluate the ethical implications of technology and solve problems independently. By fostering these skills, education systems aim to ensure that students engage thoughtfully with AI tools, protecting their cognitive development and promoting responsible technology use.

Policies and Guidelines for Responsible AI Usage Among Youth

In response to concerns about AI's impact on cognitive development and social behavior, governments and educational authorities are implementing policies to promote responsible AI use among youth. One key policy area is regulating AI in education, which includes ensuring that AI-driven learning platforms are ethical, transparent, and accessible to all students, while preventing biases and protecting data privacy. Another important focus is limiting the time young people spend on AI-driven entertainment platforms, such as gaming or social media, to reduce negative psychological effects like dependency and shortened attention spans. Research indicates that excessive screen time can be detrimental to mental health. Policies may include screen time limits, regular breaks, and age-appropriate guidelines for using AI-powered tools. These regulations aim to protect youth from the potential harmful effects of AI while fostering responsible and developmentally appropriate usage.

Initiatives That Can Help Counteract AI's Negative Cognitive Impact

To mitigate the negative cognitive impacts of AI, several initiatives can balance digital engagement with activities that promote critical thinking and creativity. One effective approach is promoting offline activities such as physical games, hands-on projects, and community engagement, which require problem-solving, collaboration, and creativity. These activities foster skills like resilience, teamwork, and patience that AI tools do not emphasize. Additionally, mindfulness practices can improve cognitive functioning and reduce digital distractions. Incorporating mindfulness into curricula can help students manage stress, enhance focus, and regulate emotions.

Promoting AI literacy is another crucial initiative, teaching young people not only how to use AI but also how to critically evaluate its algorithms and understand ethical concerns. Collaborative learning environments also counteract the isolating effects of AI, encouraging creativity and interpersonal skills. By integrating digital literacy, critical thinking, and mindfulness, educational systems can ensure that students are proficient in using AI tools while nurturing independent thought. Policies should prioritize the ethical use of AI, while promoting initiatives like offline activities and collaborative learning to safeguard young people's cognitive growth and creativity in an AI-driven world.

FUTURE IMPLICATIONS: A DOUBLE-EDGED SWORD

As AI continues to evolve and integrate into various aspects of life, its potential impact on society and cognitive development becomes increasingly significant. While AI offers numerous benefits in terms of efficiency, convenience, and innovation, its long-term effects on cognitive agility—particularly among the youth—are becoming a growing concern. The future implications of AI on mental skills, decision-making, and problem-solving are complex, and understanding these dynamics will be key to ensuring that AI serves as a tool for human enhancement rather than a hindrance.

The Potential Long-Term Effects on Society if AI Continues to Undermine Cognitive Agility

If AI continues to undermine cognitive agility, society may face serious challenges. Increasing reliance on AI for tasks like information retrieval, problem-solving, and content creation risks the atrophy of critical thinking, creativity, and problem-solving abilities (Khogali & Mekid, 2023). Over time, this could lead to a generation that lacks the intellectual resilience needed for deep, independent thinking, making it difficult to solve complex or novel problems without technological aid. This dependence may erode cognitive skills like adaptability, resourcefulness, and critical reasoning. Additionally, AI's role in replacing face-to-face interactions could diminish empathy and social skills, such as emotional intelligence and teamwork, which are vital for personal and professional success. As AI continues to shape daily life, fostering a balance between technology and human interaction will be crucial to preserve essential cognitive and social abilities.

The Balance Between Harnessing AI's Benefits and Maintaining Cognitive Skills

The key challenge is balancing AI's benefits with maintaining cognitive skills. AI can enhance education and productivity but may hinder critical thinking if overused. To preserve intellectual creativity, AI tools should complement, not replace, human cognitive processes. They can aid learning but should encourage active engagement, critical thinking, and creativity. For instance, AI can assist with basic subject elements, while teachers foster problem-solving and deeper engagement. Additionally, promoting responsible AI use through digital literacy and critical thinking in education is essential. This approach ensures students leverage AI's strengths without compromising their cognitive abilities.

Future Developments in AI and How They Can Be Designed to Foster, Not Hinder, Cognitive Development

Looking ahead, AI holds tremendous potential to promote cognitive development, transforming education and human interaction in positive ways. Future AI technologies can be more adaptive, personalized, and interactive, offering tools that foster creativity, critical thinking, and problem-solving. AI-based educational tools could go beyond content delivery, encouraging active learning experiences such as virtual labs where students experiment with science and math concepts. These tools could also assess students' thinking processes, offering feedback on problem-solving strategies and enhancing creative approaches.

AI systems could be designed to provide cognitive challenges tailored to individual learners. These systems would adapt to a learner's intellectual abilities, presenting progressively complex tasks and guiding students through problems rather than simply solving them. This process would help develop resilience, mental agility, and analytical skills, with AI acting as a coach to promote creative thinking.

Additionally, ethical AI design will be critical in supporting cognitive development. Ensuring AI tools encourage breaks, offer diverse perspectives, and minimizing harmful biases can help maintain a healthy balance of digital engagement. AI could promote offline interactions, mindfulness practices, and cognitive activities outside the digital realm.

To ensure AI contributes positively, developers and policymakers must create frameworks that guide responsible AI use, especially in educational contexts. These frameworks should focus on promoting critical thinking, problem-solving, and creativity. With the right balance, AI can enhance human potential, encourage cognitive growth, and foster resilience, while preventing the erosion of essential skills such as independence and social interaction. The future of AI lies in how it complements human cognition and contributes to overall societal well-being.

CONCLUSION

In conclusion, while AI tools offer significant benefits in education, entertainment, and daily life, they also carry hidden costs that can undermine the cognitive development of young people. Over-reliance on AI can diminish critical thinking, creativity, memory retention, and problem-solving skills, potentially leading to a generation that struggles with intellectual resilience and social interaction. It is essential to promote mindful AI use, ensuring that these tools enhance learning without replacing the fundamental cognitive skills that shape a well-rounded individual. Educators, parents, and policymakers must work together to foster balanced and critical engagement with AI, teaching young people to use technology responsibly and independently. By emphasizing digital literacy, critical thinking, and offline activities, we can mitigate the negative impacts of AI while harnessing its potential to improve learning and productivity. The future of youth lies in the careful integration of AI tools that complement, not replace, human cognition, ensuring a generation that thrives in an increasingly digital world without sacrificing intellectual and emotional growth.

REFERENCES

Al Shloul, T., Mazhar, T., Abbas, Q., Iqbal, M., Ghadi, Y. Y., Shahzad, T., & Hamam, H. (2024). Role of activity-based learning and ChatGPT on students' performance in education. *Computers and Education: Artificial Intelligence*, *6*, 100219.

Aliabadi, R. (2023). *The Impact of an Artificial Intelligence (AI) Project-Based Learning (PBL) Course on Middle-School Students' Interest, Knowledge, and Career Aspiration in the AI Field*. Robert Morris University.

Banerjee, R. (2024, August). EDUCATION 4.0: USE OF AI TOOLS IN CLASSROOM. In *ARTIFICIAL INTELLIGENCE IN EDUCATION* (p. 108).

Baruah, A. (2024). The Impact of Computer-Mediated Communication on Relationships and Social Interactions. *International Journal of Human-Computer Interaction*, •••, 1–7. DOI: 10.1080/10447318.2024.2442755

Bhambri, P. (2025). Innovative Systems: Entertainment, Gaming, and the Metaverse. In *Managing Customer-Centric Strategies in the Digital Landscape* (pp. 483–514). IGI Global.

Bojadjiev, J. (2024). in Education: Transforming Learning. *Reimagining Intelligent Computer-Assisted Language Education, 1*.

Byrnes, J. P., & Bernacki, M. L. (2013). Cognitive development and information behavior. In *The information behavior of a new generation: Children and teens in the 21st century* (pp. 23–43).

Champandard, A. J. (2003). *AI game development: Synthetic creatures with learning and reactive behaviors*. New Riders.

Chan, C. K. Y. (2023). A comprehensive AI policy education framework for university teaching and learning. *International Journal of Educational Technology in Higher Education*, *20*(1), 38. DOI: 10.1186/s41239-023-00408-3

Chan, L., Hogaboam, L., & Cao, R. (2022). AI in Media and Entertainment. In *Applied Artificial Intelligence in Business: Concepts and Cases* (pp. 305–324). Springer. DOI: 10.1007/978-3-031-05740-3_20

Chandramouli, K., & Margetis, G. (2024). Entertainment and Interactive Media. In *Human-Computer Interaction in Various Application Domains* (pp. 214–233). CRC Press. DOI: 10.1201/9781003490692-8

Cho, Y. (2022). Effects of AI-Based Personalized Adaptive Learning System in Higher Education. *Journal of The Korean Association of Information Education, 26*(4), 249–263. DOI: 10.14352/jkaie.2022.26.4.249

Dandotiya, A. S., Gupta, S. K., Dandotiya, N., & Sharma, M. P. (2024). *AI IN EVERYDAY LIFE: TRANSFORMING SOCIETY*. Navi International Book Publication House.

De Wever, B., Hämäläinen, R., Nissinen, K., Mannonen, J., & Van Nieuwenhove, L. (2023). Teachers' problem-solving skills in technology-rich environments: A call for workplace learning and opportunities to develop professionally. *Studies in Continuing Education*, *45*(1), 86–112. DOI: 10.1080/0158037X.2021.2003769

Duenas, T., & Ruiz, D. (2024). The risks of human overreliance on large language models for critical thinking. *Research Gate*, 2024e. http://dx.doi.org/DOI: 10.13140/RG.2.26002.06082

Facione, P. A. (2011). *Critical thinking: What it is and why it counts*. Insight Assessment.

Filimowicz, M. (Ed.). (2023). *AI and the Future of Creative Work: Algorithms and Society*. Taylor & Francis. DOI: 10.4324/9781003299875

Fitria, T. N. (2021). Grammarly as AI-powered English writing assistant: Students' alternative for writing English. *Metathesis: Journal of English Language, Literature, and Teaching*, *5*(1), 65–78. DOI: 10.31002/metathesis.v5i1.3519

Gardner, H. (2021). *Disciplined mind: What all students should understand*. Simon & Schuster.

Greiff, S., Wüstenberg, S., Csapó, B., Demetriou, A., Hautamäki, J., Graesser, A. C., & Martin, R. (2014). Domain-general problem solving skills and education in the 21st century. *Educational Research Review*, *13*, 74–83. DOI: 10.1016/j.edurev.2014.10.002

Hmelo-Silver, C. E. (2004). Problem-based learning: What and how do students learn? *Educational Psychology Review*, *16*(3), 235–266. DOI: 10.1023/B:EDPR.0000034022.16470.f3

Kaswan, K. S., Dhatterwal, J. S., & Ojha, R. P. (2024). AI in personalized learning. In *Advances in Technological Innovations in Higher Education* (pp. 103–117). CRC Press. DOI: 10.1201/9781003376699-9

Khalil, M. (2023). Artificial Intelligence: Transforming Industries and the Global Economy. *Innovative Computer Sciences Journal, 9*(1).

Khogali, H. O., & Mekid, S. (2023). The blended future of automation and AI: Examining some long-term societal and ethical impact features. *Technology in Society, 73*, 102232. DOI: 10.1016/j.techsoc.2023.102232

Kumar, A., & Nagar, D. K. (2024). AI-Based Language Translation and Interpretation Services: Improving Accessibility for Visually Impaired Students. In *Transforming Learning: The Power of Educational*, 178.

Kurni, M., Mohammed, M. S., & Srinivasa, K. G. (2023). *A beginner's guide to introduce artificial intelligence in teaching and learning*. Springer Nature.

Lee, J. (2025). Smart Solutions for Student Well-being: AI-driven Mental Health Support in a Polytechnic. In *The Rise of Intelligent Machines* (pp. 211–242). Chapman and Hall/CRC.

Lozano-Blasco, R., Mira-Aladrén, M., & Gil-Lamata, M. (2023). Social Media Influence on Young People and Children: Analysis on Instagram, Twitter and YouTube. *Comunicar: Media Education Research Journal, 31*(74), 117–128. DOI: 10.3916/C74-2023-10

Mahmoudi, H., Camboim, S., & Brovelli, M. A. (2023). Development of a Voice Virtual Assistant for the Geospatial Data Visualization Application on the Web. *ISPRS International Journal of Geo-Information, 12*(11), 441. DOI: 10.3390/ijgi12110441

Mounkoro, I., Rafique, T., de los Trino Tapia, E., Cadelina, F. A., Uberas, A. D., Karkkulainen, E. A., ... & Galingana, C. D. (2024). AI-Powered Tutoring Systems: Revolutionizing Individualized Support For Learners. *Library Progress International*, 344–355.

Pherson, K. H., & Pherson, R. H. (2020). *Critical thinking for strategic intelligence*. CQ Press.

Prasad, R., & Makesh, D. (2024). Impact of AI on Media & Entertainment Industry. In *Media & Journalism Transformations—Emerging Trends and Paradigm Shifts* (pp. 41–71). Emerald Publications.

Reiser, B. J. (2023, January). Why scaffolding should sometimes make tasks more difficult for learners. In *Computer Support for Collaborative Learning* (pp. 255–264). Routledge. DOI: 10.4324/9781315045467-37

Renacido, J. M. D., & Biray, E. T. (2025). Enhancing Peer Engagement and Student Motivation Through AI-Gamified Interactive Learning Tools. In *Advancing Sustainable Development Goals With Educational Technology* (pp. 277–342). IGI Global.

Sabry, F. (2023). *Narrow artificial intelligence: Fundamentals and applications* (Vol. 167). One Billion Knowledgeable.

Shah, S. S., & Asad, M. M. (2024). Impact of Critical Thinking Approach on Learners' Dependence on Innovative Transformation Through Artificial Intelligence. In *The Evolution of Artificial Intelligence in Higher Education: Challenges, Risks, and Ethical Considerations* (pp. 161–182). Emerald Publishing Limited.

Shanmugasundaram, M., & Tamilarasu, A. (2023). The impact of digital technology, social media, and artificial intelligence on cognitive functions: A review. *Frontiers in Cognition*, *2*, 1203077. DOI: 10.3389/fcogn.2023.1203077

Singh, B., & Pathania, A. K. (2024). AI-Driven Content Creation and Curation in Digital Marketing Education: Tools and Techniques. *International Journal of Engineering Science and Humanities, 14*(Special Issue 1), 14–26.

Steinberg, L. (2005). Cognitive and affective development in adolescence. *Trends in Cognitive Sciences*, *9*(2), 69–74. DOI: 10.1016/j.tics.2004.12.005 PMID: 15668099

Swargiary, K. (2024). How AI Revolutionizes Regional Language Education. scholar press.

Van Der Wal, A., Valkenburg, P., & van Driel, I. (2024). *Children, Youth and Media*. ECREA, 54.

van der Zanden, P. J., Meijer, P. C., & Beghetto, R. A. (2020). A review study about creativity in adolescence: Where is the social context? *Thinking Skills and Creativity*, *38*, 100702. DOI: 10.1016/j.tsc.2020.100702

Yekollu, R. K., Bhimraj Ghuge, T., Sunil Biradar, S., Haldikar, S. V., & Farook Mohideen Abdul Kader, O. (2024, February). AI-driven personalized learning paths: Enhancing education through adaptive systems. In *International Conference on Smart Data Intelligence* (pp. 507–517). Springer Nature Singapore. DOI: 10.1007/978-981-97-3191-6_38

Chapter 17
Multidisciplinary Approaches to AI Integration in Education and Healthcare Systems

Rajeshwari Sissodia
https://orcid.org/0000-0002-9978-0187
Galgotias University, India

Vinay Dwivedi
https://orcid.org/0009-0007-7502-3222
Galgotias University, India

ABSTRACT

The integration of Artificial Intelligence (AI) into education and healthcare systems has gained significant momentum in recent years, with the potential to revolutionize both sectors by enhancing efficiency, accessibility, and outcomes. This chapter explores the multidisciplinary approaches to AI integration, focusing on how collaboration across fields such as data science, psychology, social sciences, and policy-making can ensure the successful deployment of AI technologies.. It examines the transformative role of AI in personalized learning, administrative automation, diagnostic support, and telemedicine, while also addressing the challenges faced in data privacy, system interoperability, and resistance to adoption. Finally, the chapter emphasizes the societal impacts of AI adoption, urging continuous learning, ethical practices, and stakeholder involvement to ensure that AI serves to improve the quality of life globally in both educational and healthcare contexts.

DOI: 10.4018/979-8-3373-5072-1.ch017

INTRODUCTION

Artificial Intelligence (AI) refers to the simulation of human intelligence processes by machines, particularly computer systems. These processes include learning, reasoning, problem-solving, perception, and language understanding. AI can be categorized into narrow AI, which is designed to handle a specific task, and general AI, which is capable of performing any intellectual task that a human can do. In both education and healthcare, AI plays a pivotal role by automating tasks, enhancing decision-making, and providing insights that were previously beyond human capacity. In education, AI is transforming how students learn and teachers instruct by providing personalized learning experiences, while in healthcare, AI supports clinicians in diagnostics, treatment planning, and operational management, enhancing overall patient care and system efficiency.

The significance of AI in these sectors lies in its ability to process vast amounts of data, uncover patterns, and provide actionable insights at an unprecedented speed. It not only improves decision-making processes but also optimizes workflows, reducing human error and making systems more efficient. The integration of AI is becoming essential for tackling the complex challenges both education and health-care systems face, such as resource limitations, unequal access to services, and a growing demand for high-quality care and education.

AI Applications in Education and Healthcare

The application of AI in both education and healthcare has evolved significantly over the past few decades. In education, AI's history began with the development of intelligent tutoring systems (ITS) in the 1960s and 1970s, which aimed to provide individualized instruction to students. In the 1990s, AI was integrated into educational tools for automating administrative tasks, creating virtual classrooms, and supporting adaptive learning techniques. Today, AI continues to grow, with technologies such as learning management systems (LMS) and automated grading becoming commonplace in educational institutions. AI is also used to monitor student progress and provide real-time feedback for both students and instructors, paving the way for more personalized education experiences.

In healthcare, AI's history dates back to the mid-20th century when early attempts were made to develop expert systems to assist doctors in diagnosing diseases. The emergence of machine learning in the 1980s allowed systems to learn from data and improve over time. Since the 2000s, the use of AI in healthcare has expanded exponentially, with AI tools being used for medical imaging, drug discovery, patient monitoring, and predictive analytics. AI's ability to analyze medical data—such as images, test results, and patient records—has revolutionized diagnostic accuracy and treatment planning, particularly in areas like oncology, radiology, and genomics.

The Growing Importance of AI in Improving Efficiency, Accessibility, and Outcomes

AI is increasingly being recognized as a transformative tool in both education and healthcare due to its potential to improve efficiency, accessibility, and outcomes. In education, AI-powered systems can provide personalized learning pathways that adapt to each student's needs, preferences, and abilities, making education more tailored and efficient. These systems reduce the burden on teachers by automating administrative tasks, such as grading and scheduling, thus allowing them to focus on direct interaction with students. AI's ability to scale personalized education across large populations ensures that more students, especially those in underserved or remote areas, have access to high-quality learning materials and support.

In healthcare, AI improves operational efficiency by streamlining administrative tasks, such as patient scheduling, billing, and record management, thereby allowing healthcare professionals to focus on direct patient care. Additionally, AI systems assist clinicians in diagnosing diseases earlier and more accurately, often before symptoms manifest, thereby improving patient outcomes. AI's predictive capabilities help anticipate future health risks, enabling proactive healthcare and potentially reducing long-term treatment costs. As healthcare systems face growing demands due to aging populations and increasing chronic diseases, AI is seen as a solution to address these challenges while maintaining or improving quality of care.

Purpose of the Chapter

The purpose of this chapter is to explore how AI can be integrated into education and healthcare systems through a multidisciplinary approach. AI's potential can be fully realized when experts from various fields—including computer science, engineering, psychology, sociology, education, and healthcare—collaborate to design, implement, and refine AI applications. This approach ensures that AI systems are not only technologically advanced but also ethical, user-friendly, and beneficial for both educators and healthcare professionals, as well as the individuals they serve.

By examining the integration of AI from multiple disciplinary perspectives, this chapter will highlight how the collaboration between AI researchers, data scientists, educators, healthcare professionals, ethicists, and policymakers can drive meaningful innovation. A multidisciplinary approach also addresses potential challenges such as biases in AI algorithms, ensuring that AI tools are accessible, fair, and culturally sensitive. Furthermore, it allows for the development of more comprehensive AI systems that can adapt to complex, real-world scenarios across diverse educational and healthcare environments.

The Role of Various Fields in Enhancing AI's Effectiveness in Education and Healthcare

Various disciplines play a crucial role in enhancing the effectiveness of AI in education and healthcare. For instance, in education, cognitive science and psychology provide insights into how AI can be used to support different learning styles and motivate students, making personalized learning more effective. In healthcare, biomedical engineering, clinical expertise, and medical ethics guide the development of AI systems that support diagnostic accuracy, treatment planning, and patient care, ensuring that they adhere to medical standards and prioritize patient well-being.

The integration of AI also requires strong input from data science, as it ensures that AI systems are based on robust, accurate data. Sociologists and anthropologists contribute by evaluating the social and cultural impacts of AI systems, ensuring that they are inclusive and equitable. Policymakers and legal experts help navigate the regulatory landscape, ensuring that AI technologies comply with laws and ethical standards, particularly regarding data privacy and patient consent.

By understanding and leveraging the strengths of each discipline, AI systems can be designed to address the specific needs of both educational and healthcare environments, making them more efficient, effective, and sustainable.

Structure of the Chapter

This chapter is structured to first provide an overview of AI's role in both education and healthcare, then delve into the multidisciplinary approaches necessary for its successful integration. We begin with foundational concepts of AI, followed by a discussion of the historical context and the growing significance of AI in addressing contemporary challenges. The chapter will then explore how collaboration among different fields can enhance the design and implementation of AI systems.

Subsequent sections will focus on specific aspects of AI integration, including case studies, challenges faced, and policy considerations. Case studies from both sectors will provide practical examples of AI's impact and potential. Finally, the chapter will conclude by exploring future directions for AI in education and healthcare, emphasizing the need for continued interdisciplinary collaboration and innovation. Through this structured approach, the chapter aims to provide a comprehensive understanding of AI's current and future role in shaping both education and healthcare systems globally.

LITERATURE REVIEW

The expanding role of Artificial Intelligence (AI) across healthcare and education has attracted significant scholarly attention in recent years. This section continues the literature review by exploring studies that provide in-depth insights into AI applications, benefits, and the ethical and operational challenges faced in these critical sectors.

Smith et al. (2019) provide a foundational analysis of AI's integration into healthcare, focusing on its applications in medical imaging, diagnostics, and the creation of personalized treatment plans. While the potential for clinical enhancement is substantial, the study highlights critical concerns around data privacy and the complexities of integrating AI tools with existing healthcare systems.

Johnson and Lee (2020) explore the growing landscape of AI in education, emphasizing the effectiveness of AI-powered tools such as intelligent tutoring systems, personalized learning platforms, and adaptive technologies. Their findings suggest these tools contribute positively to student engagement and outcomes, though they call for ongoing evaluation to ensure inclusivity.

Brown et al. (2020) examine AI's role in streamlining healthcare administration. Their study reviews AI applications in areas such as patient scheduling, hospital resource management, and improving operational workflows. The authors argue that AI can significantly enhance healthcare delivery efficiency but caution that mismanagement could result in logistical issues and inequitable access.

Taylor and Zhang (2021) investigate AI's application in diagnostic decision support systems, particularly within radiology and pathology. They emphasize the potential of AI to assist clinicians in identifying anomalies more accurately. However, challenges related to clinical acceptance, trust in automated diagnostics, and system integration are highlighted.

Miller et al. (2021) focus on AI's administrative utility in education. Their research shows how AI automates repetitive tasks and supports data-driven decisions in educational institutions. However, they note that over-reliance on automation could depersonalize decision-making and reduce educator autonomy.

Williams and Roberts (2022) provide a broad ethical analysis of AI in both healthcare and education. They delve into concerns surrounding fairness, transparency, data privacy, and systemic bias. Their work calls for a regulatory framework that balances innovation with ethical responsibility, ensuring AI systems do not unintentionally reinforce inequality.

Garcia et al. (2022) highlight the transformative role of machine learning in healthcare diagnostics, especially in detecting rare diseases and predicting treatment outcomes. Their study underscores how advanced analytics can supplement medical expertise, though they stress the importance of interpretability and clinical validation.

Lopez and Martinez (2022) assess AI's contribution to remote healthcare through telemedicine platforms. They emphasize AI's role in delivering real-time, efficient care to patients in underserved or rural areas. Despite its promise, the study notes limitations in technological infrastructure and patient-provider communication.

Nguyen and Tran (2023) explore the use of AI in K–12 education, identifying significant benefits in personalized learning, real-time feedback, and increased student motivation. However, they caution that without equitable access, AI may widen existing educational gaps.

Davis et al. (2023) analyze AI's growing influence in higher education, particularly its application in personalized academic advising, curriculum design, and research assistance. The study advocates for thoughtful integration strategies that preserve academic freedom and support diverse learning styles.

Evans and Mitchell (2023) focus on AI's use in chronic disease management. Their research discusses predictive models and real-time monitoring tools that allow for earlier intervention and better patient outcomes. They emphasize the importance of patient trust and data security in scaling these technologies.

Khan et al. (2024) examine natural language processing (NLP) applications in both education and healthcare. Their study highlights how NLP improves communication, enables more intuitive user interactions, and streamlines documentation. The research stresses the need for context-sensitive algorithms to avoid miscommunication.

Singh and Patel (2024) explore the integration of AI into electronic health record (EHR) systems. Their findings show that AI can optimize patient care and administrative efficiency, but also identify barriers such as interoperability issues and user resistance.

Chen et al. (2024) present a forward-looking review of AI's role in enhancing equity, accessibility, and inclusion in education, especially for students with disabilities. Their research stresses that inclusive design and user-centered approaches are essential for AI to truly support diverse learners.

Finally, Anderson and Clark (2024) assess AI's potential to unify disparate health data for predictive analytics. They argue that AI can dramatically improve patient care outcomes, reduce healthcare costs, and enhance operational planning, but also call attention to the need for robust data governance and patient consent frameworks.

In summary, this extended literature review illustrates that while AI has the potential to greatly benefit both healthcare and education, its implementation must be approached with careful ethical, technical, and human-centered considerations. The integration of AI into these fields necessitates not only innovation but also a deep commitment to equity, transparency, and responsibility.

FUNDAMENTALS OF AI AND ITS RELEVANCE TO EDUCATION AND HEALTHCARE

Artificial Intelligence (AI) encompasses a variety of technologies and methodologies designed to replicate or simulate human intelligence. Some of the key components of AI include:

- **Machine Learning (ML)**: Machine learning is a subset of AI focused on enabling systems to learn from data without explicit programming. Algorithms analyze patterns in data and improve their performance over time. This has been crucial in both education and healthcare applications. For instance, in education, ML is used to adapt content to student needs, while in healthcare, it is used to predict patient outcomes based on historical health data. ML enables systems to identify hidden patterns and relationships within complex datasets, which can be used for a variety of purposes, such as adaptive learning or diagnostic support.
- **Natural Language Processing (NLP)**: NLP involves enabling machines to understand, interpret, and generate human language. In education, NLP is used for creating virtual assistants that can answer student queries, grade essays, or provide feedback on written assignments. In healthcare, NLP enables systems to analyze patient records, extract meaningful insights, and assist in automated transcription of medical notes. NLP helps bridge the communication gap between human language and machine understanding, facilitating tasks like language translation, sentiment analysis, and chatbots for student or patient interaction.
- **Robotics**: Robotics involves the design and use of robots that can perform tasks autonomously or semi-autonomously. In education, robotics is used for hands-on learning experiences in STEM subjects, where students can program robots and understand concepts of coding and automation. In healthcare, robotic systems assist in surgery (robotic-assisted surgery), patient rehabilitation, and even in tasks such as delivering medication in hospitals. Robotics enhances precision in surgery, improves patient recovery, and provides a way for students to engage in practical, interactive learning experiences in coding and engineering.
- **Expert Systems**: Expert systems are AI-based applications that simulate the decision-making ability of human experts. These systems use rule-based logic to provide solutions or make decisions based on input data. In education, expert systems can guide students through learning materials or help teachers make data-driven decisions about instructional strategies. In healthcare, expert systems assist doctors in diagnosing diseases, suggesting treatment

plans, or providing decision support in complex clinical scenarios. Expert systems are particularly valuable in environments where human expertise may be limited or unavailable, allowing for more consistent and accurate decision-making.

Several core AI concepts are foundational to the development of more advanced systems in education and healthcare:

- **Neural Networks**: Neural networks are algorithms modeled after the human brain, consisting of layers of nodes (neurons) that process information. These networks can be trained to recognize patterns, such as identifying objects in images or predicting student performance. In education, neural networks are used for personalized learning, adapting content based on student responses. In healthcare, neural networks are instrumental in processing complex medical images, such as X-rays or MRIs, to identify diseases like cancer. The ability to recognize patterns in vast amounts of data is a key strength of neural networks in both domains.
- **Deep Learning**: A subset of machine learning, deep learning uses multiple layers of neural networks to analyze complex data. Deep learning algorithms excel in tasks that involve large datasets and unstructured data, such as images, audio, and text. In education, deep learning can power advanced tools like automated grading systems or virtual teaching assistants. In healthcare, it plays a critical role in analyzing medical imaging, genomics, and predicting patient outcomes based on complex medical data. Deep learning has enabled breakthroughs in fields like image recognition and natural language processing, where it excels at extracting features from raw data.
- **Reinforcement Learning**: Reinforcement learning is a type of machine learning where an agent learns to make decisions by interacting with an environment and receiving feedback in the form of rewards or penalties. This type of learning is widely used in robotics for teaching machines how to perform tasks autonomously. In education, reinforcement learning can be applied to adaptive learning platforms that adjust content and difficulty based on student performance, ensuring that students progress at an optimal pace. In healthcare, reinforcement learning can be used to improve clinical decision-making by simulating various treatment scenarios and selecting the most effective approaches for patient care. It allows systems to learn from trial and error, optimizing outcomes over time.

The Role of AI in Education

AI has significant potential in revolutionizing how education is delivered, especially in personalizing learning experiences:

- **Personalized Learning**: AI can tailor educational content to meet the unique needs and abilities of individual students. By analyzing student performance data, AI systems can adjust the pace, content, and difficulty of lessons. This individualized approach helps ensure that students are challenged appropriately, neither overwhelmed by difficult material nor bored by content that is too easy. Personalized learning platforms powered by AI are increasingly being used in K-12 schools and higher education institutions to ensure each learner has the opportunity to succeed at their own pace. AI can identify areas where a student struggles and provide additional resources or exercises to support learning in those areas.
- **Intelligent Tutoring Systems (ITS)**: ITS are AI-powered platforms designed to simulate the experience of one-on-one tutoring. These systems provide immediate feedback, guide students through problem-solving, and offer customized support based on the student's progress. ITS can analyze a student's weaknesses and provide targeted lessons to improve performance, effectively supplementing traditional classroom instruction. These systems are particularly useful for students who may need extra help but cannot access a human tutor. ITS can adapt to the student's learning style, ensuring they are receiving the most effective help at the right time.
- **Learning Analytics**: AI-driven learning analytics systems analyze large amounts of educational data to identify patterns in student behavior, performance, and engagement. By tracking interactions with digital learning environments, these systems can predict students' learning outcomes and help educators intervene before students fall behind. This data-driven decision-making can improve teaching methods and inform curriculum development, ensuring that educational resources are used most effectively. Learning analytics can also help identify at-risk students and suggest interventions or alternative teaching strategies
- **Automation of Administrative Tasks**: AI can automate routine administrative tasks such as scheduling, grading, attendance tracking, and communications. For example, AI-based systems can grade assignments, providing instant feedback to students and freeing up time for instructors to engage in more meaningful interactions. Similarly, AI can handle student queries, schedule classes, and manage exam results, thus optimizing operational efficiency in schools and universities. By automating repetitive tasks, AI enables

educators to spend more time focusing on teaching and less on administrative overhead.

- **Data-driven Decision-Making**: AI helps educational institutions make more informed decisions by providing insights based on data. For example, AI can help schools assess the effectiveness of their teaching methods, understand trends in student performance, and identify areas for improvement. With AI-driven insights, decision-making becomes more data-centric, allowing educators to make adjustments to teaching strategies and curriculum based on real-time feedback from students. This leads to more informed, evidence-based decisions that can enhance the learning experience for all students.

The Role of AI in Healthcare

AI's transformative potential in healthcare lies in its ability to assist clinicians in diagnosing diseases, recommending treatments, and predicting patient outcomes:

- **Diagnostics**: AI tools, particularly those powered by machine learning and deep learning, can analyze medical images, lab results, and patient records to assist in the diagnosis of diseases. AI systems can detect abnormalities in medical imaging, such as tumors in X-rays or MRIs, with high accuracy. This reduces the likelihood of human error and speeds up the diagnostic process. AI is particularly effective in fields like radiology, pathology, and dermatology, where it can help identify conditions at an early stage when they are most treatable.
- **Treatment Recommendations**: AI systems can analyze large datasets to recommend the most effective treatment plans for individual patients. By reviewing medical literature, clinical guidelines, and patient histories, AI can suggest tailored treatment options that align with the patient's specific condition. In oncology, for example, AI algorithms can help determine the best course of action based on genetic information, past treatments, and clinical outcomes. These systems assist healthcare professionals in making evidence-based decisions, improving patient outcomes, and reducing the likelihood of errors.
- **Predictive Analytics**: AI-powered predictive analytics can help identify patients at risk of developing certain conditions by analyzing historical health data. This enables proactive care and intervention, potentially preventing the onset of severe health issues. For example, AI can predict the likelihood of a patient developing heart disease, diabetes, or other chronic conditions, allowing for earlier interventions that can improve long-term health outcomes. Predictive analytics also aids in managing hospital resources, ensuring that

staffing and equipment are allocated efficiently based on expected patient needs.

- **Electronic Health Records (EHR)**: AI can enhance EHR systems by automating data entry, flagging inconsistencies, and providing insights into patient health trends. With AI, EHRs can be used more effectively to track patient histories, identify potential health risks, and suggest preventive measures. AI systems can extract and organize critical information from EHRs, ensuring that healthcare providers have all relevant data at their fingertips, which leads to better-informed decisions and streamlined workflows.
- **Telemedicine**: AI is an integral component of telemedicine, enabling remote monitoring, diagnosis, and treatment of patients. Virtual health assistants powered by AI can conduct preliminary assessments, monitor patient vitals in real-time, and recommend next steps. This allows healthcare providers to extend their reach, particularly in underserved or rural areas, and reduces the need for in-person consultations. AI enhances telemedicine by making remote care more efficient, personalized, and scalable.

MULTIDISCIPLINARY APPROACHES TO AI INTEGRATION

The integration of AI in education and healthcare requires close collaboration across multiple disciplines to ensure successful implementation. Data scientists play a pivotal role in developing and refining AI models, algorithms, and data analytics that underpin AI systems. They provide the technical expertise needed to design algorithms that can analyze large datasets and generate meaningful insights. Educators and healthcare professionals, on the other hand, bring invaluable domain knowledge, ensuring that AI systems are aligned with the real needs of students and patients. Their input is essential for shaping AI tools that are both practical and effective. Policymakers are involved in creating regulations and guidelines that ensure the ethical and safe use of AI in both sectors, addressing concerns like privacy, data security, and equitable access to technology. Collaborative efforts ensure that AI systems are not only technologically sound but also human-centered, meeting the goals of improving education and healthcare delivery.

Successful multidisciplinary collaboration can be seen in various real-world AI implementations. For instance, in healthcare, collaborative projects between AI researchers, medical professionals, and data scientists have led to the development of AI tools for disease detection, such as cancer recognition software. In education, AI-driven personalized learning platforms have been developed through partnerships between educators and AI developers, ensuring that learning algorithms are adaptive and cater to diverse learning needs. These case studies demonstrate the power of cross-disciplinary work, highlighting the need for diverse perspectives in AI development to create solutions that are effective, equitable, and ethical.

The development of AI algorithms and tools is central to AI integration in education and healthcare. This process involves creating sophisticated models capable of learning from data and making intelligent predictions or decisions. In education, AI tools such as adaptive learning platforms and intelligent tutoring systems rely on algorithms that analyze student performance data to offer personalized learning paths. Similarly, in healthcare, AI tools are built to interpret medical images, predict patient outcomes, and assist in decision-making. The development of these algorithms requires collaboration between computer scientists, engineers, and domain experts, ensuring that the tools are not only accurate but also easy to use and integrate into existing educational or healthcare infrastructures. Engineers must also consider scalability, making sure that these systems can handle the growing amounts of data and demands of real-world applications.

While the development of AI algorithms is a critical step, their implementation in real-world settings presents numerous engineering challenges. One major challenge is ensuring that AI systems can integrate seamlessly with existing infrastructures, such as educational software or electronic health record systems. For instance, AI systems in education must work with different learning management systems (LMS), while in healthcare, AI tools must be compatible with hospital databases and electronic health records. Additionally, AI systems need to be robust and reliable, capable of functioning under diverse conditions and environments. Engineers must also address concerns related to system performance, such as the speed and accuracy of decision-making, especially in time-sensitive situations like medical diagnostics. Real-world deployment requires rigorous testing, continuous monitoring, and ongoing maintenance to ensure that AI systems remain effective and reliable in practice.

Psychology and Human Factors

Psychology plays a key role in AI integration by providing insights into human cognition and behavior, which helps in designing AI systems that are intuitive and align with how people learn or make decisions. Understanding cognitive processes such as memory, attention, and problem-solving allows AI developers to create tools that support effective learning and enhance patient care. In education, this knowledge helps in developing AI-based teaching systems that adapt to different learning styles, ensuring that the technology aligns with how students process and retain information. In healthcare, understanding human behavior helps design AI tools that assist in patient management by aligning with how patients make health-related decisions, encouraging adherence to treatment plans, and improving patient engagement in their care.

AI has the potential to deeply impact individual learning styles in education by offering personalized learning experiences that cater to each student's strengths, weaknesses, and preferences. For example, AI-driven platforms can adapt content delivery based on whether a student learns best through visual, auditory, or hands-on experiences. Similarly, in healthcare, AI can help tailor care to individual patient preferences and needs, ensuring that treatment plans align with patients' personal health goals, lifestyle, and treatment choices. This personalization can enhance patient satisfaction and improve health outcomes by focusing on patient-centered care. Recognizing the varied preferences in both learning and healthcare ensures that AI systems are not one-size-fits-all but are tailored to meet individual needs.

Ethical Considerations in AI Decision-Making

As AI becomes more involved in decision-making processes in education and healthcare, ethical considerations are increasingly important. In education, AI systems that assess student performance or provide feedback must do so in a fair and unbiased manner. There is a risk that AI tools could unintentionally reinforce existing biases or inequalities, such as favoring certain groups of students based on historical data. In healthcare, AI systems that recommend treatments or assist in diagnoses must be transparent and accountable, with clear explanations for how decisions are made. Ensuring that AI systems respect privacy, consent, and autonomy is crucial, as both students and patients must trust that AI systems act in their best interests without discrimination or exploitation.

Social Sciences and Ethical Considerations

The integration of AI in education and healthcare raises important social questions, particularly around equity, access, and privacy. AI systems have the potential to democratize access to education and healthcare by making resources available to underserved populations, especially through remote learning or telemedicine. However, there is a risk that the digital divide could deepen inequalities, as those without access to technology may be left behind. Ensuring equitable access to AI-powered education and healthcare services is a key concern. Furthermore, AI systems handle vast amounts of personal data, raising issues around data privacy and the security of sensitive information. Addressing these concerns requires a careful balance between innovation and social responsibility, ensuring that AI systems promote inclusion and protect individuals' privacy rights.

Examining Bias, Fairness, and Transparency in AI Systems

AI systems are only as good as the data they are trained on, and if the data reflects existing biases, AI systems can perpetuate these biases in decision-making. In education, this could mean that AI-based grading systems or personalized learning tools might favor certain demographics over others. In healthcare, biased AI could lead to disparities in diagnosis and treatment recommendations, particularly for marginalized groups. Addressing bias in AI involves ensuring that training data is representative and that AI algorithms are designed to be fair and transparent. Transparency in AI decision-making allows educators, healthcare providers, and patients to understand how and why decisions are made, promoting trust in these systems.

Ethical Dilemmas in AI-Driven Decisions in Education and Healthcare

AI-driven decisions in education and healthcare can sometimes present ethical dilemmas, such as whether to prioritize efficiency over human judgment or how to balance autonomy with automation. In education, for instance, an AI system may suggest a particular learning path for a student based on data, but the teacher might feel that a more holistic, human-centered approach would better serve the student's needs. Similarly, in healthcare, AI tools may recommend a course of treatment that is statistically optimal but does not align with the patient's personal preferences or values. These ethical dilemmas highlight the need for careful consideration of how AI is used and the importance of human oversight to ensure that AI complements, rather than replaces, human expertise.

Policy and Governance in AI Implementation

As AI technologies become more integrated into education and healthcare, there is an increasing need for regulatory frameworks to ensure their safe, ethical, and effective use. These regulations should address issues such as data privacy, security, and fairness, while ensuring that AI applications are transparent and accountable. In education, policies might govern the use of AI to track student progress, protect student data, and ensure that AI systems do not inadvertently reinforce inequities. In healthcare, regulations must focus on patient consent, data security, and ensuring that AI systems meet safety standards for clinical use. Developing and enforcing these regulatory frameworks is critical to ensuring that AI benefits both sectors while minimizing potential harm.

Standardization and Accountability in AI Applications

Standardization of AI tools and processes is essential to ensure consistency, interoperability, and reliability across different systems. In education, standardized AI platforms allow for smoother integration into classrooms and curricula, ensuring that the technology is accessible and usable across various educational institutions. In healthcare, standardization ensures that AI systems for diagnosis, treatment, and patient management can be seamlessly integrated into hospital networks and clinical workflows. Accountability is also important, particularly in cases where AI decisions have significant impacts, such as in healthcare diagnostics. Developers and users of AI systems must be accountable for ensuring that AI tools are used responsibly and do not cause harm to individuals.

Global Perspectives on AI Policy and Governance

AI policy and governance vary significantly across countries and regions, with some countries taking a more proactive approach to regulating AI, while others are still developing frameworks for its use. A global perspective on AI policy is essential, as AI technologies are often developed and used across borders. International collaborations can help establish global standards for AI applications in education and healthcare, ensuring that best practices are shared and that AI benefits are distributed equitably worldwide. By adopting a global approach, policymakers can address challenges such as privacy, bias, and access, while promoting innovation and collaboration across the international community.

CHALLENGES AND BARRIERS TO AI INTEGRATION

Limited Access to AI Tools and Resources in Underdeveloped Areas

One of the primary challenges to AI integration in both education and healthcare is the disparity in access to AI tools and resources, particularly in underdeveloped or rural areas. In these regions, the infrastructure required to support AI technologies, such as high-speed internet, computing power, and access to trained professionals, is often lacking. This creates a significant barrier to the adoption of AI-based solutions that could otherwise improve educational outcomes and healthcare delivery. The lack of resources hampers the ability to train AI models effectively and to implement them at scale, ultimately hindering the progress of AI in these regions. Bridging the digital divide requires strategic investments in infrastructure, as well as efforts to make AI technologies more affordable and accessible to underserved communities.

Interoperability Between AI Systems and Existing Infrastructures

Integrating AI systems with existing educational and healthcare infrastructures presents significant technical challenges, especially in legacy systems. Many educational institutions and healthcare providers still rely on traditional technologies that are not compatible with modern AI systems. For example, schools may use outdated learning management systems (LMS), and hospitals might rely on paper-based records or outdated electronic health record (EHR) systems that cannot easily interface with AI tools. The challenge lies in ensuring seamless interoperability between new AI technologies and existing infrastructures to enable smooth integration. Achieving this requires careful planning, standardization, and collaboration between technology providers and institutions to create systems that work together without disrupting existing workflows.

Data Privacy and Security Concerns

AI systems in education and healthcare rely heavily on data—often sensitive personal information such as academic performance, medical histories, and health outcomes. Protecting this data is of paramount importance to maintain trust and privacy. In education, AI systems may collect detailed information about student performance, learning habits, and even behavioral data, raising concerns about how that data is stored and used. Similarly, in healthcare, patient data used by AI tools must be protected from unauthorized access or misuse. Data breaches or misuse could not only violate privacy but also lead to significant legal and financial consequences. Robust data protection measures, including encryption, secure access protocols, and clear data governance policies, are essential to ensure that sensitive information is kept secure in both sectors.

Addressing Cyber Threats and Ensuring Secure AI Deployments

With the increasing reliance on AI, there is also a heightened risk of cyber threats. Malicious actors could target AI systems used in education and healthcare to gain unauthorized access to sensitive data or disrupt services. AI systems themselves are also vulnerable to adversarial attacks, where attackers manipulate input data to deceive the AI models into making incorrect predictions or decisions. For example, in healthcare, adversarial attacks could lead to misdiagnoses or incorrect treatment recommendations. Addressing these threats requires not only robust cybersecurity measures but also continuous monitoring and updating of AI systems to identify vulnerabilities. Organizations must also train their staff to recognize potential threats and ensure secure deployment practices to safeguard the integrity and reliability of AI applications.

Resistance to Change and Adoption

One of the significant barriers to AI adoption in education and healthcare is the resistance to change from key stakeholders, including educators, healthcare providers, and patients. Many educators may be skeptical of AI-based teaching tools, fearing that they may replace human teachers or fail to understand the nuances of student learning. Healthcare providers may be hesitant to rely on AI for diagnostics or treatment decisions due to concerns about accuracy or losing control over patient care. Patients, too, may have reservations about AI-driven care, worrying about the lack of human touch or the possibility of AI making decisions that do not align with their values or preferences. Overcoming this skepticism requires clear communication about the benefits of AI, including how it can enhance rather than replace human roles. Additionally, pilots and gradual implementations can help build trust by demonstrating the effectiveness and safety of AI systems in real-world settings.

Training and Reskilling for AI Literacy in Educational and Healthcare Institutions

Another significant challenge in the adoption of AI is the need for training and reskilling in both education and healthcare sectors. Educators and healthcare providers may not have the necessary skills or knowledge to effectively utilize AI tools, and without proper training, there can be hesitation in using AI systems. In education, teachers may need to learn how to integrate AI-powered learning platforms into their classrooms effectively, understanding how to use the technology to personalize student learning experiences. In healthcare, medical professionals must be trained to work alongside AI tools, interpreting AI-generated insights in clinical practice and making decisions based on those insights. As AI technologies continue to evolve, ongoing professional development is crucial to ensure that educators and healthcare providers are equipped with the knowledge and skills needed to make the most of AI innovations.

CASE STUDIES OF AI INTEGRATION IN EDUCATION

AI Applications for Personalized Learning, Student Assessments, and Support Systems

In K-12 education, AI is revolutionizing the way students learn by offering personalized learning experiences that adapt to individual needs. AI-powered platforms analyze students' progress in real-time, identifying areas where they are excelling or struggling and adjusting the learning material accordingly. This allows for a tailored educational experience, where each student moves at their own pace. For example, AI tools such as smart tutoring systems can provide one-on-one support to students, addressing gaps in understanding without overwhelming teachers. AI is also being used to automate and enhance student assessments, enabling teachers to monitor progress more efficiently. Beyond academics, AI-driven support systems are helping identify students at risk of falling behind, offering timely interventions such as additional tutoring or behavioral support. This early detection mechanism helps educators provide targeted assistance to students who need it the most.

Success Stories and Lessons Learned

Several schools and districts have seen successful implementations of AI in the K-12 sector. For instance, schools using AI-based platforms like DreamBox Learning or Smart Sparrow have reported improvements in student engagement and academic performance. DreamBox, an adaptive math program, adjusts the learning path for students based on their responses, ensuring that each child receives content suited to their learning level. Additionally, AI-driven tools such as Carnegie Learning's MATHia software have enabled personalized, data-driven insights for both students and teachers. The success of these programs shows the power of personalized learning but also highlights challenges, such as the need for proper teacher training to integrate AI tools effectively and the potential risk of over-reliance on technology without human oversight. These case studies reveal that successful AI integration in K-12 education requires careful planning, appropriate tools, and teacher involvement.

AI in Higher Education

In higher education, AI is being utilized to streamline various administrative and academic processes, benefiting both students and institutions. One of the most notable uses is in research, where AI tools help researchers sift through vast amounts of academic literature, identify trends, and predict future areas of study. AI-powered systems like IBM's Watson are being used in academic research to analyze and summarize large datasets, offering insights that would take humans significantly longer to uncover. Additionally, AI is transforming academic advising by providing students with data-driven recommendations based on their academic performance and career goals. AI systems can analyze patterns in a student's academic record to suggest courses, extracurricular activities, or career paths that align with their strengths and interests. In learning platforms, AI is enhancing the personalization of coursework by adapting lessons based on real-time feedback from students, creating a more tailored and engaging educational experience. These applications are improving the efficiency of educational institutions and helping students achieve better academic and career outcomes.

AI-Driven Educational Tools for Online and Blended Learning Environments

The growth of online and blended learning environments has seen an increased reliance on AI to support both teaching and learning. AI tools such as automated grading systems, chatbots for instant student support, and learning analytics platforms are helping institutions scale up online education.

Challenges and Outcomes

Evaluating the Effectiveness of AI in Educational Settings

Despite the growing adoption of AI in education, evaluating its effectiveness remains a significant challenge. To truly assess the impact of AI tools, educators must consider a range of factors, including improvements in student outcomes, engagement levels, and the overall quality of the learning experience. While AI tools have shown promising results in personalizing learning and providing tailored support, there is still a need for comprehensive studies that measure long-term outcomes, such as retention rates, graduation rates, and career success after graduation. Some research has suggested that AI can help improve student learning, especially for those who struggle in traditional educational settings. However, there is also concern that without proper oversight, AI tools may exacerbate existing inequalities, particularly if they fail to address the diverse needs of all learners. Continuous evaluation and feedback from both educators and students are necessary to ensure AI systems are effective and equitable.

Addressing Challenges such as Teacher Adaptation and Curriculum Integration

One of the major challenges in the integration of AI in education is the adaptation of teachers and the integration of AI tools into existing curricula. Many educators are not yet familiar with how to use AI tools effectively, and the adoption of AI technologies can create resistance if teachers feel that their traditional teaching methods are being undermined. Furthermore, incorporating AI into the curriculum requires careful planning to ensure that it enhances learning outcomes and aligns with educational standards. Teachers need proper training to understand the potential and limitations of AI tools and to learn how to use them in conjunction with their own teaching expertise. Schools must also be mindful of how AI fits into the broader educational framework and avoid relying on technology as a substitute for valuable in-person instruction and human interaction. Collaboration between educators, administrators, and AI developers is crucial to ensuring that AI tools are seamlessly integrated into the learning environment, maximizing their benefits while preserving the essential human elements of teaching.

CASE STUDIES OF AI INTEGRATION IN HEALTHCARE

AI in Diagnostics and Treatment

AI Applications in Radiology, Pathology, and Genomics

AI is transforming diagnostic processes in healthcare, particularly in areas like radiology, pathology, and genomics, where the ability to analyze large datasets quickly and accurately is crucial. In radiology, AI algorithms are used to interpret medical images, such as X-rays, MRIs, and CT scans, assisting radiologists in detecting conditions like tumors, fractures, and other abnormalities. These systems can identify patterns that may not be immediately visible to the human eye, increasing the accuracy and speed of diagnoses. In pathology, AI tools are used to analyze tissue samples and detect diseases such as cancer, automating parts of the diagnostic process and providing pathologists with more reliable insights. In genomics, AI is aiding in the analysis of DNA sequences, helping to identify genetic predispositions to diseases, guide personalized treatment plans, and facilitate advancements in gene therapy. By improving the precision and speed of diagnostics, AI is enhancing the early detection of diseases and enabling more targeted treatments.

Impact on Clinical Decision Support and Patient Outcomes

AI-driven clinical decision support systems (CDSS) are revolutionizing the way healthcare providers make treatment decisions. These systems process large amounts of clinical data, such as medical records, lab results, and patient histories, to provide evidence-based recommendations to clinicians. AI can help identify the most effective treatment options for individual patients, predict possible complications, and even suggest preventative measures. For example, AI tools are being used to predict patient deterioration in critical care settings, allowing for timely interventions that can save lives. By enhancing decision-making, AI can lead to more accurate diagnoses, better treatment planning, and ultimately, improved patient outcomes. These systems also reduce the likelihood of human error and help healthcare providers stay updated with the latest medical research and best practices, ensuring that patient care is based on the most current evidence.

AI in Healthcare Administration and Operations

Use of AI for Patient Scheduling, Resource Management, and Administrative Tasks

AI is increasingly being used to streamline healthcare administration and operational tasks, allowing healthcare providers to focus more on patient care. In patient scheduling, AI-driven systems can optimize appointment bookings, reducing wait times and ensuring that healthcare professionals' time is used effectively. These systems can automatically reschedule appointments in case of cancellations, ensuring that there are no gaps in the schedule and that resources are efficiently utilized. AI is also being used for resource management, where it helps hospitals and clinics allocate medical staff, equipment, and supplies based on predicted patient demand. For example, AI tools can forecast patient volume based on historical data and trends, enabling hospitals to better prepare for busy periods. Additionally, AI-powered administrative tools are being implemented to handle tasks such as billing, insurance verification, and patient communication, reducing the administrative burden on healthcare workers and improving operational efficiency.

Enhancing Operational Efficiency and Cost-Effectiveness

AI is playing a critical role in enhancing the operational efficiency of healthcare systems, leading to significant cost savings. By automating administrative tasks, reducing manual errors, and optimizing resource allocation, AI is helping healthcare providers minimize waste and maximize productivity. For instance, AI systems can analyze hospital supply chain data to predict when certain medical supplies are likely to be needed, reducing overstocking and stockouts. In addition, AI can assist in managing hospital bed availability by analyzing real-time data to predict patient discharges and optimize room assignments. These improvements in efficiency reduce costs for healthcare providers while improving patient care by ensuring that resources are allocated where they are most needed. The increased efficiency also allows healthcare providers to deliver services at a lower cost, which is crucial as the global demand for healthcare rises.

Telemedicine and Remote Monitoring

AI-Driven Telehealth Systems for Remote Diagnosis and Care Delivery

Telemedicine has seen tremendous growth, especially in the wake of the COVID-19 pandemic, and AI is playing a pivotal role in improving remote care delivery. AI-driven telehealth systems allow patients to consult with healthcare providers through virtual platforms, where AI tools assist in diagnosing conditions and providing treatment recommendations. These systems can analyze patient-reported symptoms, medical histories, and data from wearable devices to suggest possible diagnoses or prioritize which patients need immediate attention. For example, AI-powered chatbots can conduct initial assessments by asking patients about their symptoms and providing guidance on whether they should seek further medical attention. Additionally, AI systems can help doctors remotely monitor and manage chronic conditions, such as diabetes or hypertension, by analyzing patient data collected through telehealth platforms. This not only improves access to care, especially in underserved or rural areas, but also allows for more frequent and timely monitoring of patient health, reducing the need for in-person visits.

Use of Ai for Continuous Health Monitoring and Chronic Disease Management

AI is also being used for continuous health monitoring, especially in the management of chronic diseases. Wearable devices, such as smartwatches or fitness trackers, collect real-time data on vital signs like heart rate, blood pressure, and blood glucose levels. AI algorithms analyze this data to detect early warning signs of health issues or changes in a patient's condition, such as a sudden drop in blood sugar or irregular heart rhythms. This continuous monitoring allows healthcare providers to intervene before conditions worsen, preventing hospitalizations and improving the overall quality of life for patients with chronic conditions. Additionally, AI can help create personalized care plans for chronic disease management by integrating data from various sources, including patient histories, lab results, and lifestyle factors. By providing real-time insights into a patient's health, AI tools are enabling more proactive and preventative care, which is essential for managing chronic diseases effectively.

FUTURE DIRECTIONS OF AI INTEGRATION IN EDUCATION AND HEALTHCARE

Advancements in AI Technologies Such as Explainable AI, Edge Computing, and Quantum Computing

The future of AI in education and healthcare is poised to benefit from significant technological advancements. One of the most critical areas of development is explainable AI (XAI). As AI systems are increasingly deployed in decision-making processes, especially in sensitive sectors like healthcare and education, the need for transparency and interpretability becomes paramount. Explainable AI enables users, whether educators, healthcare providers, or patients, to understand the rationale behind AI-driven recommendations and decisions, making AI systems more trustworthy and reliable. Another key advancement is **edge computing**, which allows AI models to process data locally on devices such as smartphones, wearables, or IoT-enabled healthcare devices, reducing the need for data to be sent to centralized servers. This increases the speed of AI operations, enhances privacy by keeping data on the device, and enables real-time analytics, which is crucial in both educational and healthcare settings. Additionally, **quantum computing** holds tremendous promise for revolutionizing AI by dramatically increasing computational power. In fields like genomics or medical research, quantum computing could help solve complex problems that are currently beyond the capabilities of traditional computing, leading to breakthroughs in personalized medicine, diagnostics, and educational research.

Future Applications of AI in Education and Healthcare

In education, AI is expected to further enhance personalized learning experiences, using even more sophisticated algorithms to tailor educational content to individual students' needs. AI-driven virtual learning assistants, powered by natural language processing, will likely become commonplace, offering real-time support and feedback to students, thus making education more accessible and inclusive. Additionally, AI will continue to improve assessment methods, allowing for more accurate and adaptive evaluation systems that assess not only academic performance but also social-emotional development and behavioral patterns. In healthcare, AI will play an even more significant role in personalized treatment plans, leveraging genomics and patient data to provide highly individualized care. AI-powered diagnostic tools will become more accurate and capable of identifying rare or complex conditions, even predicting disease progression. Moreover, AI applications in remote monitoring will advance, making it possible to manage patient health continuously from home, improving chronic disease management and reducing hospital readmissions. The convergence of AI with other emerging technologies like augmented reality (AR) and virtual reality (VR) may also revolutionize medical training and therapeutic interventions.

The Role of Interdisciplinary Collaboration Moving Forward

Growing need for Interdisciplinary Expertise in AI Development and Application

As AI continues to evolve, interdisciplinary collaboration will become even more essential. The complex nature of AI systems requires expertise not only in computer science and engineering but also in fields like psychology, education theory, healthcare, ethics, and law. For AI to be effectively integrated into education and healthcare, there is a growing need for collaborative efforts between data scientists, educators, medical professionals, social scientists, and policy experts. Educators and healthcare providers must collaborate with AI developers to ensure that the technology aligns with pedagogical goals and clinical needs, while also considering the human and societal aspects of implementation. This will ensure that AI technologies are used in ways that enhance educational outcomes and improve patient care while mitigating risks like bias, inequity, and data privacy concerns. Moreover, interdisciplinary teams will play a critical role in understanding and addressing the ethical implications of AI use in these sectors, ensuring that AI remains a force for good, particularly in sensitive contexts like healthcare treatment and education for vulnerable populations.

Collaborative Frameworks to Accelerate AI Innovation

To accelerate AI innovation, particularly in healthcare and education, institutions will need to establish frameworks that facilitate collaboration among various stakeholders. These frameworks can include partnerships between universities, tech companies, healthcare providers, and government agencies. Collaborative research initiatives focused on AI applications will be crucial in ensuring that advancements are practical, ethical, and scalable. For example, public-private partnerships can foster innovation while also ensuring that AI technologies meet regulatory standards and are designed with end-users in mind. Additionally, creating collaborative networks for knowledge sharing and best practice development will help accelerate the adoption of AI. This could involve the establishment of AI innovation hubs or consortiums dedicated to addressing specific challenges in education or healthcare, such as personalized learning or predictive health diagnostics. In the future, these collaborative efforts could lead to faster AI advancements and more seamless integration of AI into everyday systems, driving greater societal benefits.

Potential Societal Impacts

Predictions for AI's Role in Shaping the Future of Education and Healthcare

The impact of AI on the future of education and healthcare is expected to be transformative. In education, AI will likely democratize access to high-quality learning resources, breaking down barriers related to geography, income, and special needs. Virtual classrooms powered by AI may allow students to learn from anywhere in the world, with tools that adapt to their learning styles and progress. Furthermore, AI's ability to analyze vast amounts of data can lead to more efficient administrative processes, reducing costs and administrative burdens on schools. In healthcare, AI is expected to revolutionize how diseases are diagnosed, treated, and managed, particularly through predictive analytics that can prevent illnesses before they occur. Personalized medicine, powered by AI, will ensure that treatments are tailored to individual patients based on their genetic makeup, lifestyle, and health history. As AI continues to improve, it could lead to significant reductions in healthcare costs by streamlining processes and reducing medical errors, while also making high-quality care more accessible to a global population.

Long-Term Societal and Economic Implications of AI Adoption

The long-term societal and economic implications of AI adoption in education and healthcare are profound. As AI takes over more routine tasks and processes, it has the potential to create significant economic efficiencies in both sectors, reducing costs for institutions and improving resource allocation. In education, AI-driven automation could lead to savings in administrative costs, allowing resources to be directed toward improving the quality of teaching and learning. In healthcare, AI could lower the cost of medical services by improving operational efficiencies, optimizing supply chains, and reducing diagnostic errors. However, the widespread adoption of AI may also lead to job displacement in certain sectors, particularly for tasks that can be automated. This highlights the need for upskilling and reskilling workers, particularly in education and healthcare, to ensure that the workforce can adapt to the changing technological landscape. Additionally, AI adoption may widen inequalities if not implemented equitably, particularly if access to AI-powered tools remains limited in underserved regions. Policymakers must address these issues to ensure that AI benefits society as a whole and does not exacerbate existing disparities. Furthermore, as AI becomes more integrated into everyday life, societal norms and values will likely shift, raising important ethical and philosophical questions about the role of technology in shaping our future.

CONCLUSION

The integration of AI into education and healthcare is an inherently multidisciplinary endeavor. Successful AI implementation in these sectors requires contributions from a range of disciplines, including data science, healthcare, education, psychology, law, ethics, and policy. By working together, experts from different fields can ensure that AI systems are not only technically sound but also ethically aligned, socially responsible, and accessible. The combination of diverse perspectives allows for a more holistic understanding of both the potential and limitations of AI. A collaborative, multidisciplinary approach is essential for addressing the complex challenges AI presents and ensuring that its integration improves outcomes for all users, whether students, patients, educators, or healthcare providers.

Case studies from both the education and healthcare sectors illustrate the transformative potential of AI but also highlight the obstacles faced in its implementation. In education, AI has shown promise in personalizing learning experiences, automating administrative tasks, and supporting educators. However, challenges such as resistance to technology, the need for proper teacher training, and concerns about equity and access remain significant barriers. Similarly, in healthcare, AI applications have enhanced diagnostics, personalized treatment plans, and operational efficiency. Yet, challenges such as data privacy concerns, integration with existing infrastructure, and the need for continuous monitoring of AI-driven systems persist. These case studies reinforce the notion that while AI has vast potential, its successful deployment requires careful consideration of both technical and human factors.

For educators, it is crucial to embrace AI as a tool that can enhance learning experiences and administrative efficiency. Teachers should be equipped with the skills to use AI-driven tools and understand their potential to personalize education for diverse learners. Healthcare professionals must stay informed about AI developments and be proactive in integrating AI into patient care while maintaining a focus on the human aspect of healthcare. For policymakers, there is a need to create clear regulations that balance the potential benefits of AI with concerns about data privacy, equity, and accountability. Policies should promote access to AI technologies while ensuring ethical practices in their application. Researchers should continue to explore the possibilities of AI in education and healthcare, focusing on addressing current limitations and creating solutions that can be scaled globally. Collaboration between stakeholders is key to driving forward innovation while ensuring that AI deployment remains ethical and equitable.

AI technologies are rapidly evolving, making continuous learning and innovation critical. All stakeholders must stay updated on the latest developments in AI to fully leverage its potential and stay ahead of emerging challenges. Ongoing professional development for educators, healthcare providers, and policymakers will ensure that they are equipped to make informed decisions about AI tools. In addition, ethical considerations must always be at the forefront of AI deployment, particularly when it comes to issues like bias, fairness, transparency, and privacy. The adoption of AI must be done with careful thought about its social and ethical implications, ensuring that these technologies benefit society at large without compromising human rights or widening inequalities.

The future of AI in education and healthcare holds incredible promise, with the potential to revolutionize both sectors in ways that significantly improve lives around the world. In education, AI can provide personalized learning pathways that accommodate diverse learning styles, increase access to quality education for underserved populations, and help educators focus on higher-level tasks. In healthcare, AI has the ability to improve early diagnosis, personalize treatments, optimize operations, and make healthcare more accessible and affordable for people across different regions and demographics. As AI continues to evolve, its integration into these systems could bridge gaps in both education and healthcare, ensuring that people worldwide benefit from advancements in technology. Ultimately, AI has the potential to improve both individual well-being and the efficiency of large systems, contributing to a healthier, more educated global population. However, this future can only be realized through collaborative efforts, ethical oversight, and a commitment to continuous improvement, ensuring that AI serves as a tool for enhancing the quality of life for all.

REFERENCES

Anderson, G., & Clark, J. (2024). AI and health data integration for predictive analytics: Transforming patient care and healthcare efficiency. *Health Systems Review*, *22*(3), 144–159.

Brown, A., Davis, L., & Wilson, F. (2020). AI in healthcare administration: Automating patient scheduling and resource management. *Journal of Health Management*, *28*(4), 213–230.

Chen, L., Wang, J., & Yang, P. (2024). The future of AI in education: Enhancing equity, accessibility, and inclusivity for students with disabilities. *Journal of Educational Innovation*, *25*(1), 76–90.

Davis, G., & Thomas, J. (2023). The impact of AI on higher education: Applications in academic advising, research support, and curriculum design. *Higher Education Technology Review*, *30*(3), 210–224.

Evans, K., & Mitchell, D. (2023). AI in chronic disease management: Predictive models and real-time monitoring in healthcare. *Journal of Healthcare Innovations*, *16*(1), 45–60.

Garcia, D., Patel, R., & Singh, V. (2022). Machine learning applications in healthcare diagnostics: A focus on rare disease detection and predictive analytics. *Journal of Medical AI*, *11*(2), 134–150.

Johnson, P., & Lee, M. (2020). The effectiveness of AI-driven educational technologies: A review of personalized learning and intelligent tutoring systems. *Journal of Educational Technology*, *22*(2), 103–118.

Khan, S., Patel, M., & Ahmed, R. (2024). Natural language processing in education and healthcare: Applications in communication and task automation. *AI in Education and Health*, *21*(2), 67–82.

Lopez, A., & Martinez, S. (2022). AI in remote healthcare: Telemedicine platforms and real-time care delivery. *Global Health Innovation*, *13*(2), 95–110.

Miller, B., Davis, P., & Roberts, H. (2021). AI in educational administration: Automating administrative tasks and enhancing decision-making. *Educational Management Review*, *19*(3), 56–72.

Nguyen, H., & Tran, J. (2023). AI-driven personalized learning in K-12 education: Enhancing engagement and student performance. *International Journal of Educational AI*, *27*(4), 143–160.

Singh, N., & Patel, P. (2024). Integrating AI in electronic health records (EHR) systems: Benefits and challenges. *Health Informatics Journal, 18*(4), 123–139.

Smith, J., Johnson, R., & Lee, T. (2019). AI applications in healthcare: A review of diagnostics, treatment personalization, and medical imaging systems. *Healthcare Review, 15*(3), 45–60.

Taylor, E., & Zhang, K. (2021). Diagnostic decision support in healthcare: The role of AI in radiology and pathology. *Medical Informatics Review, 34*(1), 89–102.

Williams, C., & Roberts, S. (2022). Ethical considerations in AI applications: A review of fairness, transparency, and data privacy in education and healthcare. *Journal of Ethics in AI, 9*(1), 77–92.

About the Contributors

Maria Efstratopoulou is an Associate Professor of Special Education at the United Arab Emirates University. Before joining UAEU, she was a Senior Lecturer in BGUniversity in the UK, teaching at the graduate program in Special Education and Inclusion. She holds a doctoral degree in Biomedical Sciences from the Faculty of Kinesiology and Rehabilitation KULeuven, Belgium, a European Master in Psychomotor Therapy for Children (KULeuven, Belgium), and a Master in Human Performance and Health for Special Populations (Aristotle University of Thessaloniki, Greece). Her research interests are in motor behaviour and assessment for children with emotional, behavioural, and developmental disorders.

Agathi Argyriadi is a psychologist with specialization on Cognitive – Behavioral Psychotherapy and Developmental Psychology. Her PhD thesis is entitled "The effects of "Aesthetic flow experiences" in school's environment of first graders. A psycho-educational approach". She also holds a M.Ed. on Special Education and a second Master on Counseling. She is currently a Visiting Assistant Professor at the United Arab Emirates University and Lecturer in the Department of Education at Frederick University, teaching developmental and cognitive psychology. In the past she has also taught at Cyprus University of Technology (Therapeutic communication), at the East London University (Research Methods and Statistics) and at the Technological Educational Institute of Peloponnese at the department of Speech Pathology (teaching Developmental Psychology and Clinical Neuropsychology), for 3 years. She has acted as a self- employed Psychologist and for a 3-year project against violence at the Ministry of Internal Affairs of the Hellenic Republic. She has also acted for two years, as an external associate at a private school in Greece, with the aim of monitoring and supporting students with learning difficulties, psychological problems and counseling of parents. Agathi Argyriadi was also a professor at the Foundation for Youth and Lifelong Learning and specifically at the Institute for Vocational Training of the Ministry of Education.

She has published articles in international journals and she has participated in numerous of training seminars. She is the writer of 10 scientific books in the field of psychology. Her research interests focus on optimizing learning environments using positive psychology and aesthetic theories, developmental psychological issues, special education field, social inclusion issues. She teaches in the Distance Learning Program of Special Education.

Alexandros Argyriadis is an Assistant Professor at Frederick University, in the domain of Community Health with an emphasis on Mental Health and Learning Disabilities. He has previously taught at the University of East London, the University of South Wales, the Hellenic Open University and the University of Thessaly, the University of West Attica and other well-known universities. The courses he has taught are related to the inclusive education of people with disabilities, cultural and medical anthropology, mental and family health, health promotion and teaching methods, special education and social inequalities. At Frederick University, he coordinates the Distance Learning Master's Program in Community Health Care and the Practicum of the MEd in Special Education. He has authored numerous scholarly books and high impact factor articles; he has been the publisher of the scientific journal "Culture Journal" and participates in several editorial boards of international scientific journals. Indicatively, he is the Deputy Editor-in-Chief of the "Health and Research" journal as well as at the journal "Vima tou Asklipiou". His work includes numerous presentations at scientific conferences, elaboration of research programs and public activities in education. He often teaches as a visiting Professor at universities abroad and designs contemporary interdisciplinary activities. Administratively, he is a member of several committees at Frederick University but also in other international organizations such as the European Union Commission, the Assessors team of the Latvian Ministry of Education Academic Information Center (AIC) / Quality Agency for Higher Education (AIKA), a member of the Electors register of Hellenic Mediterranean University and others. His research interests focus on diversity and inclusion, people with disabilities, special education, health promotion and education and community health.

Hassan Abbas is an Assistant Professor of Marketing at Sukkur IBA University, Pakistan. He recently completed his Ph.D. in Business Management from IAE Aix-Marseille Graduate School of Management, France, where his research focused on the impact of digital content on customer involvement and brand engagement. A Corporate Gold Medalist from SZABIST, he also holds an MBA and a BBA (Hons) in Business Administration. Dr. Abbas has taught marketing and research courses at several French institutions including IPAG Business School and Aix Marseille University. His research interests include digital marketing, consumer behavior, and neuromarketing, and he has authored multiple publications in reputed international journals.

Evanthia Arvanitaki is a psychologist with an academic background and experience in the field of mental health. She holds a BSc in Psychology from the National and Kapodistrian University of Athens and an MSc in Mental Health Promotion, Prevention of Mental Disorders from the National and Kapodistrian University of Athens 1st Deparment of Psychiatry. Her professional journey includes roles as a Psychologist at a Specialized Therapy Center and as an Intern Psychologist at Sismanoglio General Hospital and the Municipality of Ilioupolis. In addition, she has received specialized training in Cognitive Behavioral Therapy, Clinical Psychopathology, Child Psychology, School Psychology, and Special Education. Her research interests focus on "Interpersonal relationships, attachment styles, and their impact on mental health in individuals with autoimmune diseases". She has also conducted research on "The psychosocial burdens of caregivers for dependent relatives in the context of mental health".

Raino Bhatia, epitomizes the essence of an educator whose life is intricately woven with a profound dedication to the betterment of society through education. As the Principal cum Associate Professor of Akal College of Education, Eternal University, nestled in the serene landscapes of Baru Sahib, Himachal Pradesh, India, she orchestrates the symphony of learning with finesse and vision. She is M.Phil. and Ph.D. in Education, along with the accolade of UGC-NET, she stands as a paragon of scholarly excellence. Spanning over two decades, her journey in the realm of education has been marked by unwavering commitment and illustrious achievements. In 2009, she was bestowed with the prestigious National Award. Her literary contributions resonate across academia, with her seminal work, "The Quest for True Happiness," serving as a guiding beacon for both educators and students.

Lara Carneiro earned her BSc in Psychology from the Faculty of Psychology and Education Science at the University of Porto, Portugal (2023). Dr Carneiro holds a BSc in Physical Education (2009), a Masters degree in Physical Education (2012) and a Doctorate in Sports Science (2017) from Portugal. Carneiro currently works as an Assistant Professor at the United Arab Emirates University (UAEU) in the College of Education. She serves as an editor of Combining Exercise and Psychotherapy to Treat Mental Health, published by IGI Global, which earned a 5-star rating from Doody's Review Service. She also has experience in designing, implementing, and managing randomized controlled trials (efficacy of exercise and psychotherapy). Dr. Carneiro is also a Management Committee Member of funded research projects (e.g. CA21123 - Cancer- Understanding Prevention in Intellectual

Disabilities (CUPID). Dr. Carneiro is an external expert in the remote evaluation of proposals -COST and her research focuses on physical activity, depressive and anxiety disorders, and mental illness, including physical health co-morbidities.

Efthymia Efthymiou is an accomplished professional in the field of special education, currently serving as an Assistant Professor at Zayed University in the United Arab Emirates (UAE). With a strong background in special education, her research focuses on inclusive teaching practices, classroom discourse, and creating educational environments that support the inclusion of all students, including those with special needs. Her work centers on understanding the perspectives of various stakeholders, such as teachers and children with special needs, to develop more inclusive educational systems. She explores the role of both physical and psychological environments in shaping attitudes, positioning, and inclusion. Her research aims to identify and overcome barriers to inclusive education, with particular emphasis on leveraging technology-based teaching practices to address digital exclusion and promote inclusive teaching methods. In addition to her research efforts, Dr. Efthymia actively contributes to the advancement of inclusive education through her workshops and seminars conducted for teachers and principals in federal schools within the UAE.

Mingyue Fan holds PhD degree in Management Science & Engineering from Jiangsu University. She is currently Associate Professor in Jiangsu University. Her research areas are Digital Transformation, Big Data Analysis, Green Economy and Management Information Systems (MIS).

Ana Filipa Gomes is a Clinical Psychologist at NYU Abu Dhabi - Health Center Department. Focused on Cognitive Behavioral Therapy (CBT), with expertise in treating anxiety and trauma-related disorders. Additionally trained in Acceptance and Commitment Therapy (ACT) and pursuing a PhD with the goal of bringing a holistic, trauma-informed and compassionate approach to mental health. Contributed as the author of a Doody's rewarded book "Combining Exercise and Psychotherapy to Treat Mental Health", showcasing a commitment to advancing knowledge in the field.

Marie Grace A. Gomez is Professor 4 at the Counselor Education Area, College of Education, University of the Philippines-Diliman. She teaches counseling and research courses at the undergraduate and graduate levels. She has served as a classroom teacher, guidance counselor, and administrator in the basic and tertiary education settings. Her community extension projects involve counseling and assessment of children, persons with disability, children in conflict with the law, drug surrenderees, sexually abused children, medical personnel, women with mental health issues in institutional settings, and persons affected by COVID-19.

Deepak Gupta is a distinguished academician with over 20 years of teaching experience and expertise in Computer Science and Engineering. He holds a Ph.D. in Computer Engineering and has an extensive research portfolio, including many international journal papers, multiple conference proceedings, and several books. His research interests span machine learning, artificial intelligence, and data mining. Currently, Dr. Gupta serves as an Associate Professor and Academic Coordinator in the Department of Computer Science & Engineering at ITM Gwalior, MP, India. He has also contributed significantly to the field through patents and copyrights and actively engages as a reviewer, conference chair and editor.

S. Ida Evangeline is an Assistant Professor in the Department of Electrical and Electronics Engineering at Government College of Engineering, Tirunelveli, Tamil Nadu, India. She holds a Bachelor's degree in Electrical and Electronics Engineering from Manonmaniam Sundaranar University (2003) and a Master's degree in Power Systems Engineering from Anna University, Chennai (2005). She earned her Ph.D. from Anna University, Chennai, in 2023. She has published six research papers in international journals. Her areas of interest include optimal power flow, renewable energy, soft computing, artificial intelligence, machine learning, and deep learning.

Louiza Ioannidou is an Assistant Professor in Mental Health for Children and Adolescents at the European University Cyprus and a Registered School Psychologist. Dr Ioannidou has obtained her PhD in Psychology, her MA in School Psychology (applied program), and her BA in Psychology, all from the University of Cyprus. She has also trained in the field of Cognitive - Behavioural Therapy, Positive Psychology, Mindfulness, Solution Focused Therapy, and Business - Team Coaching. She has also a diploma in the Master Practitioner in Eating Disorders and Obesity. Her teaching and research experience focuses on school bullying, children and adolescents' mental health and resilience, and parental involvement. Her research interests also focus on developing, implementing, and evaluating psychoeducational programs to promote children's and adolescents' mental health, well-being, resilience, and a safe school climate. Her research findings are published in scientific journals and presented in scientific conferences. She is the author and editor of the books "Building Mental Resilience: Positive Psychology, Emotional Intelligence, and Play" (2024) and "Effective Practices for Mental Health Promotion in Education" (2025) published by IGI Global.

Ashfaq Jafar is a PhD scholar in Cognitive Psychology at the National Institute of Technology, Kurukshetra, India. His research, supervised by Dr. Shabnam (Assistant Professor, NIT Kurukshetra) and co-supervised by Dr. Azizuddin Khan (Professor, IIT Bombay), explores the cognitive processes in human-computer interaction. He holds an MSc in Psychology from Bangalore University and a BSc in Psychology from St. Joseph's College, Devagiri, Kozhikode, Kerala. Before his doctoral studies, Ashfaq gained experience in teaching and mentoring undergraduate and postgraduate students in Psychology. He also served as the magazine editor of the psychology department at his undergraduate institution and organized national and international conferences, demonstrating his strong communication and organizational skills.

Avantika Jain is an undergraduate BSc Psychology (Hons) student at PES University, Bengaluru India. She is aspiring to build a career as a future psychologist and researcher. Her areas of interest include psychological case studies and scales, research on cross-cultural issues, counselling, gender studies, and psychological disorders. She has gained valuable experience through internships in hospital, clinical, and counselling settings, where she had the opportunity to observe mental health care practices, take case histories, counsel a patient under supervision, and prepare detailed psychological reports. Additionally, she contributed to a habit transformation program by developing intervention modules aimed at promoting positive behavioral change. Driven by a passion for mental health and a commitment to lifelong learning, Avantika is dedicated to making meaningful contributions to the field of psychology through both research and clinical practice.

Dimitra Katsarou is an Assistant Professor of Developmental Psychopathology and Language Disorders, Department of Preschool Education Sciences and Educational Design, University of the Aegean. She has 50 scholarly publications in influential peer-reviewed journals and more than 100 conference presentations, She has authored a monography, two books, four editing books, and co editing books, as well as participating in several chapters in other scientific publications. She is academically responsible for education, training and education programs of Greek and international organizations and participates as a key researcher in Greek and international research programs, such as Erasmus Plus, Alliance edu, Cost.eu, Erasmus Sport. Her research interests focus on the special education of children with intellectual disabilities, neurolinguistics, cognitive processes, autism, developmental psychopathology, speech and language development, genetic syndromes and intergenerational activities.

Azizuddin Khan is currently Professor in Psychophysiology and Cognitive Psychology at Department of Humanities and Social Sciences at Indian Institute of Technology Bombay (IITB). He is heading Psychophysiology Laboratory. He was visiting faculty at University of Jyväskylä, Aligarh Muslim University, India and University of Warsaw, Poland. He has research interest in the field of Mental

Health, Depression, Environmental Psychology, Polar Research, Developmental Neuropsychology, Emotion regulation, Prospective Memory, and Developmental Dyslexia by using biofeedback and electrophysiological method. Dr. Khan has done his graduation and post-graduation from AMU with first division. He has completed his Ph.D. from IIT Kanpur in 2006. He has also worked as researcher at the University of Jyvskyla, Finland. Dr. Khan is an eminent psychologist, prolific writer and author of many books, credited with more than hundred peer reviewed journal articles. He is recipient several visiting researchers fellowship such DAAD, INSA, Hermes EMINTE, ICSSR.

Georgios A. Kougioumtzis is an Associate Professor in the Department of Turkish and Modern Asian Studies, at National and Kapodistrian University of Athens, Greece, in the field of Counseling, ICT, and Teaching Methodology; a Visiting Professor in the School of Psychology, at Neapolis University Pafos, Cyprus, in the field of Counseling / Educational Psychology, and Specific Learning Difficulties, and a Visiting Academic in the School of Social Sciences, at Hellenic Open University, Patras, Greece, in the field of Psychology / Counseling. He holds a Ph.D. in Pedagogics, Teaching Methodology, and Counseling / Teacher Mentoring, from the Department of Philosophy, Pedagogy, and Psychology - National and Kapodistrian University of Athens. He has published 12 books by IGI Global (USA) and Grigori Publications (Greece) in the fields of Educational Psychology, Counseling Psychology, Specific Learning Difficulties, and Teaching Methodology and ICT, and over than two hundred (200) papers. He is married and the father of three daughters.

Jagneet Kour is a Research Scholar and Faculty, Eternal University. She a dedicated scholar in the field of Education. Drawing from her extensive academic background and research expertise, Kour curates a collection of insightful contributions to educational research. Kour emerges as a beacon of academic excellence. As the proud recipient of the prestigious gold medal in postgraduate studies from Eternal University, she stands at the pinnacle of her academic prowess. Kour's achievements don't end there; she reigns as the all-around champion in her 2022 batch, leaving an indelible mark on her college's Master's in Education program. Jagneet Kour is pursuing her Ph.D. in Education, having previously obtained degrees in B.Ed. and M.A. in Education. Her academic journey is marked by notable achievements, including qualifying for the UGC NET JRF on her first attempt and successfully clearing the CTET examinations. Her journey is one of continuous growth and achievement.

Nataly Loizidou Ieridou is an associate professor in the Department of Psychology and Social Sciences at Frederick University, where she has been a faculty member since 2006, teaching undergraduate and postgraduate students at the School of Education and Social Sciences. Since February 2024, she has been the head of the Department of Psychology and Social Sciences. She completed her Ph.D. in Psychology, at the University of Essex, her Master's Degree at the Institute of Education, University of London (Master in Child Development) and her undergraduate studies at the University of Nottingham (BA in Psychology). Her research activity that has been published in scientific journals and presented in scientific conferences, covers several areas of her scientific domain. Her research interests lie in the area of developmental and school psychology, specifically in the development of literacy skills and the psychological perspective of special education, as well as factors affecting school life (both academic and socioemotional and the interaction between them).

Yogita Deepak Mane is an Associate Professor in the Department of Artificial Intelligence and Data Science at Thakur College of Engineering and Technology. She holds a Master's degree in Computer Engineering from the University of Mumbai and earned her Ph.D. from the same institution in April 2022. Dr. Mane has published over 25 research papers in renowned national and international Journals, Conferences and holds a patent to her name. Dr. Mane has contributed as a reviewer in various National and International conferences and also serve as session chair. With 18 years of experience, she has demonstrated exceptional expertise and leadership in education, excelling in both academic and administrative roles.

Evangelos Mantsos is a Post Doctorate Researcher in physical activity and disabilities

Kalliopi Megari is a Postdoctoral researcher of Aristotle University of Thessaloniki, Greece, Academic Director of MSc in Clinical Psychology and Clinical supervisor at City College, University of York, Europe Campus. She is Adjunct lecturer at University of Western Macedonia in Florina, Greece. Dr. Megari is a psychologist with a history of working in the hospital & health care industry, skilled in Clinical Neuropsychology, Clinical Research, Medical Education, Psychological Assessment and Learning Disabilities. She works both in clinical and in research practice and she provides strong professional healthcare services, graduated from Aristotle University of Thessaloniki, and attended further education from Department of Educational and Social Policy, University of Macedonia, in people with special needs and disabilities. She holds undergraduate degrees in Nursing and Psychology, as well as a Master' s and a PhD in Neuropsychology from Aristotle University of

Thessaloniki. She has some years of occupational and research experience working with patients who have neurological, psychiatric, and cognitive disorders, as well as chronic disease patients suffering from cancer and cardiovascular diseases. She is the head of the Centre of creative activities of children and adults with disabilities and she also works as a counseling psychologist in Prison, Diavata Thessaloniki, at the school of second chance. She was the Global Engagement Representative of SLC International Neuropsychological Society from 2018-2021 and she was a research fellow in the Department of Cardiovascular Surgery in AHEPA Hospital. Currently she is a Global Membership Committee member of International Neuropsychological Society and leader of Rehabilitation of COVID-19 patients working group of NeuroCOVID International Neuropsychology Taskforce SIG. In addition, she is the General Secretary of the board of directors of Hellenic Neuropsychological Society and Ethics Committee president of Hellenic Neuropsychological Society. Since 2021, she is a member of PIAC Community Outreach Subcommittee of AMERICAN PSYCHOLOGICAL ASSOCIATION Membership and a member of Engagement Committee of American Group Psychotherapy Association (AGPA). Her work has earned her many prestigious international awards and was an Ambassador of National Academy of Neuropsychology (NAN), USA Leadership and Ambassador Development Program (2022-23). She has given lectures at Aristotle University of Thessaloniki, University of Warsaw and Norwegian University of Science and Technology in Oslo. She is committed to leadership skills and issues on equity, diversity, and inclusion as her clinical and research work states.

Veena, a Professor in the Department of Psychology at PES University, Bengaluru, India, has over two decades of experience in teaching and education. She has taught undergraduate, postgraduate, and Ph.D. programs at various colleges and universities across Bengaluru and has also worked as a freelance educator with different institutions. She has authored research articles published in esteemed international and national journals and presented papers at numerous conferences. As a research supervisor, she has guided M.Phil. and Ph.D. students. Dr. Veena is a peer reviewer for several national and international journals and serves on the editorial board of the International Journal of Applied Psychology. Her research interests focus on Clinical, Educational, and Positive Psychology, as well as Child and Adolescent Mental Health and Well-being. Dr. Veena has conducted and been invited as a resource person for numerous lectures and workshops covering topics such as life skills, group dynamics, stress management, team building, self-esteem, goal setting, learning strategies, study habits, relaxation techniques, and mental health awareness, particularly during the lockdown and pandemic periods.

Sonia Najam Shaikh is pursuing her Ph.D. in Management Science and Engineering at Jiangsu University, China. She holds an MBA in Human Resource Management. Sonia's research focuses on HRM, artificial intelligence, and Big Data Analytics Capability, with a particular interest in leveraging emerging technologies to enhance organizational performance.

Suman Najam Sahikh holds MBA degree from Sukkur IBA university, Pakistan. Currently, she is phd scholar at 4Putra Business School, University of Putra Malaysia, Selangor, Malaysia

Erum Naseer: Holds MS degree from Sukkur IBA University. Currently she is PhD scholar atUniversiti Kebangsaan Malaysia. Her main research areas are HRM, GHRM, Green Behavior.

Neeta Prashant Patil is an Associate Professor in the Department of Information Technology at Thakur College of Engineering and Technology. She holds a Master's in Engineering and a Ph.D. in Technology from the University of Mumbai. Dr. Patil has authored over 18 research papers in esteemed national and international journals and has actively participated in numerous conferences at both levels. As a reviewer for reputed international journals, she contributes significantly to the academic community. With more than 16 years of experience teaching undergraduate and postgraduate students, she has excelled in various academic and administrative roles, showcasing remarkable expertise and leadership in the field of education.

S. Pavithra is an esteemed Assistant Professor at Sri Venkateshwaraa College of Engineering and Technology, Puducherry. Holding a Master's degree in Data Science from Puducherry Technological University and a Management degree from Pondicherry University. She has established herself as a prominent expert in her field. With a passion for research and a commitment to lifelong learning, Ms. Pavithra has bridged theoretical concepts with practical applications in cutting-edge technological domains. Her expertise spans both industry and academia, contributing significantly to technological advancements and knowledge dissemination. Her research accomplishments include holding Patents, Publishing Journals. Additionally she has authored book and chapters, further showcasing her expertise in current technologies.

Shabnam is currently working as Assistant Professor in the Department of Humanities and Social Sciences, National Institute of Technology (NIT) Kurukshetra (Haryana) India. She has more than ten years of teaching experience of teaching graduation, post-graduation and doctoral level courses. She has also received Young Scientist Award for her doctorate research. She has presented many research papers in

International Conferences in India and Overseas. She has published more than 30 research papers in journals of international repute. Her research interests include Neuropsychology, UX Research, Visual Search, Sleep Studies and Sign Language.

Saeed Abbas Shah Assistant Professor Email: s.abbas@iba-suk.edu.pk Dr. Saeed Abbas Shah is an Assistant Professor of Marketing at Sukkur IBA University, Pakistan, where he has been serving since 2015. He specializes in the field of Marketing and teaches various courses including Strategic Marketing Management, Brand Management, Advertising Management, and Services Marketing. He completed his Master's in Digital Marketing from University College Dublin, Ireland (2016–2017), and earned his Ph.D. from the Universitat Autònoma de Barcelona under the IDEM (International Doctorate in Entrepreneurship and Management) program. His doctoral research focused on the role of the digital divide in the context of the Sharing Economy, particularly platforms like Uber and Airbnb. Dr. Shah's academic interests lie at the intersection of digital marketing, consumer behavior, and platform-based economies.

Sonia Najam Shaikh is pursuing her Ph.D. in Management Science and Engineering at Jiangsu University, China. She holds an MBA in Human Resource Management. Sonia's research focuses on HRM, artificial intelligence, and Big Data Analytics Capability, with a particular interest in leveraging emerging technologies to enhance organizational performance.

Ritika Sharma holds a B.Tech and M.Tech in Computer Science, with a strong foundation in advanced computing concepts. She possesses specialized skills in the domain of Machine Learning Image Processing and is passionate about leveraging data-driven technologies to solve real-world problems.

Gurtek Singh is an Assistant Professor of Social Sciences at Akal University, Punjab. He has completed his Ph.D. thesis in history at Lovely Professional University (2021-2024). His research focuses on culture and traditions. Dr. Singh has published numerous peer-reviewed articles in top-tier journals, including Scopus-indexed publications. He has presented his work at various prestigious national and international conferences. As an educator, Dr. Singh is dedicated to innovative teaching methods and mentoring students. He has received accolades for his teaching, examination, and research excellence. Dr. Singh serves as a reviewer for Shodhkosh, IGI Global, and is the Program Officer of the Red Ribbon Club (RRC) at Akal University, Punjab.

Rajeshwari Sissodia is a assistant professor. Her research domain is Cloud Computing and IoT.

Maria Sofologi is an Adjunct Ass. Professor at the Department of Early Childhood and Education at the University of Ioannina in Greece. She delivers the courses "Cognitive Psychology", and "Developmental Psychology". She is also a postdoctoral researcher at the University of Ioannina in Greece. She holds a Ph.D. in Cognitive Psychology from the Aristotle University of Thessaloniki. She also holds a Master of Science degree in Cognitive Psychology from the Aristotle University of Thessaloniki. During her master's degree years she trained and practiced different assessment cognitive tools to evaluate all cognitive functions like memory, attention, language, executive functions both in adults and children. She is the key speaker in many European and Hellenic conferences concerning cognitive psychology, educational psychology, special education in children and adults, as well. Her academic work includes a series of many scientific publications, books, and book chapters concerning Cognitive Psychology, Special Education, Educational Psychology, and Cognitive impairments in children and adults as well.

Jan Muhammad Sohu Department of Business Administration Sukkur IBA University Email: jan.sohu@iba-suk.edu.pk Dr. Jan Muhammad Sohu is a distinguished academic and researcher with extensive expertise in digital marketing, big data analytics capability, digital transformation, environmental sustainability, value co-creation, digital platform capability, and corporate governance. Currently Dr. Sohu is assistant professor of digital marketing at Sukkur IBA University, Pakistan (only AACSB Accredited public sector university in Pakistan). Holding a PhD in Management from Jiangsu University, Dr. Sohu has published 45 plus papers in numerous impactful and high-ranking journals (WOS, SCOPUS, ABDC, CABS) and has contributed scholarly book chapters with well-known publishers that address critical intersections of sustainability, digital technologies, and business practices. With a rich background in both academic and industry settings, he brings valuable experience in editorial roles, contributing as a peer reviewer and advisory board member for several impact factor journals. His expertise in big data analytics and corporate governance, combined with his international network, makes him a strong researcher for any role related to academic research. Dr. Sohu is dedicated to fostering innovative research and ensuring the highest standards of academic rigor and inclusivity in scholarly publications. Dr. Jan Muhammad Sohu has actively contributed as an editor and peer reviewer for a wide range of reputable international journals, focusing on AI, sustainability, digital transformation, artificial intelligence, Digital Marketing, Big Data Analytics, HRM, green innovation, and higher education. His review expertise spans both theoretical and empirical research, using advanced methods such as SEM, ANN, fsQCA, and hybrid models. His total reviews completed 2021–2025 are over 52 and a few are included here.

Safia Soomro hold B.Ed (Hons) degree from Sukkur IBA University, currently she is Mphil Scholar at Sukkur IBA University, her research areas are Leadership, Education Psychology

Sanam Soomro holds MS degree in Human Resource Management from Sukkur IBA University Currently, she is PhD scholar at School of Management, Jiangsu University, Zhenjiang, China. Her research areas are Artificial intelligence, Human Resource management, Work-life Balance and Employee Well-being

Niki Tzioumaki is a psychologist with an academic background and experience in the field of mental health. She holds a BSc in Psychology from the National and Kapodistrian University of Athens and an MSc in Aging and Chronic Diseases Management in Hellenic Open University. In addition, she has received specialized training in Cognitive Behavioral Therapy, Child Psychology, School Psychology, and Special Education. Also, she works as Second Lieutenant in Hellenic Air Force.

Shantha V is an undergraduate student pursuing a BSc (Hons.) in Psychology at PES University, Bengaluru. Her academic and research interests span various domains within psychology, with a primary focus on clinical and counselling psychology. Shantha has previously published a chapter with IGI Global and presented a research paper at an international conference, showcasing her early but growing contribution to the field. She has also completed a certified four-month internship in counselling psychology, where she gained hands-on experience in therapeutic practices and client engagement. Passionate about understanding the human mind and supporting mental well-being, she aspires to pursue advanced studies and a career in clinical psychology. Her work reflects a commitment to integrating theory with empathetic practice, and she continues to explore opportunities that bridge academic knowledge with real-world impact.

Efthimia Xiraka has been studying Psychology at the European University of Cyprus, and Cognitive Behavioral Psychotherapy at the Alypia Training Center for CBT

Li Zhen is a Professor at the School of Management, Jiangsu University, China, specializing in Management Science and Engineering. With a Ph.D. and postdoctoral experience, her research focuses on construction and supply chain management. Dr. Li has contributed significantly to academia through her publications and supervision of doctoral research.

Index

A

B

C

D

E

J

M

N

V

W

www.ingramcontent.com/pod-product-compliance
Lightning Source LLC
LaVergne TN
LVHW080349011026
849161LV00009B/2236